DIABETES
SELF-MANAGEMENT
Answer Book

DIABETES
SELF-MANAGEMENT
Answer Book

501 TIPS AND SECRETS TO
KEEP YOU HEALTHY

DIABETES SELF-MANAGEMENT BOOKS
NEW YORK

Note to the reader:
The information contained in this book is not intended as a substitute for
appropriate medical care. Appropriate care should be developed in discussion
with your physician and the rest of your diabetes care team. This book has
been published to help you with that discussion.

Library of Congress Cataloging-in-Publication Data

Diabetes self-management answer book: 501 tips and secrets to keep you
healthy.
      p. cm.
  Includes index.
  ISBN 0-9631701-7-1
  1. Diabetes—Popular works. 2. Diabetes—Miscellanea. I. Diabetes Self-
Management Books.
  RC660.4. D557 2004
  616.4'62—dc22   2004013787

PROJECT EDITOR
JAMES HAZLETT

DESIGN AND ILLUSTRATION
RICHARD BOLAND

Diabetes Self-Management Books is an imprint of R.A. Rapaport Publishing, Inc.,
150 West 22nd Street, New York, NY 10011.

Printed in the United States of America.

10 9 8 7 6 5 4 3 2 1

Contents

Preface

Because diabetes—probably more than any other chronic disease—is managed in large part by the patient, the most important resource someone with diabetes can have is solid, reliable information. Whether you have just been diagnosed with diabetes or have been intimately involved in your own treatment for many years, you need information you can trust. Information you can apply right away to the management of your diabetes. And ideas and techniques to help you take better care of yourself right now and for many healthy years to come.

One of the best ways to get the information you need is to ask questions. That's what we do in this book. We take the most frequently asked questions on specific topics—important, sometimes pressing questions—and give you expert answers in down-to-earth language.

To get those answers, we have gathered diabetes experts who have counseled and treated people with diabetes for many years. With this book, you'll share the collective knowledge of physicians, diabetes educators, researchers, and writers from some of the nation's top health-care institutions and universities. Whatever topic is on your mind, their answers get to the heart of your question quickly to help you achieve and maintain physical well-being and peace of mind.

I hope you find a prominent spot on your shelf for this handy reference book. Every time you use it, you'll come away with information you can use right away. Use this book often, and use it in good health.

For the staff and authors who made this book possible,

James Hazlett
Editor, *Diabetes Self-Management*

Contributors

Amy P. Campbell, M.S., R.D., C.D.E., is Education Program Manager for Affiliated Programs and the Office of Disease Management at Joslin Diabetes Center in Boston, Massachussetts.

Karen A. Chalmers, M.S., R.D., C.D.E., is Director of Nutrition Services at Joslin Diabetes Center in Boston, Massachussetts.

Sheri Colberg-Ochs, Ph.D., is an Assistant Professor at the Department of Exercise Science, Physical Education, and Recreation at Old Dominion University in Norfolk, Virginia.

Nancy Cooper, R.D., C.D.E., is a Diabetes Nutrition Specialist at the International Diabetes Center in Minneapolis, Minnesota. She is a Contributing Editor of *Diabetes Self-Management*.

Virginia Peragallo-Dittko, R.N., B.C.-A.D.M., M.A., C.D.E., is a diabetes nurse specialist and Director of the Diabetes Education Center at Winthrop-University Hospital in Mineola, New York. She is member of the Editorial Board of *Diabetes Self-Management*.

James T. Fitzgerald, Ph.D., is Associate Director for Education and Evaluation at the Geriatric Research, Education, and Clinical Center, Ann Arbor VA Center; Associate Director for Education at the Geriatrics Center, University of Michigan Medical School; and Associate Professor, Department of Medical Education, University of Michigan Medical School, Ann Arbor, Michigan.

Marion J. Franz, M.S., R.D., C.D.E., heads Nutrition Concepts by Franz in Minneapolis, Minnesota. She co-chaired the work group that drafted the American Diabetes Association Position Statement, "Nutrition Principles and Recommendations in Diabetes."

Jennifer Merritt Hackel, R.N., M.S., C.S., C.D.E., is a Nurse Practitioner and diabetes educator at the University of Michigan Geriatric Center, Ann Arbor, Michigan.

Charlotte A. Hayes, M.M.Sc., M.S., R.D., C.D.E., is a diabetes nutrition and exercise consultant in private practice in Atlanta, Georgia. She is certified by the American College of Sports Medicine as an exercise specialist.

Robert Hogikyan, M.D., is a Clinical Associate Professor at the University of Michigan, Ann Arbor, Michigan, and is Medical Director for the Extended Care Center at the VA hospital in Ann Arbor, Michigan.

Kathryn Palanci, B.S., is a Program Coordinator in the Department of Medical Education at the University of Michigan in Ann Arbor, Michigan.

Shauna S. Roberts, Ph.D., is a medical writer and editor based in New Orleans, Lousiana.

Barbara R. Shay, M. Ed., is a Program Associate at the University of Michigan in Ann Arbor, Michigan, and the Geriatric Research, Education, and Clinical Center, Ann Arbor VA Center.

Peter Vaitkevicius, M.D., is a geriatrician and cardiologist who specializes in cardiac care of the older adult. He is an Assistant Professor at the University of Michigan School of Medicine and a staff physician at both the University of Michigan Medical Center and the VA Ann Arbor Healthcare System.

Linda Ann Wray, Ph.D., is Assistant Professor of Biobehavioral Health at Pennsylvania State University, University Park, Pennsylvania.

1
Getting Started

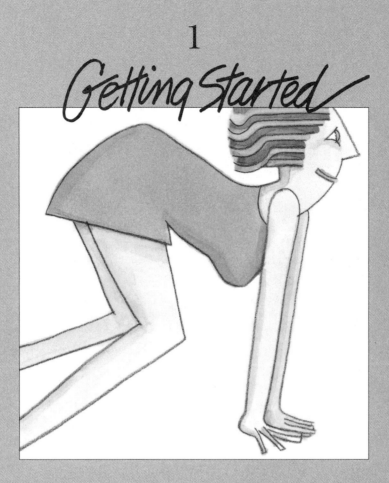

Living With Diabetes

1. How can my family help me with my diabetes? Are there community resources that could also help me?

2. Can I find good information about living with diabetes on the Internet?

3. I live alone. Where can I find help with my diabetes?

4. Do I need to tell my boss that I have diabetes? What about other people?

5. I've seen those medical alert bracelets. Should I get one because of my diabetes?

6. Sometimes my family isn't very helpful at all when it comes to my sticking to a healthy meal plan. What can I do about that?

7. My diabetes meal plan doesn't include very many of my favorite dishes. Is there anything I can do about that?

8. I get discouraged sometimes trying to follow a meal plan. What can I do?

9. There are just too many things to think about with diabetes. How can I keep track of all the things I need to do? What can I do to reduce my stress?

10. It's depressing to think that my diabetes won't let me lead the life I used to or the way I'd like. What can I do about that?

11. My eyes aren't as good as they used to be, so I have a hard time seeing my feet to check them every day. How am I supposed to check my feet?

12. I can't see well enough to measure my insulin. What can I do about that?

13. How often should I be getting dilated eye exams?

14. I don't see as well as I used to, so getting out and exercising every day is difficult. What can I do?

15. What about holidays and special occasions? It's not the same if I can't indulge my sweet tooth every so often.

16. I know smoking isn't really good for me, but since I need to lose weight because of my diabetes, is it all right to keep smoking to keep from eating junk food?

17. My sex life isn't what it used to be. Does diabetes have anything to do with that? What can I do about it?

18. I feel like my diabetes is taking over my life and it's getting me down. How can I deal with that?

19. I am having a hard time adjusting to the switch from pills to insulin. Why is this switch necessary? Can I do anything to make it easier?

20. Sometimes I feel like I'm losing some of my marbles. Does diabetes have anything to do with that? Is there anything I can do about that?

21. My doctor wants me to switch from seeing just him at each visit to seeing a whole team of people. Is this really necessary?

Day-to-Day and Long-Term Care

22. I keep hearing the term "lipids." What is a lipid?

23. Why am I at a higher risk for heart disease?

24. What is the HbA_{1c} test?

25. What happens if my blood glucose drops too low?

26. Will diabetes shorten my life expectancy?

27. Will I go blind?

28. I have been told to check my feet daily. What am I looking for?

29. What is the best way to prevent ingrown toenails? Most of what I read says to cut them straight across.

30. How can I prevent damage to my kidneys?

31. My hands and feet tingle. What causes this?

32. I have heard that impotence can be a complication of diabetes. Why?

33. What medical tests and other things do I need to take care of myself?

34. Sometimes I leave my doctor's appointment more confused than when I arrived. Any suggestions?

35. There are times when I seem to urinate more often. What causes this?

36. I have several different health concerns that I take drugs for. How can I be sure these drugs won't cause problems when I take them together?

37. Why is it important to have an annual eye exam?

38. I feel fine. Is diabetes really that serious?

39. My gums are red, sore and bleeding. Is this happening because I have diabetes?

40. What is the relationship between diabetes and my oral health?

41. What are the risks to my oral health because I have diabetes?

42. How does ethnicity affect diabetic complications?

43. Does treatment differ for each ethnic group?

Getting Physical

44. What does exercise have to do with diabetes? Why do I need to exercise if I have diabetes?

45. Should I talk with my doctor before starting to exercise?

46. What kinds of exercise should I be doing?

47. Are there types of exercise I shouldn't be doing?

48. How do I know how often and how long I should be exercising?

49. Is it possible to exercise too much? What happens if I do?

50. I really don't like to exercise if it means jogging and stuff like that. Is there something I can do that's not so hard?

51. It is hard to do regular exercise, particularly if it means long workouts. Will shorter workouts be all right?

52. What happens if I skip a day or two of exercise?

53. My feet hurt when I exercise. What should I do about this?

54. My legs hurt when I exercise. What should I do about that?

55. Should I eat before I exercise? Why is that important?

56. Should I carry a snack with me when I exercise?

57. Is it better for me to check my blood glucose before or after I exercise? And why?

58. Is it all right to exercise before going to sleep?

59. What kind of exercise can I do if the weather is bad or if I worry about dangers in my neighborhood?

Q A *Living With Diabetes*

1.
How can my family help me with my diabetes? Are there community resources that could also help me?

Families can be an important source of support in managing your diabetes. The first thing you need to do is educate yourself and your family about your diabetes. Next, determine the areas where you need and want assistance and/or support. Then communicate these needs to your family. Encouragement and support from your family can help you in maintaining your diabetes, particularly in maintaining your diet and exercise programs.

Family members should also be aware of the warning signs of high and low blood glucose and know what to do to help you. Symptoms of high blood glucose include frequent urination, dry mouth, and excessive thirst. Symptoms of low blood glucose include shakiness, sweating, irritable mood, numbness around the mouth, nausea, blurred vision, and weakness, but not all of these signs need to be present.

There are many community resources available to help you. Contact your local American Diabetes Association affiliate, health department, or hospital for advice on sources of diabetes information, exercise programs, weight-loss programs, smoking-cessation programs, and diabetes support groups in your area. The Internet is another source for locating community and information resources.

2.
Can I find good information about living with diabetes on the Internet?

As with most topics on the Internet, there are an enormous number of sites offering information and advice on diabetes and its treatment. Finding reputable and unbiased sites is essential for any search for information using the Internet. The following sites are recommended for information regarding diabetes:

- MEDLINEplus, a service of the National Library of Medicine
  http://www.nlm.nih.gov/medlineplus/diabetes.html
- Centers for Disease Control and Prevention Public Health Resource
  http://www.cdc.gov/diabetes/

Q A

- American Diabetes Association
  http://www.diabetes.org/
- American Association of Diabetes Educators
  http://www.aadenet.org/
- University of Michigan Diabetes Research and
  Training Center
  http://www.med.umich.edu/mdrtc/

3.

I live alone. Where can I find help with my diabetes?

There are many diabetes resources that can provide you with information and assistance. Determine the areas of information or the type of assistance you want. Talk to your doctor or nurse about these needs; they should be able to make suggestions and direct your efforts. You can also contact your local American Diabetes Association affiliate or your local health department (city, county, or state). Coping with diabetes can sometimes be difficult, and it is important to seek help and support when you need it; discuss your feelings with relatives living nearby, friends, or your minister, priest, or rabbi. Some people find diabetes support groups useful in caring for their diabetes.

4.

Do I need to tell my boss that I have diabetes? What about other people?

Who you tell about your diabetes is a personal decision. With regard to your employer, you cannot lie about having diabetes (this could be grounds for dismissal), but you don't have to volunteer such information. People with diabetes are protected from job discrimination under the Americans with Disabilities Act; however, your employer must know you are "disabled." To learn more about diabetes and your rights in the workplace, we suggest you go to the American Diabetes Association's website http://www.diabetes.org/main/community/advocacy/workplace_discrim.jsp.

Our advice is that you tell at least some fellow employees so they are aware of the warning signs of high and low blood glucose and can get appropriate assistance if you experience either of these problems.

Q A

5.

I've seen those medical alert bracelets. Should I get one because of my diabetes?

Yes. In an emergency situation it can quickly provide important information to health-care personnel; knowing an individual has diabetes is important when providing emergency care. However, there are many options for medical alert identification besides wrist bracelets; there are also ankle bracelets, necklaces, and wallet cards to name just a few. Choose the identification product that appeals to you and best fits your lifestyle.

6.

Sometimes my family isn't very helpful at all when it comes to my sticking to a healthy meal plan. What can I do about that?

Diabetes affects the entire family; some of your family members may be going through some of the same emotions as you (anger, denial, minimizing the seriousness of your diabetes). Some may react by trying to take charge (the food police), while others may deny the seriousness of your diabetes and tempt you with food. Remember, the fact that you have diabetes can be very stressful for your family as well as for you. An open discussion with your family about their feelings, worries, and expectations—as well as what you need and want from them regarding your diabetes—may be helpful. Tell them how they can be supportive. And tell them which behavior you find less than supportive. Remind them that you are ultimately responsible for your diabetes management even though they may not agree with some of your decisions. Be patient and take these opportunities to educate them.

7.

My diabetes meal plan doesn't include very many of my favorite dishes. Is there anything I can do about that?

A diabetes meal plan is nothing more than a healthy eating plan and should contain selections from all six food groups. However, there are foods to avoid; foods high in fat and cholesterol should be used sparingly. If possible, substitute the ingredients of your favorite dishes with healthier choices (for example, use skim

Q A

or 2% milk instead of whole milk). Try low-fat or sugar-free versions of your favorite foods. You can also try alternative cooking methods (baking rather than deep frying, for instance). Try experimenting with healthier dishes that are similar to your favorites; maybe establish new favorite dishes. If you do indulge in your favorite dishes, limit the frequency and amount you eat.

8.
I get discouraged sometimes trying to follow a meal plan. What can I do?

Changing your diet can be a challenging endeavor. Altering patterns developed over a lifetime can be very difficult. It's made harder by the fact that food has many different functions and associations for people aside from nutrition. Nonetheless, nutrition therapy (following a diabetes meal plan) is usually an integral component of diabetes care. So you are not alone; many people find diabetes meal plans tough to follow.

There are two recommendations we can make, though. First, determine the source of discouragement; is it a lack of variation in your diet, is the diet too complex, are you unable to maintain your diet? Once you have identified the source, contact a dietitian, a certified diabetes educator (C.D.E.), or your physician to help you address your concerns or problems.

Second, you might find more success by making a more gradual change to your diet; for example, switching from whole milk to 2% milk and then to skim milk. You will probably have lapses in your diet management along the way. But try not to be overly critical of yourself and your efforts.

9.
There are just too many things to think about with diabetes. How can I keep track of all the things I need to do? What can I do to reduce my stress?

Managing diabetes is a complex activity. You may find caring for it overwhelming. You are asked to do many new things and to alter your lifestyle. Trying to balance your diet, exercise, and medicine and keeping

Q A

an eye on your blood glucose level can be very stressful at the onset. Try focusing on short-term goals—what you have to do for tomorrow or this week. Acknowledge that you will have good days and bad days, but keep on trying.

Stress can affect your blood glucose levels, so it is important to be able to identify symptoms of stress; headaches, muscle tension, sleeplessness, and less interest in sex are some symptoms that can indicate stress. There are many ways to handle your stress. Some ways people have found to be effective include exercise, prayer, visual imagery, deep breathing, massage, and talking with their spouse, a relative, or a friend about their difficulties. Joining a diabetes support group may also help you manage the stress you feel. If you are overwhelmed and feel unable to cope, it's important to discuss your feelings with your doctor or nurse. They can assist you directly or help locate another professional or program that can.

10.
It's depressing to think that my diabetes won't let me lead the life I used to or the way I'd like. What can I do about that?

Feeling depressed about having diabetes is a common problem. Having a chronic disease to contend with can be daunting. However, having diabetes doesn't mean you can't have a full and rewarding life. Nor does it necessarily mean that you have to restrict or forgo your normal activities, interests, or hobbies. What is it that you feel you can't do anymore? Talk with your doctor or nurse to see if that is actually the case.

When you are sad or depressed about your diabetes, talking about your feelings may be helpful. Discuss your feelings with your spouse, a relative, a friend, your doctor, or your religious leader (minister, priest, rabbi, imam). You can join a diabetes support group (call the American Diabetes Association, your local health department, or your local hospital about groups in your area). If your feelings of depression last for two or more weeks or if they keep you from managing your diabetes, it would be a good idea to contact your doctor. You may need extra help or your depression may have a physical cause.

Q A

11.
My eyes aren't as good as they used to be, so I have a hard time seeing my feet to check them every day. How am I supposed to check my feet?

It is very important that you check your feet every day. People with diabetes have decreased circulation to their extremities, are more susceptible to infections, and have less feeling in their feet. When you check your feet, look for sores, cuts, or infections that you may or may not feel.

If you are not able to see your feet, ask your spouse, relative, or friend do it for you. If this is not an option, use a magnifying glass or a magnifying mirror with an extension to clearly see the entire foot area. If you find a foot problem or concern, contact your doctor or nurse. Also, remember to have your doctor or nurse check your feet at every office visit.

12.
I can't see well enough to measure my insulin. What can I do about that?

There are various dosage aids available to assist people with visual limitations. Some such devices include systems that allow you to measure by touch, devices that give an audible indication (such as a click) for each measure, and syringe magnifiers. Devices for people who are blind may also be of assistance. (If you have trouble measuring insulin, you may also have trouble reading your blood glucose meter. There are blood glucose meters that have voice units that let you hear the results of your test.)

Other options for measuring your insulin dose include having someone do it for you—your spouse, a relative, or a friend, for instance, if they are available and willing. You may want a contingency plan, however, that includes one of the products mentioned above in case nobody is available to measure your insulin for you. Talk to your doctor or nurse about your vision difficulties and the possible options to determine the best choice for you.

Q A

13.
How often should I be getting dilated eye exams?

Whether you should have your pupils dilated during a particular examination depends on several key considerations: (1) the specific eye conditions that you have, (2) the reason you're being evaluated at each examination, and (3) how well you're managing your diabetes, including blood sugar levels, blood pressure, and blood lipids.

Diabetes affects many different parts of the eye, not just the light-sensitive retina. People with diabetes also commonly have problems with the cornea (the front surface of the eye), the internal lens (where cataracts can form), the optic nerve (which can be damaged by glaucoma, or chronic, progressive damage to the optic nerve usually associated with increased internal eye pressure), and the nerves responsible for controlling eye muscles. Diagnosis and continuing management of some of these conditions do not require dilation of the pupils at each visit. For example, people with diabetes are two to four times more likely to develop glaucoma, and proper management of this disease does not require dilated pupils at all visits to the eye doctor (although it does require dilation at least annually), but it does include regular measurements of internal eye pressure (every 1–6 months depending on the severity of the condition).

The most serious diabetes-related eye disease is diabetic retinopathy, which has several different stages of severity. Although it often does not cause symptoms in earlier stages, diabetic retinopathy may result in blindness if left untreated. The American Diabetes Association recommends that people with diabetes receive dilated retinal examinations at least annually, because dilation allows the doctor to see more of the internal eye, more easily, and in stereo (3-D). Some forms of retinopathy can only be detected with three-dimensional examination techniques. More serious stages of retinopathy are often followed more closely by eye doctors (in particular, severe nonproliferative diabetic retinopathy [leaking of fluid from blood vessels in the eye], proliferative diabetic retinopathy [the development of fragile, new

Q A

blood vessels in the eye that can cloud vision by bleeding or cause blindness by detaching the retina from the back of the eye], and macular edema [swelling at the part of the retina that gives sharpest vision, causing blurred vision]), with dilated eye exams as often as every 2–6 months. Laser treatment or drug therapies typically are used when the degree of retinopathy reaches a certain threshold. (Research has shown that treatment at earlier stages is not beneficial.)

The Diabetes Control and Complications Trial (DCCT) and the United Kingdom Prospective Diabetes Study (UKPDS), two large studies involving people with Type 1 and Type 2 diabetes, respectively, clearly showed that tight control of blood glucose and blood pressure reduce the risk and progression of diabetic retinopathy. It is widely believed that uncontrolled blood glucose and high blood pressure, as well as abnormal blood lipids (commonly seen in people with diabetes) increase the risk of all types of diabetic eye disease. Eye doctors will often follow patients with poor control of these factors more closely.

14.

I don't see as well as I used to, so getting out and exercising every day is difficult. What can I do?

Being physically active is important for controlling your diabetes. Exercise burns calories and reduces your blood glucose levels. It is important for you to exercise regularly. The usual recommendation is 20 to 30 minutes of exercise 3–5 times per week (not every day).

Your vision problems should not prevent you from exercising. There are many types of physical activity appropriate for people with poor vision. Flexibility exercises (stretching) and weight machines for strength training do not require good vision. Walking with a friend, dancing with a partner, and water exercises are a few other activities where poor vision is not a problem. Try out a number of activities to find those that you enjoy. Ask your doctor or nurse for recommendations. And remember, before you start any new exercise program, discuss it with your doctor or nurse to make sure it is safe for you.

Q A

15.
What about holidays and special occasions? It's not the same if I can't indulge my sweet tooth every so often.

Many holidays and celebrations have strong associations with food—for example, Thanksgiving and roasted turkey, Fourth of July and barbeques, and birthdays and cake. For many people, these events wouldn't be the same if these foods were missing.

Small indulgences are probably fine, but limit these indulgences to special occasions and small portions. As with many things, moderation is the key. Try using sugar-free and fat-free substitutes in your traditional recipes (this may take some experimentation to determine the appropriate measures) or try to find low-fat, low-sugar recipes for your favorites foods.

16.
I know smoking isn't really good for me, but since I need to lose weight because of my diabetes, is it all right to keep smoking to keep from eating junk food?

No, it's not all right. Smoking is much more harmful than gaining a few extra pounds. The negative effects of smoking (for example, cancer and heart disease) are well documented. For people with diabetes, the dangers of smoking are increased. Smoking raises blood glucose levels and makes it more difficult to control your diabetes. Smokers are also at increased risk for diabetes complications, such as kidney disease, foot problems and heart disease.

Not all people gain weight when they stop smoking, and there are things you can do to minimize potential weight gain. Before you stop smoking, become more physically active and improve your diet. Increasing your physical activity can be as simple as climbing stairs rather than taking an elevator, raking leaves in your yard, or walking to a mailbox rather than driving. Improve your diet by choosing low-fat and low-calorie foods and beverages, by increasing your intake of fruit, grains, and vegetables, and by cutting back on the amount of meat you eat.

Smoking is a difficult habit to stop, but there are many programs and products available to help you

Q A

to stop. Ask your doctor or nurse about these programs and products to determine what would be best for you.

17.
My sex life isn't what it used to be. Does diabetes have anything to do with that? What can I do about it?

Yes, diabetes can have a negative impact on your sex life. A common problem for men is impotence (inability to achieve or maintain an erection, also called erectile dysfunction). Women with diabetes may experience difficulty achieving an orgasm, have vaginal dryness, and are more susceptible to vaginal infections. The good news is that there are many effective treatments for male impotence due to physical causes; ask your doctor about such treatments. For women, lubricants (for example, K-Y jelly) can assist with vaginal dryness, and there are many over-the-counter products that treat vaginal infections. However, if these problems persist, seek further medical advice from your doctor or nurse.

Sexual problems are not a normal part of aging. While some people find it embarrassing to discuss such issues, there are effective treatments that can resolve many of these problems. If you are having difficulties, please discuss these difficulties with your doctor or nurse.

18.
I feel like my diabetes is taking over my life and it's getting me down. How can I deal with that?

It is not unusual for people to feel angry or depressed about having diabetes. Diabetes is a life-long disease requiring many lifestyle changes. For people who have just been diagnosed with diabetes, the sudden requirement for attentive self-care can be overwhelming. Most people are asked to start a regular exercise program, change their diet, monitor their blood glucose levels, and begin medications (either pills or insulin injections). Thankfully, there are some coping strategies and programs that can help you adjust and get used to your diabetes. Ask your doctor or nurse about these. Find one that is best for you and your lifestyle.

Q A

It might help to talk about these feelings. Discuss your feelings with someone close to you (your spouse, a relative, or friend). Many people find diabetes support groups helpful in understanding and coping with diabetes. Call the local affiliate of the American Diabetes Association, your local health department, or your local hospital to find out about groups in your area. If these feelings last for two weeks or more or if they interfere with the management of your diabetes, it would be a good idea to talk with your doctor. You may need extra help. Alternatively, your feelings may be caused by something physical.

19.
I am having a hard time adjusting to the switch from pills to insulin. Why is this switch necessary? Can I do anything to make it easier?

The ideal goal of diabetes treatment is to achieve a normal level of blood glucose. Getting your blood glucose level as near to normal as possible helps prevent or slow down the progression of diabetes complications. Oral medicines and/or insulin injections, along with a meal plan and exercise, help in achieving this goal. Over time, some oral medicines may no longer help you achieve or maintain normal blood glucose levels. When this happens, your doctor may switch you to insulin injections to achieve the best control possible. Most people are anxious and wary about giving themselves insulin shots, but those injections are helping them avoid complications. If you need further assurance, talk with your doctor about your feelings or seek the advice and experience of insulin users.

20.
Sometimes I feel like I'm losing some of my marbles. Does diabetes have anything to do with that? Is there anything I can do about that?

Uncontrolled diabetes (consistently high blood glucose levels) over an extended time may result in a decline in mental processes, including concentration, reasoning, language ability, and memory. However, it is more likely that you are feeling the anxiety and stress of treating and coping with your diabetes. Deal-

Q A

ing with a lifelong, chronic disease such as diabetes can be stressful and feel overwhelming. Many people with diabetes feel this way at one time or another. There are many ways to reduce stress. Try to find several methods that you find effective and best fit your lifestyle. Discuss your feelings with someone close to you (your spouse, a relative, a friend, or your clergyman, for instance) or join a support group (call the American Diabetes Association, your local health department, or your local hospital to find groups in your area). If you think that what you are experiencing is not stress-related, if it continues for an extended period of time, or if it prevents you from caring for your diabetes, contact your doctor or nurse and discuss your concerns.

21.
My doctor wants me to switch from seeing just him at each visit to seeing a whole team of people. Is this really necessary?

Type 2 diabetes is a complex, multifaceted disease. Providing appropriate and effective treatment (getting and maintaining your blood glucose levels at or as near to normal levels as possible) is also complex and multifaceted. Seeing more people at your medical visits means more comprehensive care for you. It is difficult, if not impossible, for your doctor to provide all the components necessary for treating your diabetes; the team approach is a way to provide you with all the support and information you need to manage your diabetes. Each of these health professionals will focus on different aspects of your diabetes care. For example, the doctor may focus on the effectiveness of different medicines, the dietitian will provide you with an appropriate diet plan, and the social worker can help you find local support services. A diabetes health-care team usually consists of a doctor, a nurse, and a dietitian. However, it may also include a pharmacist, a health educator, a podiatrist, and/or an eye doctor. The most important team member, though, is you.

Q A

Day-to-Day and Long-Term Care

22.
I keep hearing the term "lipids."
What is a lipid?

A lipid is a term for fat or blood fat. These fats include cholesterol and triglycerides, which are both produced by our body. They are also found in animal foods that we eat. Your body uses cholesterol to build cell walls and to help create certain vitamins and hormones. Triglycerides are stored fats that your body uses for energy, much in the manner that a car has a reserve fuel tank. When your body needs energy, it breaks down these lipids into fatty acids and burns them for fuel.

There are three kinds of blood fats that affect blood vessels: (1) high-density lipoprotein, (2) low-density lipoprotein, and (3) very-low-density lipoprotein. High-density lipoprotein (HDL) cholesterol carries cholesterol away from the blood vessel walls to the liver. The liver then breaks up the cholesterol and sends it out of the body. The more HDL you have in your blood, the better for your blood vessels. Low-density lipoprotein (LDL) cholesterol carries cholesterol to parts of your body that need it. Unfortunately, LDL cholesterol can stick to blood vessel walls, and cholesterol on blood vessel walls can lead to cardiovascular disease. So the less LDL you have in your blood, the better. Very-low-density lipoprotein (VLDL) carries triglycerides, cholesterol, and other fats to fat tissue. VLDL then forms itself into LDL.

It is important to have your lipids tested annually to make sure that you are maintaining healthy levels of blood fats. Target goals are as follows:
- Total cholesterol under 200 mg/dl
- LDL cholesterol under 100 mg/dl
- HDL cholesterol over 40 mg/dl for men and over 50 mg/dl for women

23.
Why am I at a higher risk for
heart disease?

People with diabetes are more likely to develop blood vessel disease, also known as atherosclerosis or "hardening of the arteries," which leads to heart disease. Unhealthy cholesterol levels contribute to this. When blood vessels become narrowed by a buildup of plaque, blood flow slows. This slow blood flow can damage the heart (coronary artery disease), the brain

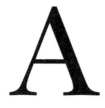

(cerebrovascular disease), or the feet and legs (peripheral vascular disease). The lack of blood flow to the feet and legs can lead to amputation. A complete blockage, caused by a blood clot in a narrowed artery, can cause a heart attack or stroke.

You are at greater risk for heart disease if you have any of the following characteristics:

- You smoke
- You have high blood pressure
- You have high cholesterol levels
- You are overweight

Your risk is significantly increased if you have more than one of these characteristics.

24.
What is the HbA$_{1c}$ test?

Hemoglobin (Hb) is a protein of red blood cells that carries oxygen from the lungs to the cells throughout your body. The bond between oxygen and hemoglobin is fortunately a loose one, which allows oxygen to be released to the tissues where it is most needed. But hemoglobin also bonds to glucose, and that is a very tight bond, lasting for the life of the red blood cell (approximately four months). By measuring the amount of glucose attached to the hemoglobin component called A$_{1c}$, your doctor can get an accurate picture of your average blood glucose control over the preceding few months. Thus, the HbA$_{1c}$ test is an indication of how well your diabetes is being controlled. To perform this test, a sample of your blood is taken and sent to a lab. The blood sample can be drawn at any time of the day, regardless of what you recently ate or what your blood glucose levels are at the time of the test. A nondiabetic HbA$_{1c}$ level is between 4% and 6.5%: discuss with your doctor what your HbA$_{1c}$ goal should be. In general, the American Diabetes Association recommends that the goal be below 7%. Keeping your blood glucose as close as you can to nondiabetic levels will help you prevent or slow the development of long-term complications of diabetes.

25.
What happens if my blood glucose drops too low?

A drop in blood glucose levels can occur when a person with diabetes injects too much insulin, doesn't

Q A

eat enough food, or exercises without eating extra food. A person with low blood glucose (hypoglycemia) may feel nervous, shaky, weak, or sweaty and have a headache, blurred vision, and hunger. Taking small amounts of sugar (four teaspoons), juice (four ounces), or food with sugar (three graham crackers) will usually help you feel better within 15 minutes. Check your blood glucose level. If it is below 70 mg/dl, eat again. Continue this pattern of eating, waiting, and checking your blood glucose until your blood glucose rises above 70 mg/dl. Contact your doctor if you experience frequent hypoglycemia. If left untreated, low blood glucose can cause you to lose consciousness. At the worst, untreated low blood glucose can cause seizures, coma, and even death.

26.
Will diabetes shorten my
life expectancy?

Uncontrolled diabetes increases your chances of developing complications that could affect your life expectancy. The complications associated with diabetes (eye diseases, kidney disease, nerve damage, and blood vessel disease) occur more often in people with diabetes than in people without diabetes. Your best defense against these complications and for a normal life expectancy is to keep your blood glucose levels as close to normal as possible. Normal blood glucose levels are the levels of people who do not have diabetes. The closer you can get to and maintain normal blood glucose levels, the more likely you are to prevent or delay complications and enjoy a normal life expectancy.

27.
Will I go blind?

Uncontrolled diabetes can result in blurred vision, glaucoma, cataracts, or other eye problems that could eventually lead to blindness. People with diabetes are more likely to develop an eye disease than people without diabetes. However, these problems are usually avoided or kept minimal with proper diabetes management and care. The keys to prevention are to keep your blood glucose at a healthy level, control high blood pressure, quit smoking, lower high cholesterol, and get yearly eye exams.

Q&A

The three main eye diseases associated with diabetes are retinopathy, cataracts, and glaucoma. Of the three, retinopathy is the most common. Retinopathy refers to damage in the small blood vessels that bring oxygen to the retina. The retina is the lining at the back of the eye that receives the image formed by the lens. There are two types of retinopathy: nonproliferative and proliferative. In nonproliferative (or background) retinopathy, the small blood vessels in the retina bulge and form pouches. These bulges weaken the blood vessels and may cause them to leak fluid. This leaking does not usually harm your sight and often never gets worse. However, nonproliferative retinopathy may progress to proliferative retinopathy. In proliferative retinopathy, the small blood vessels are so damaged they close off. In response, new blood vessels grow and branch out to other parts of your eye. Although these new vessels are growing in the eye, they lack the ability to nourish the retina as well as the original vessels. In addition, the new vessels have the tendency to break easily, thus releasing blood into the eye. This can cause dark spots and cloudy vision.

Diabetic retinopathy is the leading cause of blindness in people ages 20–74. Currently, it occurs in 90% of persons with Type 1 diabetes and in 65% of persons with Type 2 diabetes. Damage from diabetic retinopathy can occur before any outward signs of the disease. It is important that you have an eye exam by a professional once each year and that you immediately report unusual symptoms such as cloudy vision, dark spots in your vision, fluctuating vision, and episodes of temporary blindness.

28.
I have been told to check my feet daily. What am I looking for?

You need to examine both feet each day and you need to examine the entire foot. If you cannot see well enough to do this, have a friend or relative who can see well do it for you. You are looking for the following conditions:

■ Cuts, cracks, and breaks in the skin
■ Ingrown toenails
■ Redness
■ Changes in shape

- Changes in color
- Cold spots or hot spots
- Ulcers
- Punctures
- Blisters
- Calluses
- Swelling
- Pain
- Loss of feeling
- Corns
- Dryness or peeling

If you notice any of these symptoms, contact your doctor or nurse no matter how minor you think it is.

29.
What is the best way to prevent ingrown toenails? Most of what I read says to cut them straight across.

Although heredity may play a part in the occurrence of ingrown toenails in some individuals, here are some good nail-care practices that will lessen your chances of getting ingrown toenails.

- Your information about trimming the nails straight across is correct. This provides shape and support to the nail. Never cut deeply into a toenail's corners; a nail splinter can be created along the side, which may grow into the skin and cause an infection. It is better to smooth the edges and corners with an emery board, which can also prevent jagged edges that may catch on your socks. You should also leave a small bit of nail growth at the end of the toe, never cutting the nails too short or into the "quick."

- Avoid ill-fitting shoes, socks, and nylons, which can place undue pressure on your feet and toes. If footwear is too snug or narrow in the toe box, it can crowd the toes and interfere with the proper growth of the nails. Take care to wear shoes with ample room for the toes to move freely, and be sure your socks or nylons are not pulled tightly against the toes.

- See your foot doctor immediately if you suspect you may be developing ingrown toenails. Delaying treatment may result in infection. Symptoms of an ingrown toenail may include pain, redness, and swelling around the nail or a change in the usual shape of the nail. Your physician can prescribe a

Q A

number of treatments or even therapeutic footwear as needed.

Ingrown toenails should not be taken lightly. They can lead to infection and serious complications if not cared for properly. Good nail grooming, well-fitting footwear, regular foot checks by your health-care professional, and prompt attention to unusual signs and symptoms should provide you with the best prevention tools available.

30.
How can I prevent damage to my kidneys?

The key to prevention is proper management of your diabetes and keeping in contact with your doctor. When you have high blood glucose, you overwork your kidneys because your body needs to flush out the excess glucose. Years of overuse can damage your kidneys. Do your best to keep your blood glucose levels normal, eat healthy, and exercise.

There are steps you can take to prevent or slow down kidney disease:
■ Keep your blood glucose levels as close to normal as possible.
■ Have your doctor check your kidneys periodically. This should include the following lab tests: blood urea nitrogen, serum creatinine, creatinine clearance, and albumin excretion rate.
■ Keep your blood pressure under control.
■ Limit the amount of protein in your diet.

31.
My hands and feet tingle. What causes this?

This could be nerve damage. Many people who have had diabetes for a long time have nerve damage. Although nerve damage can affect many parts of the body, it is very common for people with diabetes to have pain in their feet and legs or for those areas to tingle or feel numb. This is called distal symmetric polyneuropathy. This can be the beginning signs of nerve damage, so let your doctor know. To prevent or lessen nerve damage keep blood glucose levels in control, stop smoking, drink less alcohol, keep blood pressure and cholesterol levels under control, and have a yearly check for nerve damage. Other signs of nerve damage may include coldness, burning, sensations of

Q A

bugs crawling over your skin or of walking on a strange surface, deep aching, overly sensitive skin, or jabs of needlelike pain. The signs of nerve damage to the feet, legs, or hands tend to worsen at night. Signs often get better if you get out of bed and walk around a bit.

**32.
I have heard that impotence can be a complication of diabetes. Why?**

The nerve damage and circulatory problems encountered by people with diabetes can lead to a gradual loss of sexual feeling or response in both men and women. However, these problems do not affect sex drive; this remains unchanged. About half of men with diabetes become impotent; they become unable to have erections or may reach sexual climax without ejaculating normally. For men, the most common cause is damage to either the nerves or the blood vessels in the penis.

Physical impotence usually happens slowly and gets progressively worse. Signs include a less rigid penis and fewer erections. Eventually, there are no erections.

For women, poor vaginal lubrication is a common complaint. And long periods of high blood glucose can lead to damage that can interfere with the ability of the vagina to expand and lubricate on arousal.

Keeping your blood glucose under good control is the best way to avoid the nerve damage and circulatory problems that lead to these problems.

**33.
What medical tests and other things do I need to take care of myself?**

Here are some suggestions:
- Visit your doctor or nurse at least every 3–6 months if stable, or more frequently if needed.
- Get a yearly medical checkup (a medical history and physical exam).
- Get an HbA_{1c} test every 3–6 months.
- Get a yearly eye examination.
- Make sure your doctor or nurse examines your feet at each visit.
- Get a fasting lipids test yearly.
- Get a urine test yearly.

Q   A

34.
Sometimes I leave my doctor's appointment more confused than when I arrived. Any suggestions?

Yes. First, don't be afraid to ask questions. And repeat the explanations and/or the care instructions you get back to your doctor to ensure that you heard or understood correctly. Some people take notes during their office visit or have the doctor write things down for them. You could also ask a relative or trusted friend to accompany you during the visit to help you remember the conversation.

If you are confused after your visit, talk with the nurse or the C.D.E. (certified diabetes educator) in the office as soon as possible. They will be able to answer your questions or refer you to the person who can. Often a pharmacist can help answer questions, especially those about your medications. Just keep asking; you need to be a knowledgeable consumer of medical care.

35.
There are times when I seem to urinate more often. What causes this?

Any of a number of things may be causing this. One is autonomic neuropathy. Autonomic neuropathy is a complication of diabetes that often affects the organs that control urination. Nerve damage can prevent the bladder from emptying completely, allowing bacteria to grow more easily in the urinary tract (bladder and kidneys). This can lead to a urinary tract infection. One of the symptoms of urinary tract infection is the need to urinate often. When the nerves of the bladder are damaged, a person may have difficulty knowing when the bladder is full or controlling it (urinary incontinence). Other signs of a urinary tract infection include pain or burning when you urinate, cloudy or bloody urine, low back pain or abdominal pain, fever, and chills. When your blood glucose level is high, you are more likely to get a urinary tract infection. These infections can be treated with antibiotic drugs.

Q A

36.

I have several different health concerns that I take drugs for. How can I be sure these drugs won't cause problems when I take them together?

A talk with your doctor is in order. Tell him your worries and have him explain what each pill is for and why you need to take it. Ask about possible drug interactions that you should be concerned about. Also talk with your pharmacist; he can also describe the purpose of each pill. He will also be able to let you know of any side effects or possible drug interactions. You also want to let your doctor and pharmacist know of any over-the-counter medicines and/or supplements you are taking. Both over-the-counter medicines and vitamin/mineral/herbal preparations can have side effects and can interact in a negative way when combined with your other medications. Your best defense against harmful interactions is open communication with both your doctor and pharmacist.

37.

Why is it important to have an annual eye exam?

An annual exam is essential because of the potential for eye problems associated with diabetes: retinopathy, glaucoma, and cataracts. Proper management of your diabetes will minimize the risk of getting these problems. Here are some guidelines to help you keep your eyes free of disease:

■ Keep your blood glucose levels as close to normal as possible.

■ Control your blood pressure (high blood pressure can make eye diseases worse).

■ Quit smoking (smoking damages blood vessels).

■ Lower high cholesterol (high cholesterol can also damage blood vessels).

■ Get yearly eye exams by an eye doctor. (Many eye diseases can do damage without symptoms. An eye doctor has the tools and tests to find problems early.)

38.

I feel fine. Is diabetes really that serious?

Yes, diabetes is a very serious, life-threatening disease if left untreated or uncontrolled. Many of the symp-

Q   A

toms of diabetes appear only after an extended period of time, so it is important to address your diabetes before the symptoms appear. It is very important that you see and be treated by a doctor to make sure that you avoid or minimize the risk of diabetes complications. Such complications include glaucoma, cataracts, periodontal disease, heart disease, kidney disease, and nerve damage.

39.
My gums are red, sore and bleeding. Is this happening because I have diabetes?

That could be. Like other complications of diabetes, gum disease is linked to diabetes control. People with poor blood glucose control get gum disease more often and more severely, and they lose more teeth than do persons with good control. In fact, people whose diabetes is well controlled have no more gum disease than those people who don't have diabetes. You can protect yourself by knowing the symptoms of gum disease and contacting your doctor and dentist if they appear. These signs include the following:

- Red gums
- Swollen or tender gums
- Gums that bleed when you brush or floss
- Gums that pull away from your teeth
- Pus between your teeth and gums when you press on the gums
- Bad breath
- Loose teeth
- Teeth that are moving away from each other
- A change in the way your teeth fit together when you bite
- A change in the way your partial dentures fit

40.
What is the relationship between diabetes and my oral health?

Diabetes puts you at risk for gum disease and other oral infections. Infections can make your blood glucose levels go up, and a high blood glucose level can make your oral infections even worse. People with diabetes have tooth and gum disease more often if their blood glucose level stays high.

You can protect yourself by knowing the signs of gum disease (gingivitis) and other oral infections and

Q A

contacting your doctor and dentist if they appear, by taking care of your teeth, and by having regular dental exams. These are clear signs of gum disease:

- Red, sore, and swollen gums
- Bleeding gums
- Gums pulling away from your teeth
- Loose or sensitive teeth
- Bad breath
- Dentures that do not fit well

41.
What are the risks to my oral health because I have diabetes?

There are a number of oral health risks associated with diabetes:

- Gingivitis
- Periodontal disease
- Dental cavities
- Thrush
- Dry mouth
- Tooth loss

Reduce the risks by controlling your blood glucose, keeping your teeth and mouth clean, and visiting your dentist at least every six months.

42.
How does ethnicity affect diabetic complications?

Belonging to any of the following ethnic groups places you at greater risk for diabetic complications and death due to their complications: African-American, Latino, American Indian, Alaska Native, and Asian and Pacific Islander.

Genetics do play a role in diabetes, so ask your doctor about the relationship between your particular ethnic heritage and diabetes.

43.
Does treatment differ for each ethnic group?

Yes, treatment can vary for different ethnic groups based on complication patterns and cultural practices and preferences, but the goal remains the same: to keep blood glucose, lipids, and blood pressure at healthy levels. The closer that you can get to healthy levels, the more likely you are to prevent or delay complications.

Q A
Getting Physical

44.

What does exercise have to do with diabetes? Why do I need to exercise if I have diabetes?

Regular exercise helps to burn calories and increases your metabolic rate, which in turn helps you to control your weight. Engaging in a regular exercise program will also help your body to use insulin more effectively. This, in turn, will help to lower your blood glucose. Maintaining a healthy blood glucose level will help to reduce your risk of long-term diabetes complications such as nephropathy, neuropathy, and cardiovascular disease. Here are some additional reasons why you should exercise:

■ Regular exercising increases your vitality and helps combat fatigue.

■ Exercise helps you to sleep more soundly at night.

■ Exercise helps you to cope more effectively with daily stress.

■ Regular exercise assists in maintaining bone strength and bone density, and it helps keep you strong and flexible.

45.

Should I talk with my doctor before starting to exercise?

Yes! The first step in any fitness program is an appointment with your doctor. There are certain diabetes complications (such as peripheral neuropathy) that can make various forms of exercise difficult. Your physician or health-care provider can recommend the types of exercise that are most appropriate for you. In addition to reviewing your diabetes history, your doctor will complete a head-to-toe physical examination. Specifically, your doctor needs to check the following items:

■ Your blood pressure. If you have either high or low blood pressure, this will need to be treated before you start an exercise program.

■ Your current fitness level (to help determine a starting point for exercise and specific fitness goals).

■ Your overall health (including cardiac health, vision, pulmonary health, and vascular health). Various tests such as an EKG with or without an exercise stress test may be performed.

Q A

- Your lipid profile (cholesterol, HDL, LDL, and triglyceride levels).
- Your feet.

Once you have medical clearance from your doctor, you are ready to begin!

46.
What kinds of exercise should I be doing?

Once you have met with your doctor and received medical clearance to begin, the best type of exercise is the type that you enjoy and will do. Long-term adherence to an exercise program is strongly dependent upon enjoying the exercise activity. Walking is an exercise enjoyed by both exercise enthusiasts and people who have just started to exercise. Walking is an activity that can be performed anywhere, alone or with a partner, and is economical (the only "special equipment" is a good pair of walking shoes). Walking is also an ideal exercise for non-exercisers to begin with since it is easy to control the intensity, duration, and frequency. Experiment with other forms of exercise such as biking, aerobic dance, strength training, and recreational sports. You may want to work with an exercise specialist who can write an exercise prescription. An exercise prescription is an individualized plan based on your current fitness levels and fitness goals. It includes a warm-up and cool-down, aerobic and strength training activities, and stretching for flexibility. Your doctor will be able to recommend an exercise specialist for you.

47.
Are there types of exercise I shouldn't be doing?

The answer to this question is a little more complicated than a simple "yes" or a "no." Diabetes by itself does not place limits on the types of exercise that you can do. However, other medical conditions (such as cardiovascular disease) or complications stemming from diabetes may make some forms of exercise inappropriate. For example, peripheral neuropathy that affects the feet may make exercises such as walking or jogging difficult. Non-impact activities such as swimming, chair exercises, or rowing may be more suitable in that case. Be sure to check with your doctor regarding any limitations you may have.

Q   A

One good rule of thumb is that exercise should not cause pain. Pain is an indication that something is wrong; it is a different sensation from muscle fatigue. If you experience pain when you are exercising, stop what you are doing. The old adage "no pain, no gain" is simply not true.

48.
How do I know how often and how long I should be exercising?

If you haven't been exercising on a regular basis, it is crucial that you start out slowly. Walking for 5–10 minutes at a time, three times per week may be a good starting point. If walking is difficult for you, you may want to begin by performing exercises while sitting in a chair. Videotapes demonstrating chair exercises are available commercially. While exercising, you should not feel shortness of breath or feel "winded".

For proper fat metabolism and to increase your level of cardiovascular fitness, you will need to exercise aerobically (increasing your heart and breathing rates and thereby increasing your intake of oxygen). Oxygen is the component that helps to prevent lactic acid production and buildup. It is lactic acid that causes you to feel muscle fatigue. While exercising in a laboratory setting, there are instruments to measure your oxygen consumption to know whether you are staying in an aerobic zone; naturally, most of us don't exercise in such a setting! One of the best and easiest methods to determine whether you are exercising aerobically is to use the "talk test." When you exercise, make sure you are able to carry on a conversation during the exercise. This is the proper aerobic zone. If, during this time, you are able to sing a song, you aren't exercising hard enough. Ultimately, you will want to work toward exercising aerobically 20–30 minutes, 3–5 times per week. Be sure to add a 5-minute warm-up and a 5-minute cool-down to each exercise session.

49.
Is it possible to exercise too much? What happens if I do?

Yes, you can certainly exercise too much. How much is too much? Excessive exercise means that the benefits of exercise are outweighed by the risks of overtraining. Varying your exercise routine will help

Q   A

guard against this. For example, a mixture of walking, swimming, golf, weight training, and gardening will offer more protection from overtraining than five to seven continuous sessions of walking or jogging. Varied activities or exercises means using diverse muscle groups, tendons, and joints. Generally, it is recommended to take 1–2 days off per week from your primary exercise routine. Certainly, you will still want to maintain an active lifestyle on these "off" days; simply refrain from your primary exercise routine.

Here are some signs of overtraining:

- Muscle soreness that does not go away
- Oversleeping or difficulty falling asleep
- Irritability
- Depression
- Lack of interest in usual activities
- Greater susceptibility to colds and flu

50.
I really don't like to exercise if it means jogging and stuff like that. Is there something I can do that's not so hard?

Becoming a regular exerciser is about building physical activity into your daily life. It does not necessarily mean that you will need to join the local running race, unless that is your goal. You may want to start walking to your neighborhood mailbox a couple times per day, searching for the furthest parking space rather than the closest, or washing your car by hand instead of using the automatic car wash. The possibilities of exercise options are endless and range from the leisurely to very strenuous. What you choose to do will be based on your current fitness level, your interests, what's available to you, and any physical limitations you may have. In other words, your exercise regime will be completely individualized and entirely up to you. Exercise (or becoming more active) is a mindset and a lifestyle to adopt—today, tomorrow, and the rest of your life.

51.
It is hard to do regular exercise, particularly if it means long workouts. Will shorter workouts be all right?

Absolutely! There are documented fitness benefits from participating in two 15-minute exercise sessions

Q A

per day or three 10-minute sessions per day. Make sure that your sessions add up to a minimum of 30 minutes. It is not always easy or convenient to find the time for a continuous 30- to 45-minute workout and many of us may not exercise if it means interrupting our normal routine. Some types of exercise are doubly efficient, that is, they cover several aspects of fitness training at once. For example, there is a specific type of exercise referred to as *circuit training* that effectively combines both aerobic and strength training in one convenient, 30-minute session. There are many videotapes available commercially that will guide you through a circuit-training workout. The bottom line is that some exercise is better than none at all.

52.
What happens if I skip a day or two of exercise?

Skipping a day or two of exercise will not compromise the fitness gains that you have accomplished. Remember, a day or two of rest from your usual exercise routine is important for muscle recovery and overall health. However, you can still maintain a certain level of activity. If your normal routine consists of 30 minutes of biking, try walking in your neighborhood after dinner, playing 9 holes of golf, or weeding the flower gardens. While missing 1–2 <u>days</u> of exercise will not alter fitness gains, if you don't exercise for 1–2 <u>weeks</u> you may begin to lose the fitness gains you have achieved. If you are forced to take such an extended period of time off from your exercise routine, you may need to moderate your exercise intensity when you begin again.

53.
My feet hurt when I exercise. What should I do about this?

Foot pain during exercise can be caused by a number of things such as peripheral neuropathy, infection, and orthopedic problems (such as bunions, improperly cut toenails, or pressure points). It is important for you to have this evaluated by your doctor. Proper foot support and ventilation is important. First, be sure to always wear well-fitting socks, preferably made from natural fibers. Second, be sure to wear the appropriate athletic shoe for your activity, that is,

Q A

walking or running shoes for walking, basketball shoes for basketball, etc. Last, purchase your shoes from a reputable athletic shoe store. If you have an older pair of athletic shoes, be sure to take them with you. A properly trained shoe technician will look for wear patterns in your shoes, your tendency to pronate or supinate (walking on the inside or outside of the sole of your foot), and will check to see of you have a high arch or a flatfoot. All of these factors are important in determining the type of shoe to purchase.

54.
My legs hurt when I exercise.
What should I do about that?

It depends on the cause of the pain. Intermittent claudication is a cramping pain or weakness in the legs (particularly the calves) that occurs with walking but disappears with rest. This kind of pain is caused by inadequate blood supply to the working muscles and is a sign of peripheral vascular disease (a complication from diabetes). This will need to be evaluated by your doctor. Other possible causes of leg pain include muscle aches and cramps or joint pain caused by arthritis. Muscle cramps that occur during exercise can be relieved with rest and stretching. Once the muscle cramp has subsided, exercise can be resumed. Stiffness and soreness associated with osteoarthritis or muscle fatigue can be relieved by massage, warm (not hot) soaks in the bathtub, increasing water intake, and making sure that your diet contains the optimal amount of calcium and magnesium. Over-the-counter ibuprofen or some of the newer anti-inflammatory medications can also help with muscle and osteoarthritic pain. As with any continued pain or discomfort, consulting with your doctor is always recommended.

55.
Should I eat before I exercise?
Why is that important?

This depends upon your blood glucose level. Checking your blood glucose before, during, and after exercise is very important. You will want to check your blood glucose 30 minutes before and again immediately before you begin to exercise. If your blood glucose level is dropping, you will need to eat an extra snack.

Q A

In general, to avoid hypoglycemia, it is best to wait 1–3 hours after a meal before you exercise. Exercising right after eating a large amount of food can cause gastrointestinal distress by forcing blood away from the gut (where it is needed to absorb nutrients) to the exercising (working) muscles.

56.
Should I carry a snack with me when I exercise?

You should always have something with you that can be used to treat a low blood glucose reaction. Snacks that are transportable and nonperishable include regular soft drinks, juice, raisins, and glucose gel. If you are exercising with a partner or in a group, make sure at least one person knows how to treat low blood glucose. If you feel a low blood glucose reaction coming on, make sure you stop your exercise immediately and treat it. Before resuming exercise, check your blood glucose to make sure it has returned to a safe level.

57.
Is it better for me to check my blood glucose before or after I exercise? And why?

You will want to check your blood glucose before, during, and after you exercise. Monitoring is the key to avoiding blood glucose lows. If you exercise with a partner, make sure he or she knows the signs of low blood glucose and how to treat it.

In general, the guidelines for monitoring your blood glucose while exercising are as follows:

Check 30 minutes before exercising, then again just before you begin. If your blood glucose level is low or you see it's dropping, have a snack before you start exercising.

Check every 30 minutes during continuous exercise.

Check again after exercise because blood glucose can continue to drop for hours following sustained exercise. This happens because your body uses the glycogen stored in your muscles and liver as fuel during exercise. Your body replenishes that glycogen by drawing glucose from your blood. This process could continue for up to 24 hours.

If your fasting blood glucose reading is above 300, it is best to check with your doctor before exercising.

Q A

58.
Is it all right to exercise before going to sleep?

Blood glucose can continue to drop for several hours after exercising, particularly after strenuous exercise. Therefore, to avoid a low in the middle of the night or sleep, it is best not to exercise before going to bed. In addition to its impact on blood glucose levels, late-night exercise can affect how quickly you fall asleep. Exercise increases respiration and heart rate; it is an *energizer*. During the daytime hours, this effect is a positive one. However, when you are going to bed the goal is to relax and not to energize. An after-dinner walk is fine, but keep your strenuous exercise limited to the earlier parts of your day.

59.
What kind of exercise can I do if the weather is bad or if I worry about dangers in my neighborhood?

Safety is of utmost importance. Attempting to exercise outdoors during inclement weather can be very dangerous, as it is difficult to maintain solid footing in rain, snow, or on ice. Please don't exercise outdoors in your neighborhood if you don't feel safe. If you can't exercise outside there are a number of options available to you:

■ Mall walking; many malls have groups that meet and walk together before the mall opens for shopping.
■ Exercise videotapes: chair exercises, yoga, strength training, kickboxing—the possibilities are endless!
■ Exercise classes at your local Y or recreational center.
■ Stair walking at home (using a handrail).
■ Bowling.
■ Scrubbing your floors vigorously.
■ Using one piece of high-quality indoor exercise equipment (for example, a stationary bicycle or a treadmill).

If you choose to exercise outdoors, following certain precautions will help to ensure a successful and safe exercise session:

Dress appropriately for the weather. Dress in layers that can be easily added to or removed if necessary.

Make sure you stay hydrated. Drink water before, during and after exercise. For lengthy exercise ses-

Q A

sions that take you further from home, be sure to either locate water fountains, carry some water with you, or place water bottles on your route ahead of time.

If you exercise for a long period, you may want to rehydrate with a sports drink. A sports drink contains carbohydrates and electrolytes such as sodium and potassium to help maintain healthy bodily function. Electrolytes are lost by perspiring, and sports drinks help replace them while keeping you well hydrated.

2
Daily Living

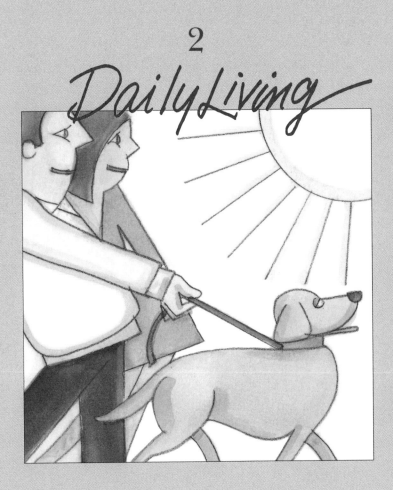

The Basics

Exercise

74. Why does my doctor want me to start an exercise program?
75. What will happen to my blood glucose when I exercise?
76. How do I know if I'm exercising at the right intensity?
77. Is there any way to make sticking to my exercise routine easier?

Avoiding Complications

78. How can I prevent diabetes complications or keep them from getting worse?
79. I have a friend with diabetes who carries an emergency kit. Should I carry one too?
80. What causes hypoglycemia, what are the symptoms, and how should I treat it?
81. How can I avoid having a low blood glucose reaction?
82. I'm so afraid of hypoglycemia that I eat all the time. What can I do?
83. What are the symptoms of high blood glucose and what can I do to bring it down?
84. Should I also check my blood pressure at home?
85. Why do I have to have a urine test for protein every year?
86. I urinate five or six times a night. Are my kidneys damaged from diabetes?
87. I have protein in my urine. What should I do?
88. Why do my feet feel cold all the time?
89. What can I do about the tingling in my feet?
90. How should I check my feet?
91. What is the best way to cut my toenails?
92. Can having diabetes affect the health of my teeth?
93. Why does my doctor make a big deal about my seeing the dentist regularly?
94. Is there anything special I need to do to prepare for my regular dental checkup?
95. If I'm healthy and my diabetes is in control, do I still need to get a flu shot?
96. Why does my doctor want me to lose weight?
97. My vision has been blurry lately. Should I have my eyes checked and get a new pair of glasses?
98. How can I calm my itchy skin?

Emotional Issues

99. What can I do to make having diabetes less stressful?
100. Sometimes I just don't want to face my diabetes anymore. How can I take a vacation from diabetes?

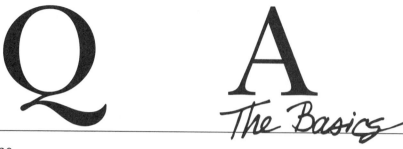

60.
What is diabetes?

Diabetes is a chronic condition that causes high blood glucose levels, but it can be managed.

When we eat food, our bodies convert some of it into glucose, which is a type of sugar. The glucose then travels through the bloodstream to the body's cells where it is used for energy. Insulin, a hormone produced by the beta cells in the pancreas, functions like a key to help glucose in the bloodstream enter the cells. When the level of glucose rises in the blood, the pancreas releases insulin so that it can move the glucose into the cells. When blood glucose levels dip, the pancreas secretes less insulin. This system keeps our energy levels on an even keel.

When you have diabetes, this system breaks down. In some people, the body does not produce insulin at all. In other people, the body either doesn't produce enough insulin or it has difficulty using the insulin properly. When insulin is not able to do its job, glucose cannot be used by the cells for energy and it builds up in the blood instead. The result is a high blood glucose level, which is the primary sign of diabetes.

Over time, this elevated blood glucose can cause damage to the body. High blood glucose levels can cause problems with the blood vessels in the body and can damage the eyes, nerves, kidneys, and heart. That is why it is important to manage diabetes through healthy eating, exercise, and, if needed, diabetes drugs. Keeping blood glucose in a desirable range can be done, with education and help from your health-care team, family, and friends.

61.
What is Type 2 diabetes?

When you have Type 2 diabetes, your body does not properly use the insulin it makes, which causes glucose to build up in your blood. Insulin acts like a key to allow glucose in your bloodstream to enter cells where it can be used as fuel. When blood glucose levels rise, such as after a meal, the pancreas releases more of it. When blood glucose levels drop, such as after exercise, the pancreas secretes less insulin. This process keeps blood glucose levels at a stable, healthy level.

Q A

When your cells are resistant to insulin, the pancreas reacts by producing extra insulin. Over time, the pancreas cannot keep up with the body's demand for insulin and the blood glucose levels rise. The liver also plays a role in regulating blood glucose. If it doesn't recognize the presence of insulin, the liver will release stored glucose, which also causes higher levels in the bloodstream. In sum, there are three main features of Type 2 diabetes: resistance to insulin, the failure of the pancreas to make enough insulin, and the release of too much glucose by the liver.

Type 2 diabetes has a genetic component, meaning that it runs in families and is found more often in certain ethnic groups such as African-Americans, Native Americans, and Latinos. The malfunction that causes insulin resistance and high blood glucose actually involves altered genes that send misguided signals to the cells that regulate blood sugar, blood pressure, blood lipids (such as cholesterol), and other complex body functions. Other risk factors such as overweight and lack of exercise contribute to insulin resistance. This connection is so strong that a weight gain of 11 to 18 pounds (especially around the abdomen) can double a person's risk of developing Type 2 diabetes.

62.
What is the difference between Type 1 and Type 2 diabetes?

In Type 1 diabetes, the body either does not make any insulin or it makes very little of it. No one is sure why this happens, but one theory is that the body's immune system attacks or destroys the cells that make insulin. People with Type 1 diabetes therefore need to take insulin by injection to replace the insulin their body does not make. It is also important for people with Type 1 diabetes to eat a healthy diet, get regular exercise, test their blood glucose at regular intervals every day, and have regular check-ups with a health-care team to make sure the diabetes is under good control. Type 1 diabetes is usually diagnosed in people under the age of 30, but it can occur at any age. The signs of Type 1 diabetes usually develop very quickly and can be severe. The symptoms include weight loss, frequent urination, excessive thirst and hunger, fatigue, nausea, and vomiting.

Q A

In Type 2 diabetes, the body still makes insulin, but either it does not make enough or the body cannot use it efficiently, or both. Sometimes people with Type 2 diabetes take insulin, but they do not require it for survival, as people with Type 1 do. Many oral drugs are also used to treat Type 2 diabetes. As in Type 1 diabetes, people with Type 2 diabetes need to follow a healthy food plan and exercise regimen.

Type 2 diabetes usually develops after the age of 40, but it may also occur in younger people who have risk factors such as obesity. In fact, Type 2 diabetes is increasingly affecting children. Type 2 diabetes tends to run in families, and being overweight and inactive may trigger its development. When someone is overweight, the body has a more difficult time using insulin properly (this is called insulin resistance), which leads to high blood glucose levels. Some people with Type 2 diabetes do not experience any symptoms, some people may have just one or two symptoms, and some people may have several. The common signs or symptoms of Type 2 diabetes include frequent urination and excessive thirst, fatigue, blurry vision, tingling or numbness in the hands or feet, infections that do not heal or take a long time to heal, and weight loss.

63.
What is blood glucose and why is it important?

When we eat food that contains carbohydrates, it breaks down to a form of sugar called glucose. This is the form of sugar that enters the bloodstream to be used as fuel by the body. It is very important because it is the body's main energy source. The body can use some of it right away and store the rest in the liver and muscles for later use.

Insulin, a hormone that is produced by the beta cells in the pancreas, works like a key to move glucose into the cells where it is used for energy. If blood glucose is too low, the pancreas releases less insulin. Diabetes is caused by a breakdown in this process. The body either doesn't make enough insulin or doesn't use it efficiently. As a result, glucose can't move into the cells, so it builds up in the bloodstream.

Having too much glucose in the blood is called hyperglycemia, or high blood glucose. Having too lit-

Q A

tle glucose in the blood is called hypoglycemia, or low blood glucose. Blood glucose that is either too high or too low can cause you to feel sick, and it can also harm your body if it is left untreated. Managing your blood glucose and keeping it within a desirable range will help you stay healthy and avoid diabetes complications.

64.
How is diabetes diagnosed and what is prediabetes?

Diabetes is usually diagnosed using a "fasting blood glucose" test. Your doctor will test your blood on two separate visits to ensure that the results are accurate. Just as when you have your cholesterol checked, you cannot eat or drink anything other than water for 8 hours before the test so that the lab can get a "clean" reading of your blood sugar. A laboratory will analyze the results. Diabetes is diagnosed when the fasting blood glucose levels are 126 mg/dl or higher.

If your fasting blood glucose levels are between 111 mg/dl and 125 mg/dl, you have prediabetes, or impaired glucose tolerance. This means that your body doesn't use insulin to process glucose as efficiently as it should, but it is not yet causing glucose to build up in the blood at levels that indicate diabetes. However, prediabetes is a serious risk factor for Type 2 diabetes and it should never be ignored. Research has demonstrated that you can delay and possibly prevent Type 2 diabetes by treating prediabetes through healthy eating and planned exercise.

If your fasting blood glucose levels are between 111 mg/dl and 125 mg/dl and you have other risk factors for diabetes, your doctor will give you an oral glucose tolerance test. In this test, your doctor will give you a sugar drink and then test your blood glucose level two hours later. A two-hour value of 200 mg/dl or higher indicates a diagnosis of diabetes. Two-hour blood glucose values that fall between 140 mg/dl and 200 mg/dl indicate prediabetes. A nondiabetic two-hour glucose reading is below 140 mg/dl.

65.
Will my diabetes ever go away?

While there is much research going on to search for a cure for diabetes, at this time a cure is not available. Although diabetes will not go away, the good news is it can be controlled and you can live a healthy life. The best ways to control your diabetes are through healthy eating and exercise. You may also need to take medicine or insulin to keep your blood glucose levels normal and stay healthy. Your diabetes health-care team will work with you to ensure that you know everything you can do to live a healthy life with diabetes.

Over time, diabetes causes changes in your body. These are natural changes that occur at different times for different people, usually over the course of many years. They generally cause your body to become more resistant to the action of your insulin, and eventually might cause your body to produce less insulin. As these changes happen, your diabetes plan will need to change, too. You may need to change the medicine you take or adjust the dose. Or you may need to add another drug and/or insulin to your treatment plan.

Because diabetes changes for everyone over time, it is important to maintain regular contact with your health-care provider. By monitoring your blood glucose records and results of other laboratory tests, you and your health-care team can adjust your treatment plan as needed. Regular diabetes care visits will help you stay in control of your diabetes and help prevent diabetes complications.

66.
Everyone says that I am in denial. What is wrong with me?

Denial is one way of trying to cope with strong, negative feelings. People who are in denial about having diabetes try to ignore the condition and may fail to seek treatment. They just want it to go away. Other people go into partial denial. They admit they have diabetes, and take some steps to treat it, but they don't go all the way. They make take their medicine, but they eat whatever they want. Or they might see the doctor but never fill the prescription. Unfortunately, wishing diabetes would go away without taking appropriate action can lead to devastating consequences, including damage to the blood vessels, kidneys, nerves, and heart.

If denial is your only way to cope with diabetes, you need to recognize this fact and do something to

Q A

change it. The first step is to realize that there is nothing wrong with you. Denial is protective, very common, and based on the false belief that there is nothing you can do to change your situation. To overcome denial, it helps to realize that there is a lot you can do and there are many people who can help you.

One important step is to accept that it is natural and acceptable to have unpleasant feelings about diabetes and make room for them in your life. After all, these unpleasant feelings won't go away if you ignore them. A better tactic is to try to uncover the hidden beliefs about diabetes that are causing you to feel so miserable. Do you believe that you have to follow your diabetes care plan perfectly, with no slip-ups? No one can do that! Or maybe you fear that nothing you do will ward off the complications of diabetes. Results from numerous studies show this isn't the case. Think about what your fears may be and learn what the real story is and how you can overcome them. Remember, knowledge is power.

You may also want to share your feelings with a friend. Sometimes just talking about your diabetes and your fears can give you peace of mind. Joining a diabetes support group or talking to a counselor or diabetes educator may help you find solutions to some of the difficulties you are experiencing as well.

Most important, get regular feedback about your own health status from your health-care providers. Seeing that the steps you are taking are keeping you healthy is empowering. Soon you'll find yourself less and less interested in turning your back on diabetes.

67.
Does stress affect blood glucose levels?

Stress can have a profound effect on blood glucose levels. Your blood glucose readings may go up or down, depending on the type of stress you are experiencing.

Physical stress can be caused by anything from a head cold or minor injury to a heart attack. With this type of stress, your blood glucose is likely to rise. This is because physical stress triggers the release of stress hormones into the bloodstream. This, in turn, causes the release of stored glucose for extra energy. This extra energy helps the body handle the physical stress

55

Q A

it is experiencing. This is why a person's blood glucose tests might show higher than normal numbers when he has a cold or the flu or is in the hospital for an injury or a heart attack. In fact, some people experience higher readings a day or so before they actually feel the symptoms of an illness.

Mental or emotional stress, which can be caused by anything from getting a traffic ticket to going through a divorce, can also raise blood glucose levels. However, it can also cause blood glucose readings to drop. To find out which way emotional stress affects your blood glucose level, you may need to keep a weeklong journal in which you describe the stress you are feeling. You can then compare it to your blood glucose readings and see how your emotional stress correlates with your blood glucose readings. Once you make this determination, you will know what to expect during times of stress and make adjustments in your diet and exercise, as appropriate. (It is possible that you may want to adjust your medication as well, but you need to check with your doctor before doing so.)

68.
What are ketones?

When your body doesn't have enough glucose to use for energy, or in the case of Type 1 diabetes, when there is too little insulin to break down the glucose, your body will burn fat instead. As fat is metabolized, it leaves behind toxic by-products called ketones, which can build up in your blood and also be passed out in your urine. Ketones make the blood more acidic, which can upset your body's chemical balance and cause you to feel sick. This is called *ketosis*. If you become dehydrated and ketone levels are high, a life-threatening condition called *ketoacidosis* can develop. Most people who experience ketoacidosis have Type 1 diabetes, but anyone with diabetes should be aware of its signs. These include dry mouth, extreme thirst, fruity-smelling breath, frequent urination, stomach pain, nausea and vomiting, labored breathing, dry skin, fever, fatigue, and drowsiness. If you experience these symptoms, it is important to seek medical attention right away. Many times, when ketoacidosis starts to set in, it can feel like the flu, so if you do feel sick, it is important to test your urine for ketones. Fortunately, ketoacidosis takes a few hours or even a cou-

Q   A

ple of days to develop, which gives you time to detect and treat it.

The risk of developing ketoacidosis rises when you are sick. The stress of fighting off an infection can raise blood glucose levels. Also, some people mistakenly cut back on their insulin when they are ill, because they aren't eating as much as usual. This can raise the risk of ketoacidosis further. Exercise can contribute to the risk of developing ketoacidosis, too, because when you exercise, your body sometimes burns fat for extra fuel. It's a good idea to test your blood glucose before you exercise. If it's high, test your urine for ketones and treat it before embarking on any activity.

To avoid ketoacidosis, it is important to devise a "sick-day plan" in advance with your doctor. That way, you will know how to take care of your diabetes and avoid rising ketone levels when you are sick. In addition, it is important to check your urine for ketones when you are sick. If ketones are present, call your health-care provider for advice on how to treat them.

There are several ways to test for the presence of ketones. Urine test strips are easy and convenient to use. You can also buy tapes and tablets for urine testing. You do not need a prescription to purchase these products and they are available at your pharmacy. The MediSense Precision Xtra blood glucose meter can also test your blood for ketones. Check with your health-care provider about what type of test kit to keep at home and how to use it.

69.
I have Type 2 diabetes. Will my children also get diabetes?

The exact cause of Type 2 diabetes is not known, but researchers know that it does run in families. If someone in a family has Type 2 diabetes, other family members are more likely to also have it. Usually another factor needs to be present to bring on the disease, however, such as being overweight and inactive; being a woman with a history of gestational diabetes during pregnancy or having given birth to a baby over nine pounds; or being of Latino, African-American, or Native American descent. Other risk factors for developing Type 2 diabetes include having impaired glucose tolerance, high blood pressure, or high cholesterol.

Q A

Although there are no guarantees, there are ways your children, siblings, and other blood relatives can reduce their risk of developing Type 2 diabetes. First, they should maintain a healthy weight and eat a healthy diet that is high in fruits, vegetables, whole grains, and lean meats and poultry, and that is low in fat. Portion size is important, too: A single serving of most foods is about the size of your palm. Staying physically active is another important way to lower the risk of diabetes. Although a structured exercise program is ideal, any regular physical activity is helpful. Walking is great, and it's free!

In addition to living a healthy lifestyle, your family members should have regular checkups with their doctor so that if diabetes does begin to develop, they can catch it early. All adults over the age of 45 should have a test for diabetes every three years, but those with a family history of the disease should have the test more often.

70.

How does menstruation affect diabetes?

Because of hormone changes, blood glucose levels may rise before and during your menstrual period. These higher levels tend to last 3 to 5 days before returning to normal. In fact, some studies have shown that two-thirds of women have premenstrual blood glucose increases, and one-third of women have to adjust their insulin dose because of it.

Other factors can affect your glucose levels at this time, as well. For instance, food cravings may cause you to eat things that are not on your meal plan, especially foods that have a high carbohydrate count. Some women experience symptoms before or during their periods, such as upset stomach, cramping, and back pain, too. You may feel sick, your appetite may change, or you may not feel like exercising. All of these symptoms can raise your blood glucose.

It is important to be aware of how your period affects your diabetes control. You can do this easily by testing your blood glucose and keeping a log of your levels that corresponds with your menstrual cycle. If you do experience high blood glucose during this time, you and your doctor can use this information to make adjustments in your diabetes treatment plan.

Q A

71.
Can I donate blood?

The American Red Cross accepts blood donations from people with diabetes if they meet certain conditions. As with nondiabetic blood donors, you need to be healthy and feel well at the time of donation, be at least 17 years old, weigh at least 110 pounds, and have not given blood in the past 56 days.

People who take oral drugs to control their diabetes may donate as long as their blood glucose levels are in control. If you take insulin, you must wait two weeks after starting insulin or changing your dose. People who have lived in the United Kingdom for more than three months since 1980, have been in Europe for six months or more since 1980, or have taken beef insulin made from United Kingdom cattle after 1980 cannot donate blood. This requirement has been put in place to prevent the risk of contamination with variant Creutzfeldt–Jakob disease, or mad cow disease.

If you have high blood pressure, you may still donate if your blood pressure is within certain limits on the day you donate. People with heart disease must have had no symptoms, such as chest pain, in the past six months, and cannot be taking any heart medicines except aspirin. If you've had an organ transplant, you must wait 12 months before donating blood.

When you go to donate blood, the nurse or technician there will discuss your health history before taking blood. You will receive a brief exam and have your temperature, pulse, blood pressure, and blood count measured at this time. If you are making a blood donation for use during your own surgery, the rules for eligibility are less strict.

72.
What is the link between Type 2 diabetes and heart disease?

Many people are surprised to learn that treating diabetes involves more than keeping blood glucose levels within range. In fact, treating diabetes also includes monitoring and treating HDL cholesterol, LDL cholesterol, triglycerides, blood pressure, and weight.

One of the most important underlying causes of Type 2 diabetes is insulin resistance. In the initial stages of this syndrome, which precedes the diagnosis

Q A

of Type 2 diabetes, the cells become resistant to the action of insulin. That means a given amount of insulin will lower blood glucose levels less than would be expected. The pancreas reacts by making two to three times more insulin than the non-insulin-resistant person requires just to keep the blood glucose within a healthy range. In addition, the liver may release more stored glucose because it isn't receiving signals from insulin to stop. Once the pancreas is unable to keep up with the high demand for insulin and blood glucose levels start to rise, Type 2 diabetes is diagnosed.

Insulin resistance associated with a number of conditions that are linked to both Type 2 diabetes and heart disease. In addition to high blood glucose levels, impaired glucose tolerance, and impaired fasting glucose, insulin resistance is characterized by high blood pressure, high triglyceride levels, and low HDL cholesterol levels. These conditions are also the primary risk factors for heart disease. That's why insulin resistance syndrome is the link between diabetes and heart disease.

Insulin resistance can be treated with exercise, a healthy diet, and certain drugs, all of which help to ward off heart disease. If you also have very high cholesterol levels or blood pressure, those conditions can be treated with medicines as well.

73.
I have heard that people with diabetes have heart attacks more often than people without diabetes. What can I do to reduce my risk of a heart attack?

In addition to controlling your blood glucose, it is also very important to take care of your heart when you have diabetes. This is because people with diabetes have a much higher risk of developing heart disease. High cholesterol levels and high blood pressure, which are characteristic of insulin resistance, also add to that risk.

The good news is that everything you do to control your blood glucose level also helps keep your heart healthy. Keeping your blood glucose in a healthy range can help lower your LDL cholesterol and triglyceride levels, Controlling your blood glucose

Q A

also helps make the LDL cholesterol you do have less likely to stick to the inside walls of your blood vessels.

Controlling your blood pressure is another important way to reduce your risk of heart disease. High blood pressure makes your heart work harder, putting extra strain on your heart as well as on the small blood vessels in your eyes and kidneys. Work with your doctor to control your blood pressure by eating a healthy diet, exercising, reaching and maintaining a healthy weight, and taking medicine, if necessary.

And don't smoke. Please. Smoking narrows blood vessels and increases blood cholesterol, which increase your risk of a heart attack by two times compared to nonsmokers.

Eating a healthy diet that's low in fat, especially saturated fat, and cholesterol is especially important. This can help in lowering your LDL cholesterol. A fat-reduced diet can also assist in weight control. Losing even a little weight can improve blood cholesterol, blood pressure, and blood glucose levels.

Get regular physical activity. Physically inactive people have a greater risk of heart attack than people who are active. Regular activity can raise your levels of beneficial HDL cholesterol as well as help control blood pressure and weight. Your heart can get the most benefit from aerobic activities like walking, biking, and swimming. Start slow and gradually increase the length of time and frequency of exercise, with the ultimate goal of 20 to 30 minutes of exercise on most days of the week.

Try to alleviate stress. Stress can raise blood pressure, and many people find that it can also cause blood glucose levels to rise. Relaxation or meditation classes, exercise, reading, and participating in hobbies or other special interests may help keep stress at a tolerable level. If you are struggling with stress from your diabetes or from other aspects of your life, it may also help to talk to someone you trust. A family member, friend, clergy member, or counselor can help you find ways to overcome the problems that are causing stress.

You may want to talk to your doctor about taking drugs to lower your cholesterol level or blood pressure. Even when you are careful with your diet and

Q A

exercise, it might not be enough to keep your heart healthy. You may want to discuss taking a low dose of aspirin regularly, as well. Studies have shown that taking a low-dose aspirin daily can lower the risk of heart disease.

Finally, be alert to the signs and symptoms of a heart attack. These include pain, pressure, squeezing or tightness in the chest; pain that spreads to the neck, jaw, shoulders, or arms; shortness of breath, dizziness, or fainting; and sweating or nausea.

Exercise

74.
Why does my doctor want me to start an exercise program?

Becoming more physically active is one of the most important tools you have for controlling your diabetes. Activity is any type of action that requires energy expenditure, such as washing the car, walking the dog, or climbing the stairs. Exercise is more intense: It raises your heart rate, makes you breathe more heavily, and causes you to break a sweat. Both are beneficial, as long as you do them regularly.

First, exercise brings down blood glucose levels temporarily. When you exercise, you have to burn more glucose to fuel your body. Exercise also tends to have an "insulin-like" effect. That means it increases cells' sensitivity to insulin to let that glucose in. So exercise can improve the insulin resistance that comes with Type 2 diabetes and thus improve your blood glucose levels.

In addition, people with diabetes have a very high risk of developing cardiovascular disease and often have additional risk factors such as high blood pressure, high total cholesterol and triglycerides, low HDL cholesterol, and poor circulation. Exercise will make improvements in every one of these risk factors.

Another benefit is weight reduction. Most people with Type 2 diabetes are overweight. Exercise burns calories, which helps you lose weight and keep it off. Losing weight also reduces insulin-resistance and lowers your risk factors for heart disease.

Finally, exercise can simply make you feel better and more energetic.

Q A

Starting a fitness program doesn't have to be difficult or expensive. You don't have to join a gym or buy a fancy Lycra outfit. Rather, put on some comfortable clothes and a sturdy, supportive pair of walking shoes or sneakers, and get moving. Take a daily walk around your neighborhood or the local mall. Try to increase the length of your walks over time. Take up a sport, such as tennis or cycling, that you enjoy. Use the push mower instead of the riding mower to cut the grass. Take the stairs. Your doctor or diabetes educator can help you devise a fitness program that works for you.

75.
What will happen to my blood glucose when I exercise?

Exercise usually makes your blood glucose go down. Your body uses the glucose in the blood for energy during exercise. At the same time, exercise also makes your body's cells become more sensitive to insulin, which improves their ability to use and store glucose and thereby lowers blood glucose levels. If you use diabetes pills or take insulin, be aware that exercise could make your blood glucose go too low.

Be aware, however, that if your blood glucose level is high before starting to exercise, exercise can actually make it go even higher. The best way to determine how exercise affects your body is to test before, during, and after exercise.

First, test before starting your exercise routine. If your blood glucose is within target range, you're good to go. If it's high (over 250 mg/dl), wait until it drops before beginning your program.

You might want to test during exercise if your activity lasts more than one hour (test every 30 minutes if possible), or if you are doing an activity for the first time and you are not sure how it will affect your blood glucose. Also, be aware of the signs and symptoms of a low-blood-glucose reaction, which could set in as a result of your exercise. Keep a source of fast-acting carbohydrate nearby in case you need to treat hypoglycemia.

When you are done exercising, test your blood once more to see what happened to your blood glucose level. Remember that the blood-glucose-lowering effect of exercise can last up to 24 hours after you

Q A

have stopped exercising, so watch for signs of hypoglycemia during the rest of the day or during the night after you exercise.

76.
How do I know if I'm exercising at the right intensity?

There are several differences between physical activity and exercise. Activity means any action that expends energy. Washing the car, vacuuming, or walking the dog all count as physical activity. Exercise is more intense. It is usually planned, sustained over at least 20 minutes, and more vigorous. Exercise raises your heart rate and usually causes you to break a sweat.

To benefit from aerobic exercise, you need to do it hard enough to make your heart beat faster. Your doctor can tell you—based on your age and other factors—what pulse rate to aim for. However, it's important not to overdo it. You are exercising too hard if you can't hold a conversation while exercising. If you feel dizzy or short of breath or feel sick to your stomach, you should stop exercising.

When you exercise, be aware that doing so can lower your blood sugar. Be sure to test before starting any exercise routine, and make sure your glucose level is within target range before beginning. Keep a source of fast-acting carbohydrate nearby, too, in case you begin to feel low during your workout.

77.
Is there any way to make sticking to my exercise routine easier?

Exercise can feel like a chore, but there are ways you can make sticking to a routine easier.
■ Exercise with a friend or group. It's more fun and you'll be less likely to skip your activity if your friends are expecting you to show up.
■ Choose activities that you enjoy (or at least don't dislike).
■ Schedule your exercise sessions on your calendar just as you do picking up your children and going to meetings.
■ Set short- and long-term goals and monitor your progress.
■ Reward yourself for achieving goals with a movie, a book, or some other nonfood treat.

Q A

■ Sign up for an exercise class. Classes offer structure, social support, and variety. Plus, you usually have to pay for them in advance, so you have a financial incentive to stick to it.

■ Vary the exercises you do so you don't get bored.

■ Don't expect instant results. It takes two to three months before some people notice any changes.

■ As you gain strength, energy, and better balance, be alert for the good effects on your everyday life, such as how many steps you can climb before you get winded.

Avoiding Complications

78.

How can I prevent diabetes complications or keep them from getting worse?

Complications may be the scariest part of having diabetes. Diabetes is the leading cause of blindness and end-stage kidney disease. It is also a major contributor to nerve damage and amputation. Heart disease, stroke, and other circulatory diseases are serious complications, as well.

Fortunately, studies have shown that tight control of glucose levels can prevent or slow down the progress of diabetic complications. The most important step is to keep your blood glucose levels within your target range. Most complications are caused by high blood glucose levels. Checking your blood glucose level every day will help you determine whether your diabetes treatment plan is working, and it will help your doctor make adjustments if needed.

Because hardening of the arteries (which can lead to heart attack, stroke, and other circulation problems) is a major complication of diabetes, it is important to keep your blood pressure and cholesterol levels under control. Eating a healthy diet and getting regular exercise may go a long way toward keeping these levels down, but you may still need to take medicine. Not smoking, too, is one of the most important steps you can take to protect your health and ward off complications.

Catching problems early before they become serious is also important. You should check your feet

Q A

every day, monitor your glucose levels regularly, see your dentist at least twice a year, see your eye doctor at least once a year, and see your diabetes doctor regularly. Your health-care team will give you tests that show signs of oncoming problems, such as kidney disease, well before they become serious. That way you can make adjustments in your treatment plan and begin drug therapy if necessary to stop complications from progressing.

79.

I have a friend with diabetes who carries an emergency kit. Should I carry one too?

It is a good idea to keep some necessary diabetes supplies on hand for those times in life when things just don't go as planned. Having to work late at the office, getting caught in a traffic jam, or waiting for airplanes that don't leave on schedule can present a challenge to someone with diabetes who is unprepared. Here is a checklist of items you may want to carry in your emergency kit:

- Diabetes medicines
- If you take insulin, extra bottles of each kind of insulin you use and syringes
- Blood glucose meter with extra strips, lancets, and batteries
- Urine ketone test strips
- Alcohol wipes, tissue, and cotton balls
- Glucose tablets or another carbohydrate source for treating low blood glucose
- Diabetes medical identification (ideally, you should wear this identification on your body, such as on an ID bracelet)
- Phone numbers of your doctor's office or clinic, and your pharmacy

80.

What causes hypoglycemia, what are the symptoms, and how should I treat it?

Hypoglycemia is a reaction that occurs when blood glucose levels dip too low. It usually affects people who take insulin or diabetes pills, which lower blood glucose. The effects of these drugs are balanced by the timing and amount of food you eat. So if you eat less, or skip or delay a meal, your already lowered

Q A

blood glucose levels can fall too low. Prolonged exercise and drinking alcohol on an empty stomach can also cause your blood glucose to fall too low. If you are taking too high a dose of your medicine or insulin, you may experience hypoglycemia more often, and your dosage may need to be lowered.

Some of the early warning signs of a low-blood-glucose reaction include feeling weak, dizzy, shaky, or sweaty; having a headache or feeling tired, hungry, or irritable; a rapid heartbeat; pale, clammy skin; numbness or tingling, especially on the lips or in the mouth; and confusion, nervousness, or light-headedness. Symptoms can vary from person to person, so it is helpful for you and your close family members to know your particular symptoms and identify them quickly so you can treat your low blood glucose right away.

If possible, check your blood glucose whenever you feel symptoms of hypoglycemia. If your blood glucose is below 70 mg/dl, eat or drink something that has 15 grams of carbohydrate (if you can't test but have symptoms, eat or drink something anyway). Some examples of treatment choices with 15 grams of carbohydrate include the following:

■ Glucose tablets or gel (check the proper dose on the package)
■ ½ cup (4 ounces) fruit juice or regular soda pop
■ 1 cup skim milk
■ 1 tablespoon honey
■ 2 tablespoons raisins
■ 6 to 7 LifeSavers or other hard candies

After treating with food, rest and check your blood glucose again in about 15 minutes. If it is still low, eat another 15 grams of carbohydrate and recheck after about 15 minutes. If your blood glucose is still low after a second treatment, call your diabetes healthcare provider for additional help. If your blood glucose responds to one or two treatments of carbohydrate, follow it up with your next scheduled meal or snack within about an hour. If you are not scheduled for a meal or snack within the hour, eat a small snack containing carbohydrate to maintain your blood glucose level until it is time to eat.

Always carry a source of carbohydrate with you to

Q A

treat low blood glucose. Keep it in your purse or briefcase, in your car, in your golf bag, and anywhere else you can think of where you might need it when you are away from home.

Unfortunately, if you ignore the signs of hypoglycemia, if your blood glucose drops too rapidly, or if you delay treating it, hypoglycemia can lead to seizures or even death. Some people have no warning signs of hypoglycemia and they require frequent blood glucose monitoring and safeguards to prevent hypoglycemia.

81.
How can I avoid having a low blood glucose reaction?

If you take insulin or diabetes pills, it may not be possible to avoid low blood glucose reactions completely. But certain actions raise your risk of having a reaction:

■ Try not to skip meals or snacks or eat less than your meal plan calls for. Your medicine is designed to lower your blood glucose to keep it in balance with the food you eat. If you change what you eat, you'll throw off that balance.

■ Eating at the wrong time can raise your risk of having a hypoglycemic reaction because your medicines are timed to work at certain times of the day in concert with the foods you eat.

■ Avoid taking too much insulin. If you have frequent hypoglycemia, you may need to change your dose.

■ Exercising more intensely than usual will burn more glucose and thus lower your levels. It is important to test your blood glucose before beginning your exercise routine.

■ Drinking alcohol can lower your blood glucose as well. It may also cloud your judgment, making it more difficult to recognize and react to a low-blood-glucose reaction.

So sticking to your prescribed meal plan, exercise plan, and medication plan is the best way to keep your glucose levels from falling too low.

82.
I'm so afraid of hypoglycemia that I eat all the time. What can I do?

It is common to be fearful of hypoglycemia especially if you had an episode that was upsetting. One way some people avoid hypoglycemia is by keeping their

Q A

blood glucose elevated. The problem with that solution is that high blood glucose levels create other problems. High blood glucose levels can lead to diabetes complications such as blindness, kidney disease, and heart disease.

Recognizing that you are fearful of hypoglycemia is the first step. The next step is to work with your health-care team to slowly lower your blood glucose. Your team can also help you learn to recognize the symptoms of hypoglycemia, which can include weakness, dizziness, shakiness, fatigue, headache, a rapid heartbeat, clammy skin, numbness or tingling, confusion, nervousness, and irritability. If you experience any of these symptoms, test your blood glucose if you can, and eat 15 grams of carbohydrate. If your blood glucose doesn't rise 15 to 20 minutes after eating, have another 15 grams of carbohydrate and call your health-care team for advice. While it is probably impossible to avoid having a low blood sugar reaction ever, you can prevent them by not skipping or delaying meals and by checking your blood sugar level before exercising to ensure that it won't drop too low during your activity.

By being prepared and sticking to a schedule, you can avoid a severe reaction and take care of any reactions that do occur.

83.
What are symptoms of high blood glucose and what can I do to bring it down?

High blood glucose, or hyperglycemia, means there is too much glucose circulating in your bloodstream. Some of the most common symptoms of high blood glucose include feeling thirsty, hungry, or tired; having blurry vision, headaches, dry and itchy skin, frequent infections, poor wound healing, or numbness or tingling in the hands, legs, or feet; going to the bathroom frequently; or having a fruity-smelling breath. Some people may feel only one or two symptoms, while others may feel several at the same time when their blood glucose is too high. The only way to know for sure if your blood glucose is too high is to do a blood test.

Your diabetes treatment plan is designed to keep your blood glucose level within a certain range.

Q A

Sometimes, however, your levels rise above this range. Several factors may trigger a rise in blood glucose: These include eating more food than usual, getting less activity than usual, forgetting to take your diabetes medicine or taking too low a dose, and being under physical stress (such as being ill) or emotional stress.

If you notice a pattern of frequent high blood glucose levels, you need to change something in your diabetes care routine. You may need to alter your eating or exercise habits. Or you might need to change the type or dose of your diabetes medicine (or start taking a new one). It's a good idea to check your blood glucose level regularly and jot down the numbers. You may notice a pattern to your high numbers that is easy to take care of. Talk with your health-care team about the best way to help you bring your blood glucose levels down. If you have just an occasional or random high blood glucose, it is not usually something to worry about. A little extra exercise or adjustment in the amount of food eaten at a meal or snack might be all you need to bring it down again. However, if you have chronically high blood glucose levels, it is important to work with your doctor to bring them down. Keeping your blood glucose within target range is the best way to avoid diabetes complications in the future.

84.
Should I also check my blood pressure at home?

High blood pressure is characteristic of insulin resistance, and controlling it is an important aspect of treating Type 2 diabetes. Although high blood pressure has no symptoms, it can overwork and damage your blood vessels, heart, and kidneys. If left untreated, this can lead to heart disease, stroke, and kidney failure. That's why periodic blood pressure monitoring is part of your self-management program. A healthy blood pressure goal is 130/80 mm Hg or less. Some people require two or three blood pressure drugs to reach this blood pressure level.

Your doctor should check your blood pressure at every visit. However, some people have higher blood pressure readings when in the doctor's office because they are nervous. In fact, this effect is so common it's

Q A

now known as "white coat syndrome." If you suspect your readings may be elevated at the doctor's office, it may be helpful to check your blood pressure at home when you are more relaxed. If you choose to do this, however, it is important to make sure that the blood pressure cuff is the right size for your arm. If the cuff is too small, the blood pressure reading will be inaccurate.

85.
Why do I have to have a urine test for protein every year?

The presence of protein in your urine is an early warning sign of kidney disease. Diabetic nephropathy, a type of kidney disease, is a major complication of diabetes. Although it can take years to develop, if left untreated it can lead to end-stage renal disease, or kidney failure.

The kidneys filter waste products, water, and chemicals out of the blood. These are then excreted through the bladder in the urine. High blood glucose levels and high blood pressure can overwork the kidneys, causing them to leak a protein called albumin into the urine. Because kidney disease has no symptoms until the late stages, it is important to have an annual test for protein in the urine to detect and treat it quickly.

There are three ways to collect urine for this test. One way is to collect urine in a container provided by the laboratory over a 24-hour period to measure the ratio of protein to a substance called creatinine. Another method is to collect urine in a small container first thing in the morning, then measure the ratio of albumin to creatinine. A third method is to collect urine over a specific time frame such as four hours or overnight. The 24-hour test is considered the most accurate.

In 24-hour clearance tests, healthy people have less than 30 milligrams of albumin per milligram of creatinine in the urine. A small amount (30–300 milligrams of albumin per milligram of creatinine) is the first outward sign of kidney damage. Keeping your HbA_{1c} value below 7% and your blood pressure less than 130/80 mm Hg are two important ways to protect your kidneys. If early kidney damage is discovered in your annual urine test, there are ways to

Q A

slow down kidney disease. Studies have shown that taking a class of blood pressure drugs called angiotensin-converting enzyme (ACE) inhibitors can slow kidney disease progress. A low-protein diet may also help.

86.
I urinate five or six times a night. Are my kidneys damaged from diabetes?

Urinating frequently, especially at night, can be a sign that your blood glucose level is too high. It can also be a symptom of several other conditions, such as an enlarged prostate, a urinary tract infection, or simply the result of drinking too much or having caffeine before bedtime.

Frequent urination is not, however, an early symptom of kidney disease. Indeed, kidney disease does not have any symptoms until it has reached a very late stage. Normally, kidneys filter waste and chemicals out of the bloodstream and into the urine. Kidney disease occurs slowly, as high blood glucose levels and high blood pressure overwork these filters and cause them to become leaky. The first sign of kidney damage is the presence of protein in the urine. That's why it is so important to have an annual urine test for protein. Late-stage kidney disease is marked by water retention and swelling, called edema, as well as anemia, fatigue, nausea, vomiting, weakness, and difficulty sleeping.

If you do have to urinate frequently in the night, the first step is to check your blood glucose level when you wake in the night. If your levels are high, that may be the problem. Then talk to your health-care provider to determine if any other underlying cause may be at work.

87.
I have protein in my urine. What should I do?

Kidneys are designed to filter the waste products out of your blood. They help the blood retain useful nutrients; dispose of chemicals, toxins, and waste products through the urine; and regulate your blood pressure. High levels of blood glucose and high blood pressure can overwork your kidneys, causing the filters to leak a protein called albumin. A small

Q A

amount of protein in the urine is the first outward sign of kidney damage.

There are many effective treatments for early kidney damage. The first step is to ease the workload of the filters by keeping your blood glucose level within target range and your HbA_{1c} level below 7%. The second step is to keep your blood pressure under 130/80 mm Hg. You may require medicines to achieve these target goals.

The third step is to take medicine that has been shown to protect the kidneys from further damage. There are two categories of blood-pressure drugs, ACE (angiotensin-converting enzyme) inhibitors and ARBs (angiotensin receptor blockers), that have been shown to reduce the level of protein in the urine and slow down the progression of kidney disease. These drugs may be prescribed even if you don't have high blood pressure, because they are so effective in protecting your kidneys.

The fourth step in treating diabetic kidney disease is controlling the amount of protein-containing foods that you eat. Large amounts of dietary protein can overwork the filters in your kidneys. If you have kidney damage, your goal is to reduce their workload. You will need the guidance of a dietitian to learn the right amount of protein for you, because a restriction that is too severe can also be harmful.

88.
Why do my feet feel cold all the time?

People with diabetes can experience a variety of problems with their feet. One of the best ways to prevent foot problems is to keep your blood glucose levels in good control. Elevated blood glucose levels can affect your blood circulation by narrowing and hardening your blood vessels, which can limit the flow of blood to different parts of your body, including your feet. Poor blood flow to your feet can make them feel cold, numb, or tingly, and appear blue or swollen. Without enough blood, your feet might also not be able to fight infection well, so wounds may heal slowly or not even heal at all.

The best way to warm up your feet is to wear warm socks, even at night when you sleep. Avoid heating pads or electric blankets and hot water bottles, as they could burn your feet without you even realizing it. Always test bath water before placing your feet in the bathtub to make sure it is not too hot. To increase the flow of blood to your feet, avoid sitting with crossed legs, stop smoking (smoking restricts blood flow to the feet), and participate in some exercise (check with your health-care team about safe exercises for people with foot problems).

Nerve damage associated with diabetes can also make your feet less sensitive to pain, heat, or cold. This type of damage can also cause tingling or burning sensations. That is why it is important to always wear shoes and avoid going barefoot if you have lost feeling in your feet. Nerve damage can affect the nerves that cause sweating, so your feet could become dry and the skin could crack or peel. Calluses, corns, and foot ulcers are other potential foot problems associated with diabetes. If you have discomfort that results from nerve damage, certain drugs and over-the-counter pain-relieving creams may be soothing.

In addition to keeping blood glucose levels in good control, and stopping smoking, check your feet daily for signs of infection or injury. Have someone else check them for you if you cannot see them well. When you see your doctor, take your shoes and socks off so you won't forget to have your feet checked for visual signs of blood vessel, muscle, and nerve damage. And call your provider if you have a foot problem, even if it seems to be a minor problem to you.

89.
What can I do about the tingling in my feet?

Tingling in your feet is likely a sign of nerve damage, or sensory neuropathy. Nerves send and receive signals. If you stub your toe, a pain signal is sent to your brain and you quickly move your foot away. Untreated high blood glucose can damage the nerves' signaling system, which can cause numbness, tingling, burning, aching, hypersensitive skin, electric shock–like sensations, pain when you come into contact with sheets or clothing, and the sensation that you are walking on a strange surface. These symptoms may affect your hands or feet, or just your fingers or a toe. They may come and go, and often they get worse at night.

Q A

If you have any of these symptoms, tell your doctor. Many people make the mistake of ignoring these early signs and delaying treatment because the symptoms are not constant. However, it is important to treat them right away so that you can prevent them from getting worse.

Keeping your HbA_{1c} below 7% may help to ease the symptoms, because high blood glucose levels can irritate your nerve endings. If you have pain from neuropathy, pain relievers such as acetaminophen or nonsteroidal anti-inflammatory drugs (such as aspirin or ibuprofen) may help. Some people find relief from tricyclic antidepressants such as amitriptyline (Elavil). Nonmedical treatments such as biofeedback, guided imagery, and meditation can also be helpful to some people. Over-the-counter pain-relieving creams that contain a substance called capsaicin (which is found in red peppers) has shown good results in treating neuropathy, too. Speak to your doctor before trying any over-the-counter products.

If you have nerve damage in your feet, it is important to take steps to protect against injury. You may not feel an injury, which can lead to infection. Take the time to buy shoes that fit, always wear a comfortable shoe or slipper even when indoors so that you are not barefoot, and inspect your feet every day for cuts or blisters.

90.
How should I check my feet?

When you have diabetes, nerve damage and poor circulation can cause numbness and poor healing in your feet. To avoid infections, it is important to check your feet every day. Look at both the tops and bottoms and between the toes. To check hard-to-see spots, use a mirror or ask a relative to help. You should also feel each foot with your hand.

Be alert for anything that looks or feels out of the ordinary. This includes areas that are hot, cold, swollen, or red; areas that have lost sensation or feel funny; and blisters, scratches, patches of hard skin, and cuts or breaks in the skin.

Call your doctor right away if your foot has an open sore; an infection; an ingrown nail; a tender, red toe; a puncture wound; or pain, tingling, numbness, burning, or other changes in the way your foot feels.

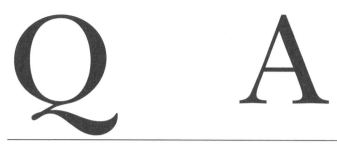

91.
What is the best way to cut my toenails?

To avoid problems with ingrown toenails, it is best to trim the nails straight across. If you are unable to safely trim them yourself, ask a family member or a member of your health-care team for help.

It is also a good idea to check your feet every day. Look them over thoroughly—on the top, bottom, and between the toes. Use a mirror to help you see hidden places. Look for corns, calluses, ingrown nails, cuts, blisters, and cracked skin. If you notice an infection, call your health-care provider as soon as possible for advice on the best treatment. (Signs of an infection include redness, red streaks, swelling, feeling hot, pain, and drainage or oozing). Avoid using chemical treatments, sharp scissors, or pumice stones to treat foot problems.

Always keep your feet clean and dry. Wash with mild soap and don't forget to dry between your toes. Use lotion if your skin is dry (but not between the toes) and wear socks and shoes made from materials that "breathe," such as cotton, wool, or leather. And don't wear a brand new pair of shoes for a whole day; wait until they are broken in. Make sure your toes have room to wiggle in your shoes!

92.
Can having diabetes affect the health of my teeth?

Elevated blood sugar can raise the risk of developing gum disease and other infections of the mouth. Diabetes can also hinder your ability to heal. That's why it's important to watch for signs of gum disease such as sore, swollen, or red gums that bleed when you brush or floss; gums that have started to pull away from your teeth; and areas between your teeth and gums that are filled with pus. Check for loose teeth or teeth that seem to not fit together when you bite, changes in the way your dentures fit, and bad breath, too.

Signs of other mouth infections include swelling in any other area of your mouth, pain in your mouth or sinuses—especially with chewing—discoloration on your teeth or in your mouth, and indents or holes in your teeth. Sensitivity to heat, cold, and sugar are signs of infection, as well.

Q   A

The good news is there are many ways to protect your teeth from infection:

■ First, keep your blood glucose under good control. This will reduce your risk for gum disease and other mouth infections, and it will also improve the healing process of any problem areas you might already have.

■ Brush your teeth at least twice a day or, ideally, after every meal. Use a soft toothbrush that is gentle on your gums and replace it every few months when the bristles begin to wear out. Floss your teeth daily and/or use dental picks or sticks to clean food from between your teeth.

■ See your dentist every six months for teeth cleaning and a checkup with your dentist. Tell your dentist you have diabetes so he or she can also watch for signs of gum or mouth disease.

93.
Why does my doctor make a big deal about my seeing the dentist regularly?

Diabetes, oral health, and overall health are all interrelated. Elevated blood glucose levels can raise the risk of infections, while infections can raise blood glucose levels, and both will affect your health. Because of these connections, certain dental problems, such as gum disease and mouth infections, occur more often in people who have diabetes. Diabetes can also cause dry mouth, which in turn can lead to cavities and infections. In addition, high blood glucose can slow healing so infections may last longer. As a result, you may experience pain, difficulty chewing, and loose teeth. Uncontrolled infections can lead to tooth loss.

Not only do infections raise blood glucose levels, but discomfort or dry mouth may make it difficult for you to follow your diabetes meal plan or take your medicine.

Having regular checkups with your dentists will allow you to find and treat any infections or other problems quickly and prevent problems from developing.

Q   A

94.
Is there anything special I need to do to prepare for my regular dental checkup?

First, make sure your dentist knows you have diabetes so he will know to watch for any problems that may have arisen as a result of your diabetes.

Having dental work done can be stressful for many people, and that stress can affect your blood glucose control. It's a good idea to check your blood glucose level just before your appointment so you can take any necessary precautions to prevent low blood glucose during your checkup. Make sure you carry some source of carbohydrate with you, such as LifeSavers or a commercial glucose preparation.

If possible, schedule your appointment for a time when you are least likely to experience a problem, such as shortly after a meal. If your appointment requires you to alter your meal or medication schedule, be sure to have your dentist consult with your physician first to make sure you get appropriate care and avoid a low blood glucose reaction.

Finally, try to relax during your checkup; stress can raise your blood glucose level. And remember that taking good care of your teeth and gums allows you to head off elevated blood glucose, so getting regular checkups is part of a good diabetes management plan.

95.
If I'm healthy and my diabetes is in control, do I still need to get a flu shot?

The flu isn't fun for anyone, but if you have diabetes, it can be more than a nuisance. People with diabetes who get the flu are six times more likely to need hospitalization, and the death rate from complications, such as pneumonia, is three times higher. Illness can also raise your blood glucose levels and greatly disrupt your diabetes care routine.

The best way to avoid these complications is to have a flu shot. Everyone who has diabetes and is more than six months old should have the shot every fall, ideally in October or November. It's necessary to have the shot every year, because each year's vaccine guards against the newest strains that last year's shot may not protect against. Also, since the flu shot isn't

Q A

100% effective, it's a good idea for your family members to get immunized as well, so they don't bring the flu home.

Certain people may not be able to get the flu shot. People who are allergic to eggs may have an allergic reaction to the shot because the virus that is used to make the vaccine is grown in eggs. People who have had reactions in the past, those who are allergic to the preservative thimerosal (which is used to make some types of flu vaccine), and people who have had Guillain–Barré syndrome should not have the shot. Check with your doctor if you think you might be at risk for a reaction.

96.
Why does my doctor want me to lose weight?

First and foremost, excess weight can make your blood glucose harder to control. Being overweight contributes to insulin resistance, one of the underlying characteristics of Type 2 diabetes. When you lose weight—sometimes, just 10% of your weight is enough—your blood glucose levels fall. Keeping your blood glucose level in your target range lowers your chances of getting complications. If you have Type 2 diabetes, you may even be able to reduce your dose of insulin or diabetes pills, just by shedding some pounds.

Overweight also raises your risk of having high blood pressure and bad cholesterol levels. This in turn raises your risk of heart and blood vessel diseases, the leading killer of people with diabetes. Losing weight can reduce these risks.

Finally, excess weight has bad effects unrelated to diabetes. It has been linked to gallstones, breathing problems, gout, osteoarthritis, and some forms of cancer. Extra weight also makes it more difficult to exercise, which is an important component of diabetes control.

97.
My vision has been blurry lately. Should I have my eyes checked and get a new pair of glasses?

Blurry vision can be a symptom of high blood glucose. If you were recently diagnosed with diabetes and are experiencing blurry vision, and if your blood

Q A

glucose levels are still elevated, you might want to wait a few weeks for your blood glucose levels to improve before changing your glasses or getting them for the first time. This is because blurry vision associated with elevated blood glucose, especially at diagnosis, usually improves as blood glucose control is established.

If you develop blurry vision when your blood glucose is not particularly elevated (especially if you have had diabetes for a while without previous vision problems), you should have your eyes checked by an eye doctor. Blurry vision can be a symptom of another eye problem related to diabetes, called retinopathy. An eye doctor can examine your eyes and see the signs of retinopathy and recommend appropriate treatment.

All people with diabetes should have an eye exam with an ophthalmologist (a medical doctor who specializes in the diagnosis and treatment of the diseases of the eye) on an annual basis. Be sure your eye doctor knows that you have diabetes when you have your appointment.

98.
How can I calm my itchy skin?

Dry, itchy skin can be a problem if you have diabetes. The good news is there are many ways to soothe this annoying problem. The first step is to make sure your blood glucose level is within your target range. High blood sugar can cause your skin to feel dry and irritated.

To soothe your skin, follow these tips:
- Bathe or shower in warm, not hot, water. Hot water can dry and irritate your skin.
- Limit your baths or showers to five minutes or less. Spending too much time under water can wash away the natural oils that keep skin supple.
- Choose a mild soap or cleanser.
- Don't scrub your skin; wash gently to avoid irritation.
- Towel off with gentle pats instead of brisk rubs.
- Moisturize your skin immediately after stepping out of the bath or shower, while your skin is still damp. Moisturizers add a protective oil layer to your skin and decrease the amount of moisture lost to the air.

80

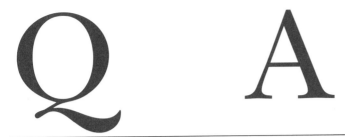

- Wash new clothes, towels, and sheets before using them to clean off the sizing that keeps these products looking crisp in the store.
- Protect your skin from harsh winter weather with gloves and a scarf.
- Consider using a humidifier during the heating season to increase the amount of moisture in the air.
- Drink plenty of water (but avoid caffeinated beverages).
- Try not to scratch. It worsens the itch and makes your skin even more irritated.
- Protect your hands with rubber gloves when washing dishes.

These hints should stop your itch in a week or two. If they don't, then schedule an appointment with your health-care professional.

Emotional Issues

99.
What can I do to make having diabetes less stressful?

Managing stress is important when you have diabetes. Not only does stress make life more difficult in general, but it can also raise your blood glucose levels. Fortunately, there are many things you can do to manage stress.

- Join a diabetes support group. By talking to people with the same concerns that you have, you can learn new ways to deal with the many issues that come with having diabetes. In addition, sometimes just talking about your concerns with people who truly understand what you are going through can be therapeutic in and of itself.
- Join a club, start a new hobby, take a class, or do some volunteer work. Diabetes shouldn't be the focus of your life! Find an activity that you love and put your thoughts and energy into that. You'll find you'll have less time to worry about diabetes and more enjoyable things to think about.
- Go for a walk, take a bike ride, or do something else that's active. Exercise raises levels of brain chemicals called endorphins, which make you feel good. Many people find exercise relieves stress. It can also make you feel healthier and improve your self-image.

Q A

■ Talk to someone about what is bothering you. Having someone you trust listen to you and offer support and advice is an important way to handle stress. Sometimes just airing your problems can help you sort through them and put things in perspective. You may just want to talk to a close friend or family member. Or you may find talking to a counselor or clergy member more helpful.

■ Carve out time for yourself. All of us are overextended, and taking care of diabetes takes even more time out of the day. You deserve some time to relax. That may mean saying no to things you don't want to do, hiring a babysitter to give you a free afternoon, or getting away for the weekend. And don't feel guilty about it!

100.
Sometimes I just don't want to face my diabetes anymore. How can I take a vacation from diabetes?

You are wise to realize that the constant demands of diabetes can be overwhelming. Diabetes is with you all the time, 24 hours a day, seven days a week. And as stress mounts in your life, taking care of diabetes can become more and more of a chore. There is a decision associated with every meal, blood glucose reading, and activity. Sometimes the decisions are so automatic, they take very little effort. Other times, those decisions are demanding and you may realize that you need a break.

But you can't ignore your diabetes altogether. Doing so will cause you to lose all the benefits of your efforts at self-management and raise your blood glucose levels. You can, however, take mini-vacations from some of the many tasks and limits that diabetes may require. For example, you might skip a noncritical blood glucose check or pick anything you want for dinner on a special night out at a restaurant. Yes, you may still have to pay for that break later (through a high blood glucose reading, for instance), but sometimes that short period of enjoyment is worth it. Periodic mini-vacations from the demands of diabetes keep you mentally healthy.

If you find yourself feeling overwhelmed and needing a break from diabetes all the time, you may need

Q A

to take a look at what is bothering you and make some changes in your life. Look for "sticking points" in your self-management, such as periods of the day when you can't resist the urge to snack, or times when you just can't handle having to do that blood test. What is causing you to feel that way? Do you have the munchies at night when no one is home and you are feeling lonely? Perhaps babysitting for your grandchild once or twice a week or starting a book club with some friends will ease that loneliness and take away the urge to splurge in the kitchen. Think about times when you didn't have this problem and what was different, and then make a change. Your health-care provider can give you guidance, too, if you need help making changes in your self-care routine.

101.
Sometimes I feel angry and depressed about having diabetes. What can I do to feel better?

Diabetes can cause a variety of emotions in people, including anger and depression. Sometimes when people are first diagnosed with diabetes they also feel a sense of denial, helplessness, or guilt as well. It is important to realize that these feelings are normal and experiencing them can actually help a person come to the point of being able to accept diabetes. A person who accepts diabetes is someone who takes responsibility to manage his diabetes and live a full, active life. Someone who has accepted diabetes might still feel angry or depressed sometimes, but prepared and able to manage these emotions.

■ Tell your family and friends about how you are feeling and let them know how they can help you. Also, talk with your health-care team about the feelings you are experiencing. Ask them for help in dealing with them. They can also refer you to a mental health professional for assistance, if necessary. You may also want to join a diabetes support group, where you can meet with people who are grappling with the same feelings and concerns that you are having.

■ Information is empowering, so learn as much about diabetes as you can. Again, talk with your health-care provider or ask him or her to direct you to diabetes classes or other educational resources.

Q A

Your local chapter of the American Diabetes Association can send you educational materials and direct you to a diabetes support group. The local library should have plenty of information about diabetes, as well.

■ Make lifestyle changes gradually. Don't expect yourself to be perfect all the time. Allow yourself to make a few mistakes along the way, and pat yourself on the back when you do something well!

■ Practice stress management techniques like deep breathing, exercising, and journaling. And don't forget to laugh—having a sense of humor can sometimes be the best medicine for us all.

■ Keep active in your usual activities such as work, sports, and hobbies. This will help remind you and others that you are still the same person you always were, even though you have diabetes.

■ Realize that you are in control of your diabetes— your diabetes does not control you. You are the one to make decisions about diet, exercise, testing, medication, and everything else about diabetes.

102.
A member of my family has diabetes and won't eat, can't sleep, and just sits around. What's wrong?

Everyone feels blue at times or feels overwhelmed by life's demands. Even the symptoms of high blood glucose, such as feeling tired and irritable, can mimic depression. A sad mood generally passes with a change of scene, a meeting with friends, or a day spent having fun.

Clinical depression is more than the blues. It's more serious, and it can get worse if it isn't treated. Although the exact cause of depression isn't known, it is triggered by a mix of genetics, brain chemistry, and life experience. Some people may be genetically more predisposed to becoming depressed, although that doesn't necessarily mean they will. Low levels of a chemical in the brain called serotonin can cause clinical depression, but this deficiency can be treated with drugs. People who have had bad experiences in their life or who use poor coping skills to manage the stress in their lives (including diabetes) are also at risk for becoming clinically depressed.

Q A

Symptoms of clinical depression include changes in appetite and sleep needs, lack of joy in life, feelings of hopelessness, and crying spells. People who are clinically depressed have difficulty carrying out day-to-day activities, such as getting up on time, making meals, going to work, or meeting with friends.

Fortunately, there are effective ways to treat clinical depression. New antidepressant medicines are very effective at lifting mood. Some people also benefit from therapy, where they can air their fears and issues in a safe environment and learn new ways to look at life and new ways to cope with problems. Once depression starts to lift, exercise and improving blood glucose levels may also help. The one thing to avoid is self-medicating, especially with drugs and alcohol. Not only is this very dangerous, but it can wreak havoc on diabetes control.

103.
My family is constantly worrying that my blood glucose will drop. How can I change that?

Diabetes affects the whole family. It's natural for your loved ones to be concerned about your health and safety and even be a bit protective of you. Sometimes, however, this concern can go too far. While loving concern and care can be helpful and supportive, criticism and constant questioning and nagging can be unhealthy and stressful for everyone involved.

If your family members are becoming overbearing, the first step is to convince them that you can manage your diabetes. You might want to enroll in a self-management course at your local hospital or American Diabetes Association chapter, and then apply what you learn. By gaining confidence in your ability to self-manage your diabetes, you may influence their image of your competence.

Sometimes family members feel helpless or guilty when a loved one has diabetes. They want to help ease your burden, but they just don't know what to do. If this is the case, take advantage of it. Give them jobs! Recruit your sister for a morning walking program. You'll be less likely to skip your exercise and have more fun doing it. Or ask your husband to participate in cooking healthier meals or take charge of afternoon snacks. By directing their energy, family

Q A

members can focus their concern on activities that actually help you.

Of course, if you are having frequent episodes of hypoglycemia, your family is right to worry. Heed their concerns and seek help from your health-care team. You may need to make changes in your treatment plan to keep your blood glucose levels in better control.

**104.
I can't afford to have diabetes. It's just too expensive! What can I do?**

You are right. Self-management of diabetes is expensive, especially if you do not have health insurance. Talk to your health-care team about ways you can cut costs. You might be able to use generic drugs, which are less expensive, or change your blood glucose monitoring schedule so that you use fewer test strips. You may also want to shop around and investigate mail-order suppliers. Some suppliers contract with your insurance company so that you won't have any out-of-pocket expenses.

Some people get angry and resentful when they have to spend their hard-earned money on health-care when they would rather spend it on a vacation. It's natural to have those feelings. They only become a concern if you give in to them and stop taking care of your health. Try to identify the real problem: Is the problem that you simply can't afford to visit the eye doctor or that you would rather spend the money on something more enjoyable? What do you have to pay for now and what things can you give up or save up money to do later? Think about your values and the expenses that are competing for your funds. Then you can decide how to spend your money based on what is most important to you.

Working With Your Doctors

**105.
Does everyone with diabetes need to see a diabetes specialist?**

Some people assume that you only need to see a specialist when you are in trouble. Clearly, specialized knowledge is needed if you are have frequent hypo-

Q A

glycemia, diabetic ketoacidosis, or are juggling the self-management of several illnesses. People with Type 1 diabetes often seek out diabetes specialists because of the complexity of their disease and the constant advances in insulin delivery systems such as insulin pump therapy. People with Type 2 diabetes also benefit from seeing diabetes specialists, since Type 2 diabetes is linked to many complications, including heart disease, and tight control of blood glucose levels can stave off those illnesses. We now know that there is no such thing as "mild diabetes."

Team management by a group of doctors and other providers who specialize in treating diabetes can offer the greatest help in controlling and caring for your diabetes. You are the most important member of the team because you are the one who makes the choices. The rest of your health-care team is there to guide and support you. You can benefit from having many health-care professionals on your team, such as diabetes nurse specialists, dietitians, pharmacists, social workers or psychologists, as well as your primary-care physician and physician specialists. Many of these providers are "certified diabetes educators," which means they have special training in helping people care for their diabetes.

Endocrinology is the medical specialty that focuses on the glands that make hormones. These include the thyroid, pancreas, pituitary, adrenals, parathyroid, testes, and ovaries. Doctors who study the workings of the endocrine glands are called endocrinologists. Since the pancreas, which makes insulin, is an endocrine gland, many endocrinologists specialize in treating diabetes.

Although everyone with diabetes would benefit from seeing an endocrinologist, not everyone has access to a specialist or needs one. Many primary-care doctors are knowledgeable and competent in delivering care to people with diabetes. *Standards of Medical Care for Patients with Diabetes Mellitus*, published annually by the American Diabetes Association, is intended as a guide for all providers of diabetes care. These standards of care outline required medical tests and diabetes treatment goals. Check with your doctor to see if he or she is following the standards of medical

Q A

care. If not, you can partner with your doctor to make sure that the standards are met. You can find out more about the standards on the American Diabetes Association's Web site, www.diabetes.org. For help finding a certified diabetes educator, call the American Association of Diabetes Educators at 1 (800) TEAM-UP4 (832-6874).

106.

My doctor looks in my eyes at every visit. Why do I need to see an eye doctor, too?

Uncontrolled high blood glucose and high blood pressure can damage the capillaries, or small blood vessels, that bring oxygen to the retina in your eye, leading to a condition called diabetic retinopathy. The retina is the lining at the back of the eye that senses light and changes the signals so that the brain can process them as sight. When those vessels are damaged, the walls can weaken and sections may pop out like little balloons. The capillary walls may also leak blood or other fluids, which can cloud vision. Untreated retinopathy is the leading cause of blindness in people with diabetes.

Diabetic retinopathy doesn't cause any symptoms until the late stages. That's why a thorough exam by a doctor who specializes in eye care is so important. Your eye doctor will use drops to dilate or widen your pupil so that the entire retina can be seen. Your primary-care doctor cannot dilate your pupils, so he'll only be able to see a small wedge of your retina when he examines you. Although looking into your eyes can give your primary-care doctor helpful information about your health, that small exam cannot replace the much more thorough exam your eye doctor gives you.

Many people don't have an annual dilated eye exam, even though it is painless and covered by insurance. For many people, fear of the results keeps them out of the eye doctor's office. But it's important to find and treat any signs of retina damage early. Because there are no symptoms, the only way that you can find out if you have any eye changes from diabetes is to have the dilated eye exam. Your eye doctor may report that your eyes are fine or that

Q A

there are some early changes. If you do have changes, laser therapy is a very effective treatment. Meanwhile, keeping your HbA_{1c} below 7% and your blood pressure less than 130/80 mm Hg are critical elements for the prevention and treatment diabetic eye disease.

107.
How can I get the most from my doctor visits?

In the age of managed care, hurried office visits are becoming the norm. Add a little anxiety to the mix, and it becomes very difficult to get all the answers and advice you need from your appointment. Planning ahead and following these tips, however, will help you squeeze the most from office visits:

■ Make a list of what you need to talk about. List your topics in order of importance, and be sure to bring them up in that order.

■ If you are seeing the doctor because of a new health problem, be prepared to answer questions about what symptoms you have and when they started, whether the problem is constant or off and on, and what things make it worse or better.

■ Take an up-to-date list of all your medicines and supplements (both prescription and over-the-counter), their doses, and how often you take each. Or drop the bottles in a bag and take that.

■ Bring your blood glucose monitoring records. Your doctor can use this information to better understand what sort of problems you may be having with your blood glucose control and be able to recommend appropriate adjustments in your treatment plan, if needed.

■ Take a notepad so you can write down instructions and other important information.

■ Be honest with your doctor. If you leave out information or fudge the truth, you might get a wrong diagnosis, or your doctor might prescribe a course of action that you can't or won't follow. In either case, your visit will be wasted. Telling the truth about a problem you're having, such as trouble keeping up with your blood glucose monitoring schedule, should not be embarrassing. Rather, it's an opportunity to talk about the problem and come up with a solution.

89

Q A

108.
When should I call my doctor?

You can't prevent every emergency, so it's important to know what to do when things go wrong. Of course, if you experience potentially life-threatening symptoms such as chest pain, shortness of breath, or profuse bleeding, you should call 911 right away. There are other situations that may be less dramatic but still merit a doctor's help. You should call your doctor right away if you experience any of the following:

■ You are sick and become increasingly drowsy, have pain in your stomach or chest, or have trouble breathing; your lips, mouth, or tongue are dry and cracked; or your breath has a fruity smell. These are symptoms of ketoacidosis, a life-threatening buildup of toxins in the blood.

■ Your blood sugar is 240 mg/dl or higher and you have ketones in your urine. Ketones in your urine are an early warning sign of ketoacidosis.

■ You have been vomiting and have not kept any liquids down for at least 4 hours. Vomiting can lead to dehydration and will also affect your glucose control.

■ You've been sick for a day or two and are not getting any better. You may have an infection that requires medicine.

■ You have a cut, blister, or ingrown nail on your foot. While these problems may not seem serious, when you have diabetes, it isn't safe to treat them by yourself.

Talk to your doctor about coming up with a sick-day plan, and discuss any other circumstances when you may need assistance. By being prepared and knowing what to do, you will be able to handle these situations.

109.
Should I worry if my insurance company insists I see a nurse practitioner instead of a doctor?

Some insurance companies try to save money by having nurse practitioners instead of doctors provide routine care to their policyholders. A few brief studies have been done to compare care given to people with diabetes by nurse practitioners with that given by doctors. These studies found patients received similar

Q A

care. However, no studies have followed people with diabetes under the care of nurse practitioners for long stretches of time.

No matter who handles your care, it's in your best interest to take an active role. Know what tests you should have and how often, and make sure you get them. Prepare your questions and concerns in advance and be sure you get the answers you need. Bring in your blood glucose monitoring log, too, to use as a guide in your treatment.

Fat and Cholesterol

110.
What are HDL and LDL cholesterol?

Cholesterol is a fat, or lipid, that is produced by the body and is also found in some foods. Cholesterol combines with protein to form a small particle called a lipoprotein, which then travels through the bloodstream, carrying cholesterol to different parts of the body where it helps the body to perform certain functions.

LDL (low-density lipoprotein) and HDL (high-density lipoprotein) are the two main types of cholesterol. When you have your blood cholesterol measured, the number for your total cholesterol includes both your LDL and HDL levels.

LDL cholesterol is often called the "bad" type of cholesterol because it contributes to the formation of fatty plaques on the walls of blood vessels. These plaques can eventually restrict blood flow through the vessels, leading to coronary artery disease and heart attack. It is best to keep your levels of LDL cholesterol low; the target level for people with diabetes is below 100 mg/dl.

HDL cholesterol, on the other hand, is often called the "good" cholesterol because it removes cholesterol from the blood and carries it back to the liver where it is disposed of. Having a high level of HDL is protective against heart disease; the target level for people with diabetes is at least 40 mg/dl in men and at least 50 mg/dl in women.

A healthy, low-fat diet and regular exercise can help keep cholesterol levels within target ranges, but

Q A

you might need medicine to bring them down if your LDL cholesterol and total cholesterol levels are too high.

111.
Do I need to worry about my cholesterol if it's only a little high?

Yes! Heart and blood vessel diseases (such as heart attack and stroke) are two to four times as common among people with diabetes. These diseases also start earlier in life if you have diabetes. In fact, about two-thirds of people with diabetes ultimately die from cardiovascular disease. High cholesterol is a risk factor for heart disease, and one that can be controlled. That's why when you have diabetes it is especially important to pay extra attention to your cholesterol level and other aspects of heart health.

When you get your cholesterol test results, look at the levels of low-density lipoprotein (LDL, or "bad") cholesterol and high-density lipoprotein (HDL, or "good") cholesterol. These numbers give you a more accurate view of your overall risk. It's most important to bring down your level of LDL cholesterol, because this is the type that contributes to the formation of plaque in the blood vessels, which can block or restrict blood flow. The target level for LDL cholesterol is below 100 mg/dl. HDL cholesterol is protective, because it sweeps cholesterol from the blood and deposits it in the liver. The target goal for HDL cholesterol is at least 40 mg/dl in men and at least 50 mg/dl in women.

Exercise and a healthy, low-fat diet may help bring cholesterol levels in check. If this doesn't work, however, you may need to take cholesterol-lowering drugs as well.

112.
What can I do to lower my cholesterol?

Perhaps the best thing to do to improve your blood cholesterol level is to establish blood glucose control. When blood glucose levels are out of control, blood fats tend to be elevated as well. So first keep your diabetes well managed, then try the following strategies to reduce your total cholesterol and LDL cholesterol and raise your level of HDL cholesterol:

Q A

■ Stay physically active. Regular exercise helps to increase HDL levels. It also helps to reduce blood pressure and body weight, lower blood glucose levels, and manage stress.

■ Stop smoking. Smoking can reduce your good HDL cholesterol, raise blood pressure, and increase the risk for a heart attack.

■ Eat less fat, especially animal fat. Animal fats tend to raise blood cholesterol levels.

■ Eat more high-fiber foods. These include whole grains and foods made from whole grains, oats and oatmeal, beans, fruits, and vegetables. Fiber may help reduce cholesterol levels, especially LDL cholesterol.

■ Limit the amount of high cholesterol foods you eat. These include egg yolks, liver, and other organ meats.

■ Control your weight. Moderate weight loss can also help to reduce cholesterol levels and improve blood glucose control.

113.
Why is LDL cholesterol so important?

Fats, including triglycerides and cholesterol, are part of every cell in your body. Your body makes both cholesterol and triglycerides, but you can also get them from foods you eat. Your body uses cholesterol to build cell walls and to make certain vitamins and hormones. Triglycerides are a form of fat that is carried in the blood but is mostly stored in fat tissue. Because fats do not mix well with water, they have to be packaged with water-soluble proteins to form lipoproteins so that they can travel through the body. High-density lipoprotein (HDL) and low-density lipoprotein (LDL) are two lipoproteins of concern in the treatment of diabetes and heart disease.

When discussing blood fats or lipids, there are four numbers that are important for you to know. For total cholesterol, the target goal is less than 200 mg/dl. LDL cholesterol should be under 100 mg/dl and HDL cholesterol should be greater than 40 mg/dl for men and 50 mg/dl for women. Triglycerides should be less than 150 mg/dl.

Keeping your LDL cholesterol under 100 mg/dl is so important because LDL cholesterol is a major contributor to the plaque buildup that causes coronary artery disease. When left untreated, high levels of

Q A

LDL cholesterol can lead to heart attack and stroke. Foods that are high in cholesterol, *trans* fats, and saturated fat raise LDL cholesterol. Saturated fats are most often found in meats, baked goods, and full-fat dairy products, such as hard cheese, butter, cream cheese, cream, whole milk, whole-milk yogurt, and ice cream. *Trans* fats are often found in cookies, crackers, fast foods, and margarine.

114.
How can I raise my level of HDL cholesterol?

HDL cholesterol is a lipoprotein (fat plus protein) that is made in the liver and intestines. It actually contains very little cholesterol. These fats collect excess cholesterol from the blood and blood vessels and carry the cholesterol back to the liver, where it can be disposed of. Because HDL cholesterol serves such an important purpose in protecting the body, high levels of it are beneficial. The target goal for HDL cholesterol is over 40 mg/dl for men and over 50 mg/dl for women.

One very effective way to raise your HDL cholesterol is to exercise regularly. Weight reduction also raises HDL cholesterol, as well as help to bring down LDL cholesterol and triglycerides. Although small quantities of alcohol have been shown to raise HDL cholesterol levels, too much alcohol can raise your triglyceride levels. Exercise is your best option.

115.
What is saturated fat?

Saturated fat is found primarily in animal foods. Meat, poultry, whole milk, and products made from whole milk such as butter, cheese, and ice cream are major sources of saturated fat in the American diet. The vegetable fats from coconut, coconut oil, and palm and palm kernel oil are also highly saturated. Saturated fats have the effect of raising blood cholesterol levels, so people with diabetes need to be careful about the saturated fat content of the diet. Saturated fats tend to be more solid at room temperature compared to unsaturated liquid vegetable oils.

People with diabetes should get less than 10% of their total daily calories from saturated fat. (Individuals with an LDL cholesterol level greater than 100 mg/dl may benefit from reducing saturated fat intake

Q A

to less than 7%.) You can lower the amount of saturated fat in your diet by limiting the total amount of meat you eat each day and by choosing foods that are lower in saturated fat. Try not to exceed about six ounces of cooked meat per day if possible. Also, trim your meat well, take the skin off your poultry, and cook your meat in ways that allow the fat to drain off. That means baking, grilling, or roasting foods on a rack, instead of frying them. Also, use leaner cuts of meat.

Liquid vegetable oils, particularly canola and olive oil, have less saturated fat than shortening, margarine, or butter. If you use margarine, use soft tub margarine instead of a stick type, because stick margarines contain more saturated fat. And look for a brand that lists a liquid vegetable oil as the first ingredient on the ingredient list.

Read the Nutrition Facts part of the food label for saturated fat information. A food labeled "low saturated fat" cannot have more than one gram of saturated fat per serving; a "saturated fat free" food has to have less than 0.5 gram of saturated fat per serving. Keep in mind that cutting back on total fat in your diet helps to reduce the amount of saturated fat as well.

116.
How can I make the leanest meat choices?

Selecting leaner cuts of meat is a great way to lower your intake of total fat and saturated fat. To choose the leanest meats, you need to pay careful attention when shopping.

First, choose hindquarter cuts, such as loin and leg cuts of pork and lamb, round and loin cuts of beef, lean ham, and Canadian bacon. These cuts are less fatty.

Second, look at each meat package and choose the one with the least visible fat. If meat is graded, pass over Prime and Choice meats and choose Select instead.

Third, limit your use of processed meats (such as hot dogs, salami, sausages, and bacon), liver and other organ meats, caviar, duck, and goose. For the more adventurous, you might want to try game meats, such as deer, turtle, buffalo, and pheasant,

Q   A

which naturally contain less fat. If you prefer tamer fare, chicken, turkey, fish, and other seafood also tend to contain less fat.

117.
How much fat should I eat in a day?

The amount of fat a person should eat every day varies according to gender, body weight, total caloric needs, and blood glucose and blood cholesterol goals. Most people eat too much fat and therefore would benefit from eating less. A registered dietitian can analyze your eating habits and determine if you need to eat less fat, and offer advice about how to go about doing it.

Many weight-loss and healthy-eating programs suggest limiting your total fat intake to less than 30% of your total daily calories. To determine how much fat this is, you need to know how many calories you eat in a day. (A dietitian can help you determine this number.) Once you know how many calories you eat, you can easily figure out the number of fat grams to aim for in your diet. For example, if you eat 2,000 calories a day:

2,000 calories × 30% = 600 calories from fat

600 calories ÷ 9 calories (per gram of fat) = about 66 grams of fat per day.

The Nutrition Facts panel on the food label provides information regarding total grams of fat per serving to help you keep track of your total fat intake.

Here are the recommended amounts daily fat grams for a variety of calorie levels:

TOTAL CALORIES	FAT GRAMS FOR 30% OF CALORIES
1,200	40
1,500	50
1,800	60
2,000	66
2,200	73
2,500	83

118.
How can I cut back on butter and margarine?

There are many ways to reduce the amount of butter and margarine in your food. In fact, using alterna-

Q A

tives not only lowers your fat intake, but adds spice and variety to your meals. For instance, instead of buttering your bread, try topping it with pureed fruit spread, nonfat cream cheese, Neufchâtel cheese, or mashed roasted garlic cloves. You can also try dipping it in a little olive oil with a dash of red pepper, the way Italians do. Olive oil contains monounsaturated fat, which is a heart-healthy form of fat.

Vegetables taste great with a variety of toppings. Try low-fat or nonfat sour cream, low-fat cottage cheese, lemon juice and garlic, or fresh salsa. Sautéing your vegetables with herbs and just a tiny bit of oil is a great way to bring out their natural flavor, too.

When baking, you can replace butter with half as much applesauce as the recipe calls for. The flavor and texture will be different when you do this, but it will still taste good.

3
Meal Planning

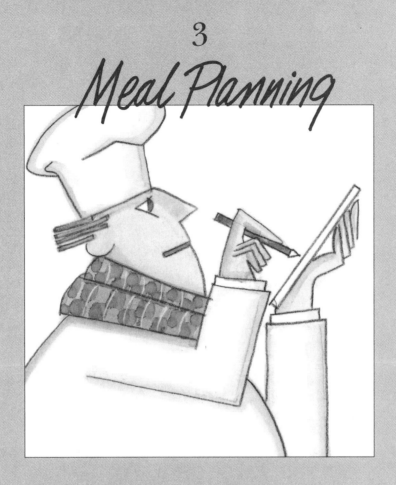

119. Why is a meal plan important? What am I supposed to do with a meal plan?

120. Why do I have to eat on a regular basis? What happens if I don't? Why is breakfast so important?

121. How do I know how much I should be eating? Why should I eat the same amount every day?

122. What times of day should I eat meals and snacks?

123. What can a dietitian do for me and how can I find one?

124. Can I take my diabetes medicines at mealtime?

125. Can people with diabetes eat sugar?

126. Is fructose better for people than regular sugar?

127. The only foods that taste good to me are sweets, especially candy. Can I eat candy and other sweets if I'm not eating much of anything else?

128. I like to have ice cream or a cookie every night. Is that all right now that I have diabetes?

129. Are artificial sweeteners safe? Are they useful?

130. How much of a sugar substitute is safe to use?

131. What is it that I have to watch for? Sugar, fat, or salt?

132. Do I need to be careful about salt because of my diabetes?

133. I'm told I need to drink a lot of water for my diabetes. Why is water so important?

134. I drink herb teas instead of soda to control my blood glucose. Is that all right?

135. I am used to having my daily sip(s) of wine. Can I continue?

136. So is it safe to drink alcohol when you have diabetes?

137. In summary, what precautions should I take when drinking alcohol?

138. What about cooking for my family? Do I need to cook more than one meal?

139. So it's all right to serve my family the same foods I eat for my diabetes meal plan?

140. How can I stick to my meal plan when I go to parties?

141. What about eating out? Can I still go out to dinner with my family and friends?

142. When I go to a restaurant, how do I figure out what menu choices are the most healthful?

143. My doctor told me to eat less protein. What foods are high in protein and how much should I eat?

144. What are whole grains and how do I work them into my diet?

145. Are low-carbohydrate diets good for people with diabetes?

146. What is carbohydrate counting? How much carbohydrate should I eat?

147. How can I determine the number of carbohydrate choices for a food by looking at the food label?

148. My family constantly comments about my food choices. How can I handle this?

149. What should I eat if I am sick and cannot eat my normal diet?

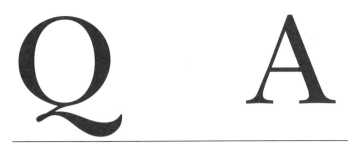

119.
Why is a meal plan important?
What am I supposed to do with
a meal plan?

Many factors affect your blood glucose levels and your risk of developing diabetes-related complications: your eating patterns, physical activity, medications, illness, and stress. As your doctor will tell you, one of the three major tools that help you to keep your blood glucose at a healthy level throughout the day is healthy eating (physical activity and medications are the other two). Eating more than usual or less than usual, eating high-sugar foods, or delaying or skipping meals can play havoc with your blood glucose and lead to complications.

Because your blood glucose increases after you eat and increases more rapidly with some foods than others, a meal plan that is individualized for your particular needs (also known as medical nutrition therapy) is a critical component of your diabetes management. According to the American Diabetes Association, the primary goals of such a meal plan are to improve metabolic outcomes (blood glucose levels, lipid profiles, blood pressure), prevent and treat diabetes-related chronic complications (obesity, heart problems, hypertension, kidney problems), encourage healthy eating and physical activity, and incorporate personal and cultural preferences.

Ask your physician for names of registered dietitians in your area or other health-care providers who have specialized nutrition training to work with you (and perhaps other family members or friends) to develop a meal plan that best fits your tastes and lifestyle. The meal plan you develop with your dietitian will include a wide selection of nutritious and tasty foods in all of the six major food groups in the familiar Food Pyramid, foods and menus that you and your family will like and are good for you too. The meal plan may also offer helpful suggestions on how to modify some of your favorite foods so that you can continue to enjoy them knowing that they not only taste great but that you are eating more healthfully. In general, your meal plan will encourage you to eat foods that are lower in fat, sugar, and sodium, and higher in vitamins, minerals, and fiber (like

Q A

grains, beans, fruits and vegetables). The specific types and amounts of food in your meal plan may vary depending on whether you want to lose some weight or maintain your weight to help manage your diabetes.

120.
Why do I have to eat on a regular basis? What happens if I don't? Why is breakfast so important?

Your goal should be to keep your blood glucose at healthy levels. Your doctor can tell you what levels are healthy for you. Because blood glucose levels vary by person, what is healthy for one person may differ from what is healthy for another person. In general, however, healthy ranges are usually about 80–120 mg/dl on waking and before meals (fasting levels), less than 180 mg/dl two hours after meals (postprandial), and 100–140 mg/dl before bedtime. Meeting the healthy level goals means maintaining consistency in your eating patterns—that is, eating at regular times (both meals and snacks), eating the right amounts of food, and balancing the types of foods you eat. For instance, eating too much can result in your blood glucose rising too high and making you sick. Other things like too little exercise, stress, and some medications can also raise your blood glucose level. If your blood glucose stays high for too long, diabetes-related complications can result. On the other hand, eating too little or skipping meals (or exercising too much) can result in low blood glucose (levels below 70 mg/dl) and make you feel dizzy or lightheaded and increase your risk of falling. It is dangerous to drive or walk when your blood glucose is low.

After a good night's sleep, eating a healthy breakfast every morning is not only an important start to your day but also critical to "wake up" your metabolism. Your parents were right when they told you to eat your breakfast! Because your blood glucose level falls while you sleep (to 80–120 mg/dl for well-managed individuals), a nutritious breakfast helps your blood glucose level to rise to a level that will help you function at your best during the rest of the day and help you prevent cravings for foods that are not good for you.

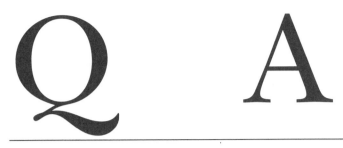

121.
How do I know how much I should be eating? Why should I eat the same amount every day?

Your dietitian or doctor will help you decide how much you should be eating based on your personal characteristics—such as your weight and height, your age, whether you're a man or woman, how much and when you exercise, how active you are every day, whether you're pregnant, breastfeeding, or anticipating pregnancy, and whether you are trying to maintain or lose weight as part of your diabetes management. A useful way to calculate your estimated daily calories is to multiply 10 calories times your present or desired body weight. You can chart your calorie intake using calorie books found commonly in libraries, grocery stores, or bookstores. It's also a good idea to become familiar with using measuring cups, measuring spoons, and food scales when cooking as well as the Food Pyramid and Nutrition Facts food labels when grocery shopping. The serving sizes associated with the Nutrition Facts labels may be different from the serving sizes you usually eat or may be different from the serving sizes recommended in your meal plan. It's also important to read the food labels to gauge total calories as well as types and levels of fats and carbohydrates to help guide your selection.

You can keep your blood glucose at a healthy level by eating about the same amounts of food at the same times every day, by adjusting your eating according to your exercise program, and by not skipping meals or snacks that are built into your meal plan. For example, skipping a meal may cause your blood glucose to go too low (particularly if you take diabetes medications or exercise too much) and may result in your overeating at the next meal and causing your blood glucose to go too high.

Eating the same amounts at the same times during the day will help your diabetes medications to work their best. However, because it is normal for your appetite to fluctuate over several days for a variety of reasons, the aim should be to eat the same amount of food on average over the course of a week.

Q A

122.
What times of day should I eat meals and snacks?

You should talk with your dietitian or doctor about the specifics of your meal plan—how many meals and snacks you should eat every day, how much you should eat during those meals and snacks, and when you should eat them—in order to keep your blood glucose at its target levels throughout the day. In general, eating more small meals rather than a few large meals will help keep your blood glucose levels constant. Consistency is the key to managing your diabetes and feeling your best.

Planned meals and snacks should be matched to your medication timing. In general, for your medications to work best, you should plan to eat some food between 15 minutes and four hours after taking your medication.

123.
What can a dietitian do for me and how can I find one?

Since good nutrition is often called the cornerstone of diabetes management, it is important to learn all you can about eating a healthy diet when you have diabetes. A dietitian is the expert who can help you do just that. A dietitian is trained in nutrition, that is, the science of foods and their effects on health. Most people with diabetes could benefit from seeing a dietitian every year. Every person with diabetes needs a personalized meal plan that takes into account lifestyle, food likes and dislikes, and diabetes goals. A dietitian can work with you to create such a plan. Later, your dietitian can help you adapt your meal plan to mesh with changes in your life or to take into account new scientific findings.

Your health-care provider, your local hospital or public health department, or your local diabetes association affiliate may be able to refer you to a qualified dietitian who works with people with diabetes. You might also try the American Dietetic Association Nutrition Information Line for a referral to a dietitian in your area who can provide a personal nutrition consultation (call 1-800-366-1655, or check their Web site at http://www.eatright.org). When choosing a dietitian, look for the initials "R.D." after his or her name. The initials indicate that

Q A

the person is a Registered Dietitian who has met standards for education and training set by the American Dietetic Association. Some people are also Licensed Dietitians (abbreviated "L.D."); licensure is a requirement set by many states. People who are Certified Diabetes Educators (C.D.E.) have specific training and experience in working with people with diabetes, are trained in diabetes care and treatment, and have passed a national examination on diabetes management.

124.
Can I take my diabetes medicines at mealtime?

You should check with your doctor or pharmacist about your schedule for taking medications. Depending on the kinds of medicines you take, the best time to take them isn't usually at mealtime but rather prior to or following meals. For example, diabetes pills, NovoLog insulin aspart, and Humalog insulin lispro are taken just before a meal, and Regular, NPH, or Lente insulin 30 minutes before eating. If you have eaten either more or less carbohydrates than usual, the rapid-acting insulins are most effective after a meal for matching your carbohydrate intake. It is important to stick to the medication schedule worked out for you by your health-care provider or pharmacist to ensure that your medicines work at their best in helping you manage your diabetes.

125.
Can people with diabetes eat sugar?

Yes, people with diabetes can eat sugar just like anyone else can. However, it should be counted as part of the total carbohydrate eaten for the meal or snack, as you would count any other carbohydrate food. Research has shown that it is the total amount of carbohydrate that you eat, rather than the source of that carbohydrate that affects your blood glucose level. In other words, 15 grams of carbohydrate from sugar should not affect the blood glucose much differently than 15 grams of carbohydrate from rice, bread, fruit, milk, or any other carbohydrate food.

Keep in mind, however, that there may be nutritional differences (in the amounts of fat, fiber, vitamins, and minerals) between foods that are high in

Q A

sugar and foods that contain other types of carbohydrate, even if their effect on blood glucose is similar. Since sugar is a concentrated source of carbohydrate (providing 15 grams of carbohydrate per tablespoon), limiting your intake of sugar and foods high in sugar will help you to control your total intake of carbohydrate, which in turn helps to control blood glucose levels. Foods that are high in sugar and low in nutrients are also often high in fat, so limiting the portions of desserts and other sweets will help control calorie and fat intake.

126.
Is fructose better for people than regular sugar?

Fructose, also called fruit sugar, is the sugar that occurs naturally in fruits and fruit juices. It has four calories per gram, just like regular sugar. In people with diabetes, fructose appears to raise glucose levels to a lesser degree when it replaces sucrose or starch in the diet. However, there is a concern that it might also raise blood cholesterol levels.

The use of fructose instead of sugar as a sweetening ingredient at the table or in cooking is not recommended, because the difference in its effect on health is not significant. At the same time, there is no reason to avoid naturally occurring fructose found in fruits, juices, vegetables, or other foods. If you use fructose or fructose-containing foods, they should be counted as carbohydrate choices in your food plan just as any other carbohydrate food would be counted (15 grams carbohydrate per carbohydrate choice).

127.
The only foods that taste good to me are sweets, especially candy. Can I eat candy and other sweets if I'm not eating much of anything else?

Unfortunately for those of us who enjoy them, sweets are full of sugars and starches that raise your blood glucose levels and raise them even more quickly if they are eaten alone. In addition to raising your blood glucose, however, most sweets are calorie-dense but nutrition-thin, don't fill you up so you're likely to eat more in response to hunger pangs, and so can ultimately foster weight gain depending on the quan-

Q A

tity you consume. In general, your dietitian or doctor will probably tell you to limit eating sweets to very small amounts (as suggested by the Food Pyramid's placement of sweets and fats in the small triangle at the very top). We all know, though, that sweets are often important foods on special occasions so, if you do indulge, make sweets a special treat.

A few helpful tips:

■ Make sure you eat a variety of the foods in your meal plan, and particularly proteins and less starchy vegetables, so you're not as hungry for sweets;

■ Consider fresh fruits or fresh fruit (no-sugar-added) sorbets as healthier alternatives to cakes, cookies, and candy;

■ Don't keep other sweets around the house where they can tempt you; and

■ When you do eat them, eat only very small portions, order "junior-size" servings, split them with someone else, or eat a bite and freeze the rest for later.

Finally, you can use low-calorie sweeteners (such as aspartame, saccharin, acesulfame potassium, and sucralose) as substitutes for sugars in many drinks (teas, hot cocoa), candies, and desserts. Your dietitian can help you identify sweets available on the market or sweets that you can prepare and incorporate into your meal plan.

**128.
I like to have ice cream or a cookie every night. Is that all right now that I have diabetes?**

Yes, if you have planned snacks built into your meal plan. Before 1994, the rule was that the sugars in ice cream, cookies, cakes, and other desserts were always bad for people with diabetes. They were considered to be worse than other carbohydrates like starches, so people were told to avoid them altogether. However, more recent studies have shown that the effect of sugars and starches on blood glucose levels is complex and that sugars do not necessarily need to be omitted entirely.

If your meal plan does not include a snack before bed, consider having a small serving of ice cream (or, better yet, fruit sorbet) or a low-fat cookie as part of your dinner meal. Remember, a blood glucose read-

Q A

ing near 140 mg/dl is the target for bedtime. You may find that a small snack is helpful if your bedtime blood glucose level is below target.

Your dietitian is your best source of information in helping you to understand your body's reaction to sugar, in determining when it is all right for you to eat sugary products, and helping you to balance sugar intake with other foods to keep your blood glucose in good control. Always check the Nutrition Facts labels to make sure the portion size and total carbohydrates (including sugars) of the snack match the amounts suggested by your meal plan. Remember, too, to use reduced-fat products to cut unwanted and unnecessary calories.

129.
Are artificial sweeteners safe? And are they useful?

Artificial sweeteners—saccharin (sold under several brand names including Sweet'n Low), aspartame (NutraSweet, Equal), acesulfame K (Sweet One, Sunett), and sucralose (Splenda)—appear to be safe in moderate amounts. None of these sweeteners affect blood glucose levels.

Certain people, however, should be wary of aspartame because it contains an amino acid called phenylalanine. People who have the condition called phenylketonuria should never use it, because it may build up in the brain and cause severe brain and nerve problems. People with advanced liver disease should talk to their doctor.

Artificial sweeteners have three benefits over sugar:
- They don't harm your teeth.
- They don't have to be counted in your carbohydrate tally for the day.
- They have far fewer calories, so you may have an easier time meeting your calorie goals for the day.

Be aware that some products labeled "sugar-free" contain sugar alcohols, such as mannitol, sorbitol, xylitol, or maltitol. These sweeteners do contain carbohydrates that must be accounted for in your meal plan. Be sure to check the Nutrition Information labels on your foods to see what you are getting.

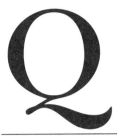 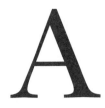

130.
How much of a sugar substitute is safe to use?

When the Food and Drug Association approves a sweetener as a food additive, it is assigned an Accepted Daily Intake level, or ADI. The ADI is 100 times smaller than the amount of the sweetener that a person could consume every day throughout a lifetime without experiencing side effects.

The ADI is different for different sweeteners and is expressed in an amount of milligrams per kilogram of body weight. For example, the ADI for the sweetener aspartame (the main sweetening ingredient in NutraSweet), is 50 milligrams per kilogram of body weight. For a person who weighs 132 pounds, this translates into 15 cans of diet soda or 86 packets of sweetener made with aspartame to reach the ADI. For the sweetener acesulfame K, consuming 25 cans of diet soda or 18 packets of sweetener would reach the ADI. These amounts of diet soda and packets of sweetener are likely to be far greater than most people would typically use in one day.

131.
What is it that I have to watch for? Sugar, fat, or salt?

Actually, you should watch out for all three.

The rule used to be that sugar was always bad for people with diabetes and so should be avoided altogether or eaten only in very small portions on special occasions. However, a number of studies show that although sugar raises blood glucose more quickly than other foods, such as meats and fats, the effect of sugar and other carbohydrates (starches) on blood glucose is complex, and sugar can be part of your meal plan. Your dietitian is your best guide to helping you determine when it is all right for you to eat sugary products and how you can balance sugar intake with other foods to keep your blood glucose in good control. In general, whole-grain starches are healthier for you than sugars are because they contain more vitamins and minerals as well as fiber (which helps you to feel fuller so you eat less and helps you to have regular bowel movements).

Fats are necessary components of your diet because they supply energy and essential fatty acids,

Q A

and absorb fat-soluble vitamins. However, many people eat too much fat, which can promote weight gain and damage blood vessels. Like sugar, fat is best eaten in very small quantities (as recommended by the Food Pyramid). Some fats—particularly saturated fats found in animal and high-fat dairy products, and *trans* fatty acids found in many fried and commercially baked goods—tend to raise blood cholesterol, which increases your risk for heart disease. Beneficial fats include unsaturated fats found in vegetable oils, most nuts, olives, avocados, cold-water fish (such as salmon and tuna), and dark-green leafy vegetables. To reduce your intake of saturated fats, you may want to use chicken broth (unsalted) instead of butter when sautéing foods, and to remove skin and extra fat from chicken and other meats. In addition, if you use oils, use them sparingly and consider olive oil as one of the better choices.

Finally, sodium (found in table salt as well as many processed and prepared foods) helps regulate fluids and blood pressure in your body. However, too much sodium may increase the amount of calcium excreted from your body, increase your risk of osteoporosis and bone fractures, and raise your blood pressure. In general, most people should consume less sodium than they currently do. Select fresh, no-salt-added, or low-sodium frozen or canned foods to reduce your intake of sodium. And try using condiments such as herb and spice combinations as replacements for salty seasonings.

132.
Do I need to be careful about salt because of my diabetes?

If you have hypertension, or high blood pressure, reducing your sodium intake may help to control your blood pressure. And since people with diabetes are at greater risk for developing high blood pressure compared with the general population, it is a good idea to learn to limit your sodium intake before your blood pressure becomes a problem.

The recommended amount of sodium for the general population is 2,400 to 3,000 milligrams of sodium per day. People with high blood pressure should not exceed 2,400 milligrams of sodium per day (which is equal to about 6,000 milligrams of salt per day).

110

Q A

Here are some tips to help you to lower your sodium intake:

- Remove the salt shaker from the table and use as little salt as possible in cooking. Use herbs, spices, pepper, lemon juice, and other low-sodium or sodium-free seasonings when you cook.
- Avoid processed foods that are highly salted, such as canned and dried soups, canned vegetables, frozen dinners, and canned or cured meats, such as bacon, cold cuts, and ham.
- Go easy on condiments that contain higher sodium levels, such as soy sauce, teriyaki sauce, salad dressings, ketchup, barbecue sauce, capers, olives, pickled onions and pickles, and seafood cocktail sauce.
- Look for reduced-sodium and no-salt-added products. Canned vegetables, canned soups, and some condiments are available now in low-salt versions, as are some snack foods.
- When you eat out, look for lower-sodium items on the menu and ask for your food to be prepared without added salt.

133.
I'm told I need to drink a lot of water for my diabetes. Why is water so important?

Water is one of those things that everybody needs to stay healthy, whether you have diabetes or not. It is necessary for the digestion of protein-rich foods like meats, to support the absorption of vitamins and minerals, and to maintain the blood viscosity that improves blood flow. Your kidneys also depend on an adequate supply of fluids. Impurities and waste products are filtered out of the blood by the kidneys, which depend on a certain amount of water for complete flushing. In addition, water helps move stool through the large intestines for elimination. You may need even more water if you drink caffeinated beverages, which act as diuretics.

Further, adequate water consumption may even be more important for people with diabetes in order to reduce the risks of diabetes-related kidney disease and other complications. In older adults, concerns about incontinence may also keep them from drinking enough water, sometimes leading to dehydration, and, in turn, to other adverse health outcomes.

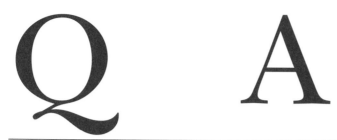

134.
I drink herb teas instead of soda to control my blood glucose. Is that all right?

Decaffeinated herb teas are great alternatives to sodas for helping you to control your blood glucose. If you like the teas sweet, use a low-calorie sweetener rather than sugar. The low-calorie sweeteners currently on the market—aspartame, saccharin, acesulfame potassium, and sucralose—have been documented as safe products for people with and without diabetes. These sweeteners provide sweetness without the calories of sugar in many low-calorie beverages as well as breath mints, chewing gums, and other foods.

Most sodas have considerable amounts of sugar in them or, even if they don't contain sugar, they have caffeine in them. Although caffeine isn't necessarily bad for people with diabetes, caffeine *can* make you less sensitive to hunger and more anxious during episodes of low blood glucose.

Other no- or low-calorie beverages that may be good alternatives to sugary sodas include plain water, sparkling water, flavored mineral waters, sugar-free flavored coffees, and hot chocolate.

135.
I am used to having my daily sip(s) of wine. Can I continue?

As in most things, moderation is the key. Your doctor will probably tell you that if you do drink, it is best to drink alcohol in moderation and to drink it with food to avoid hypoglycemia. In general, moderation translates into no more than one drink per day for women and no more than two drinks per day for men; the limits vary because of the differences in women's and men's weight and metabolism. One drink equals 12 ounces of regular beer, 5 ounces of wine, or 1.5 ounces of hard liquor (80-proof distilled spirits).

The downside of alcohol is that it has little nutritional value (it has "empty" calories), and sweet wines, beers, and mixed drinks made with sweetened sodas or juices may lead to weight gain. Further, alcohol in dry wines or hard liquor promotes the conversion of blood glucose into glycogen in the liver, which can result in an uncontrolled drop in blood glucose levels. In addition, heavy consumption of alcohol may

Q A

cause a variety of problems—from cirrhosis of the liver, damage to the heart, and high blood pressure to increased risk of motor vehicle crashes, violence, and psychological problems. Heavy alcohol use may also result in poor food habits and malnutrition.

Some recent research, however, suggests that moderate consumption of alcohol (particularly red wine) may have beneficial properties related to heart function in men over age 45 and women over age 55. Alcohol consumption has not been found to have a similar effect for younger adults. You should check with your dietitian or physician for advice about drinking wine or any other alcohol, particularly if you take prescription or over-the-counter medications, or if you have had problems with alcohol consumption in the past.

In general, if you do chose to drink a little, do so responsibly, in moderation, and in combination with nutritious low-carbohydrate foods.

136.
So is it safe to drink alcohol when you have diabetes?

People with diabetes can safely use alcohol if they follow a few simple guidelines whenever they choose to drink. This is because alcohol can affect your blood glucose level, making it go too high or too low. If you drink an alcoholic beverage mixed with a high-carbohydrate mixer like regular soda pop or fruit juice, your blood glucose may go up. Alcohol consumption can also increase your appetite, causing you to eat more. That can also lead to elevated blood glucose levels.

Conversely, drinking alcohol can also make your blood glucose drop if you drink on an empty stomach, if you are taking diabetes pills or insulin, if the amount of alcohol you drink is excessive, or if you were just exercising or just about to exercise. This can be especially risky because the symptoms of a low blood glucose reaction can be mistaken for the symptoms of having had too much to drink. As a result, you may not get appropriate treatment for hypoglycemia when you need it. And of course, you should never drink if you will be driving. The risk of having a low blood glucose reaction, added to the general effects of alcohol, could increase the chances

Q A

that you have an accident or get stopped for drunk driving.

To use alcohol safely and avoid disruptions with blood glucose control, follow these general guidelines:

■ Use alcohol only when your diabetes is under good control.

■ Never drink on an empty stomach. Consume the alcohol with a meal, or at least with a snack.

■ Limit the quantity. The Dietary Guidelines for Americans recommends no more than two drinks at a time for a man and one drink for a woman. One drink is defined as 12 ounces of beer, 5 ounces of wine, or 1.5 ounces of liquor. Also, remember that alcohol contains calories and excessive use can lead to weight gain.

■ Mix your alcohol with carbohydrate- and calorie-free beverages like water, club soda, sugar-free tonic, or sugar-free soda pop.

■ Wear medical identification that states you have diabetes. If something happens, it is important for the people helping you to have this information.

Alcohol use can worsen some of the complications of diabetes including eye disease, nerve problems, high blood pressure, and elevated blood fats. If you have any of these problems, check with your health-care team before using alcohol.

Avoid alcohol if you are pregnant, trying to lose weight, have a history of alcohol abuse, or are taking any other drugs that should not be combined with alcohol.

Check your blood glucose before, during, and after drinking, too, since alcohol can continue to lower blood glucose for several hours after you stop drinking.

137.

In summary, what precautions should I take when drinking alcohol?

Alcohol can either raise blood glucose levels or lower them, depending on the circumstances. To prevent highs and lows, it's best to drink alcohol with a meal. Although alcohol contains carbohydrate, it should be drunk in addition to the meal; it should not replace part of the meal.

Q A

If you do choose to drink outside of mealtime, keep in mind that the effects of alcohol on your blood glucose can last long after the alcohol has left your system. So testing your glucose more often the next morning is a good idea.

To reduce the overall carbohydrate content of your drinks, mix them with beverages that are carbohydrate- and calorie-free, such as water or sugar-free soda pop. And of course, drink only in moderation (not more than one drink for women, two drinks for men). One drink is 12 ounces of beer, 5 ounces of wine, or 1.5 ounces of distilled spirits. Remember, low-blood-sugar reactions can mimic drunkenness, so people around you may not recognize that you need assistance if your blood glucose drops too low.

Finally, avoid drinking alcohol if you are pregnant or nursing, if you have severe diabetic nerve disease, or if you are taking medicine that will interact with the alcohol. And never drink and drive.

138.
What about cooking for my family? Do I need to cook more than one meal?

The meals you fix to manage your diabetes are made up of healthful foods from all six major food groups, foods that are good for you and everyone in your family. So, happily, you don't need to cook more than one meal. However, if you're not already doing so, you may want to incorporate some changes into your family's diet that would be helpful to you as well as to them. For example, starches are one of the major food groups that your diet can include. However, whole-grain starches (like multigrain breads, brown rice, yams, oatmeal, and other whole-grain cereals) are much healthier for you than other "simple" starches (like white breads, rice, potatoes, and sugary cereals). This is because whole-grain starches contain more fiber, are absorbed more slowly, and balances blood glucose better. Other changes you might consider include baking (or broiling, roasting, or steaming) rather than frying your food, and using skim milk or low-fat milk rather than whole milk in your cereals or other recipes. You might also find that no-sugar jellies, salsas, and mustards are wonderful substitutes for high-sugar marmalades and high-fat sour

Q A

cream dips and mayonnaise. Your dietitian or physician can give you lots of helpful ideas about making meals that taste good and are good for you *and* your family. In addition, many good cookbooks are available (both in bookstores and through *Diabetes Self-Management,* the American Diabetes Association, and other sources) that provide recipes for tasty, nutritious, and satisfying meals that are low in fat, sugar, and sodium and high in vitamins, minerals, and fiber.

139.

So it's all right to serve my family the same foods I eat for my diabetes meal plan?

Not only is it all right, you'd be doing them a favor. The recommended diet for people with diabetes is one of the healthiest ways to eat. Not only does it provide glucose control, but very similar diets are recommended for heart health, safe and sustainable weight loss, and for good health in general. All of these diets are rich in plant foods, such as vegetables, fruits, grains, and beans, and low in fats and sweets.

There is one exception to this rule: Very young children need more fat in their diets than older children and adults. Children between 9 months and 2 years old should drink whole milk. After your children reach age 2, follow your pediatrician's advice for decreasing the amount of fat in your child's diet.

140.

How can I stick to my meal plan when I go to parties?

It's easy to succumb to the lure of all the tasty treats offered at parties. It all looks so good, and you would not want to insult the hostess, right? Fortunately, it is possible to sample the fare and stick to your plan:
- Eat before you go so that hunger does not drive you to overindulge.
- Don't start eating right away. Instead, look over all the dishes first and decide which ones you most want to try. Then sample small amounts of these foods.
- Eat your food slowly. Enjoy the taste, smell, and texture of each morsel.
- Let time with your friends or family be the highlight of the party.
- Stand or sit far from the food so you won't be tempted to keep eating "just one more piece."

Q A

■ Ask whether you can bring something to the party. If so, you'll know there'll be at least one healthful treat available.

■ If you do not use insulin, consider shifting some of your starch and fat exchanges from breakfast and lunch to your evening meal. Then you can eat a little extra at the party and still stay within your meal-plan goals for the day.

141.
What about eating out? Can I still go out to dinner with my family and friends?

Having diabetes doesn't mean you have to give up socializing with family and friends over meals or other special events! But it does mean being watchful about how the foods are prepared and how much you eat. If you have mastered the concepts of individual serving sizes and low-fat and low-sugar meal preparation when cooking at home, you should be well equipped to gauge your meal selections when eating out.

Fortunately, it's much easier these days to select menu items that are healthier for you—like baked or broiled rather than fried foods, whole-grain rolls rather than white flour rolls or high-fat muffins, and leafy green salads rather than vegetables with cheese sauces. Ask for low-starch vegetables and eliminate the mashed potatoes, select fresh fruit instead of a sugary dessert, and ask for low-fat salad dressings on the side. Since many restaurants these days serve large portions of food to their customers, you can also split meals with your friends, select "junior," "small plate," or appetizer sizes, or ask the server to put half of the meal in a doggie bag even before it gets to the table!

In addition, you can say no to alcoholic drinks or desserts that offer little nutritional value (but may affect your blood glucose levels), or you can have them as special treats. When you do indulge in drinks or desserts, remember that moderation is the key. Eat or drink only very small portions, split them with someone else, or eat a bite and take the rest home. Most restaurants are more than happy to oblige the customer who prefers and asks for heart-healthy low-fat, low-sodium, healthful dishes.

Q A

142.
When I go to a restaurant, how do I figure out what menu choices are the most healthful?

Because so many people are trying to eat more healthfully, many restaurants are striving to include lighter fare and label healthy choices on the menu. Even if the restaurant where you are doesn't do this, there are some easy ways to tell which choices will be best for you:

■ When ordering meats, avoid those prepared by some form of frying and choose instead broiled, roasted, grilled, or baked meats.

■ When ordering vegetables, look for raw, stewed, steamed, or boiled vegetables and avoid those that are fried or come with sauces. You can also ask for the sauce to be served on the side.

■ Watch out for words that signal a high fat content, such as "breaded," "cream," "cheese," "mayonnaise," "gravy," "jumbo, and "giant."

■ If the menu does not clearly say how a dish is prepared or what it contains, ask your waiter. Also ask whether the chef is open to special requests, such as using less fat or broiling instead of frying.

143.
My doctor told me to eat less protein. What foods are high in protein and how much should I eat?

If you have been advised to eat less protein, it is probably because your doctor is concerned about the health of your kidneys. Research has suggested that limiting the amount of protein in your diet may help to slow down the progression of kidney disease. That's because eating too much protein can cause the kidneys to work extra hard to remove the waste products of protein metabolism. There is no evidence, however, that restricting protein in someone without known kidney disease will delay or prevent the development of kidney disease in the future.

Protein is found in a number of foods, including meat, fish, and poultry; eggs, milk, yogurt and cheese; nuts, seeds and nut butters; and legumes, whole grains, and tofu. Since most adults in this country eat at least 50% more protein than our bodies require for good health, restricting protein intake

Q A

is not likely to cause malnutrition. The recommended amount of protein for an individual with overt nephropathy is 0.8 grams of protein per kilogram of body weight. Restricting protein to this level may slow the progression of nephropathy. For a 150-pound individual, this would translate to about 55 grams of protein per day. If you need to control the protein in your diet, check with a dietitian for help in writing a food plan to meet your nutritional needs for protein as well as other nutrients.

144.
What are whole grains and how do I work them into my diet?

Whole grains are grains that haven't had their nutrient-rich outer coating removed. As a result, they contain more vitamins, minerals, and fiber than refined grains. Foods that are high in fiber promote digestion and ease two conditions, diverticulosis (abnormal pouches in the colon, which can become inflamed) and constipation.

Whole grains include brown rice, bulgur wheat, oatmeal, popcorn, pearl barley, whole oats, whole rye, and whole wheat.

One easy way to work whole grains into your diet is to substitute them for refined foods you eat now. Use brown rice in place of white rice. When choosing noodles, breads, and crackers, look for products made from whole wheat and rye flour instead of white flour. When baking, replace one-fourth of the white flour with whole-wheat flour. When buying cereals, choose oatmeal or whole-grain cereals.

145.
Are low-carbohydrate diets good for people with diabetes?

Low-carbohydrate—in fact, fad diets in general—are a bad idea for people with diabetes. Research shows that the most healthful diet is one that is low in saturated fat and that stresses fruits, vegetables, and whole grains. But low-carbohydrate plans ignore this research. These diets, promoted in best-sellers such as *The Zone* and *Dr. Atkins' New Diet Revolution,* limit your intake of nutritious plant foods and replace them with fatty foods. As a result, low-carbohydrate diets tend to have too much saturated fat and cholesterol and far too little vitamins, minerals, and fiber.

Q A

Going on a low-carbohydrate diet may be tempting. After all, carbohydrates are what affect blood glucose levels most. In fact, some people have promoted low-carbohydrate diets specifically to people with diabetes as a way of normalizing blood glucose levels. However, these diets are too risky. According to the American Heart Association, long-term use of a low-carbohydrate diet may raise LDL (bad) cholesterol levels and raise blood pressure, which is particularly worrisome because people with diabetes already have a higher risk of developing heart disease. These diets can also cause bone loss, increase the risk of cancer, and lead to deficiencies of some vitamins and minerals. Short-term side effects may include constipation, dehydration, dizziness, fatigue, gout, kidney stones, nausea, and low blood pressure. The high levels of protein in these diets can overwork the kidneys, speeding the development of diabetic kidney disease. Finally, even though pounds may melt away when you are on the diet, they usually pile right back on as soon as you go off. The best advice is to pass these diets by and stick to a plan that is varied, low in fat, low in calories, and full of nutrients.

146.
What is carbohydrate counting? How much carbohydrate should I eat?

Carbohydrate counting is a food-planning tool that is used to help you control your blood glucose level by keeping the amount of carbohydrate in your diet consistent. It is based on the fact that all carbohydrate foods affect the blood glucose in a similar way. What affects the blood glucose level the most is the total amount of carbohydrate a person with diabetes eats at a meal, not the type of carbohydrate you eat. In other words, whether you eat 15 grams of carbohydrate from a slice of bread, or one-third cup of rice, or one tablespoon of sugar, your rise in blood glucose level will be similar with all three foods.

One carbohydrate choice contains 15 grams of carbohydrate from any carbohydrate-containing food. A typical diabetes food plan includes approximately three to four carbohydrate choices per meal (about 45 to 60 grams of carbohydrate). Amounts of carbo-

Q A

hydrate may vary between individuals depending on age, gender, activity level, medicine or insulin dose, and diabetes management goals. Some people may eat less than this, and some people may eat a little more, according to their individualized food plans. Talk with your dietitian or diabetes health-care provider about developing a food plan with the right amount of carbohydrate choices to fit your lifestyle and diabetes goals.

147.

How can I determine the number of carbohydrate choices for a food by looking at the food label?

The Nutrition Facts part of the food label will provide you with all the information you need for carbohydrate counting.

Step 1. Check the serving size. All of the information on the label is based on this portion of food. If you eat double the serving size, you need to double the carbohydrate grams also.

Step 2. Look at the total carbohydrate information. This number is the total number of grams of carbohydrate for *one serving* of food. The total number of carbohydrate grams include the grams of carbohydrate from dietary fiber and sugar, so don't add those numbers to the total number. If a food contains more than 5 grams of dietary fiber, however, you can subtract that amount from the grams of total carbohydrate. Because carbohydrate from dietary fiber is not broken down or absorbed by the body, it does not affect blood glucose. The resulting amount of carbohydrate is what you need to count

Step 3. Convert the carbohydrate grams to carbohydrate choices. One carbohydrate choice is equal to 15 grams of carbohydrate. So 30 grams is equal to two choices, 45 grams is equal to three choices, and so on. You can round to the nearest whole or half carbohydrate choice (23 grams is equal to about one and one half carbohydrate choices, for example).

Step 4. Decide how to use the food in your food plan. If your food plan calls for four carbohydrate choices at dinner, for example, and the label of a food product you are using shows about 30 grams of carbohydrate per serving (or two carbohydrate choices), you

Q A

will know that you can eat that food, and have an additional two choices from other foods to make your total of four choices for the meal.

148.
My family constantly comments about my food choices. How can I handle this?

Your loved ones care about you and want the best for you. In fact they may care so much that they're willing to take on the burden of guiding your diabetes care and meal planning, whether you like it or not. Even if you do face challenges in following your meal plan (and who doesn't), constant vigilance and comment from family members is often more of a hindrance than a help.

You may want to start off with an obvious solution: talk to them. You may need to gently describe how frustrating it is to be constantly watched and criticized. Explain the demands of diabetes, recognize that they want to help you, and then give them a job. You can tell them that it doesn't help when they comment about your food choices, but they could help you by buying healthier foods or supporting your efforts at exercise.

Unfortunately, some criticism is not generated out of kindness and you may need to talk to a mental-health specialist who can help you identify some strategies for dealing with that problem.

149.
What should I eat if I am sick and cannot eat my normal diet?

When you are sick, your body needs carbohydrate just like when you are well. Carbohydrate provides energy, helps your body heal, helps to prevent ketones from forming, and helps prevent your blood glucose from dropping too low. If you cannot eat your usual food plan due to an upset stomach, high fever, or poor appetite, try some of the following choices that might work better when you are under the weather (each item is equal to one carbohydrate choice, or about 15 grams of carbohydrate):
- ½ cup regular soda (not diet)
- ½ cup fruit juice
- ½ cup ice cream
- ¼ cup sherbet

Q A

- ½ cup cooked cereal
- 1 slice toast
- 1 cup soup
- 6 saltine crackers
- 3 graham cracker squares
- ½ cup regular gelatin (not sugar-free)
- 1 popsicle (single) or fruit juice bar

In addition to replacing the carbohydrate from your usual food plan with the above suggestions, it is important to drink plenty of sugar-free, caffeine-free liquids to replace fluids lost during illness. Try to drink about one cup of water or broth every hour.

If you have persistent nausea with vomiting and/or diarrhea for more than six or eight hours, and/or if you cannot keep any food or fluids down, call your health-care provider for assistance.

4
Blood Glucose Monitoring

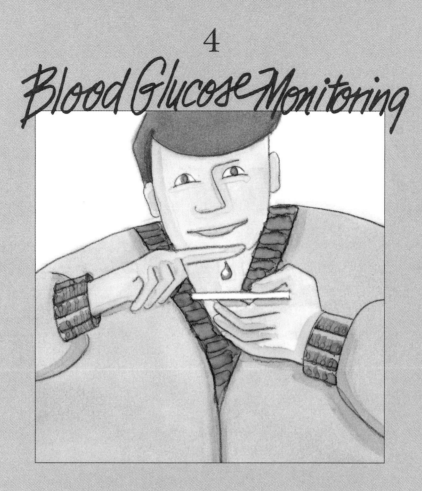

150. Why do I have to monitor my blood glucose levels?

151. What is the HbA$_{1c}$ test?

152. Can't the HbA$_{1c}$ test take the place of blood glucose monitoring?

153. How do I monitor?

154. How often should I monitor my blood glucose?

155. Why do I need to check my blood glucose more when I'm sick?

156. Does it hurt to get a blood sample?

157. How often can I use the same lancet for pricking my finger?

158. I have difficulty getting enough blood from my finger. What can I do about this problem?

159. My fingers hurt from testing my blood. What can I do?

160. What about testing my urine for glucose?

161. What about checking my urine for ketones?

162. I've been checking my blood glucose, but I don't know what the numbers mean.

163. I stopped checking my blood glucose because the high numbers scare me. What else can I do?

164. What do I do when my blood glucose is high?

165. What do I do when my blood glucose is low?

166. How long do I have to keep checking my blood glucose?

167. Do I have to use my fingers to check my blood glucose level?

168. Can someone check my blood glucose for me?

169. Why do I have to keep a record of my blood glucose readings?

170. Why does my doctor want to see my blood glucose records?

171. Can test strips be used more than once?

172. Why do test strips cost so much?

173. How do I know if my blood glucose meter is reading correctly?

174. What do I do if my meter is broken?

175. At what blood glucose level should I call my doctor?

176. I travel a lot and have learned from experience that test strips don't give accurate readings of my blood glucose level after I've left them in a hot car. I've seen advertisements for meters that operate over wide temperature ranges. Do these ranges apply just to the meter or are the strips temperature-resistant as well?

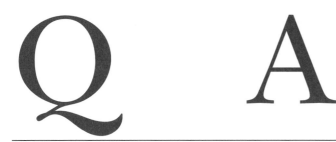

150.
Why do I have to monitor my blood glucose levels?

Monitoring provides information about your patterns of blood glucose fluctuation or control. You cannot assume that if you feel fine your blood glucose is fine. Discuss with your health-care team what blood glucose target ranges are right for you. Typically, you will have to measure your blood glucose levels at different times of the day. It is very important to check your blood glucose in the morning. If you don't, you won't know if you're in your target range at the start of the day and it will be harder to determine your medication doses later in the day. You may also want to know your blood glucose level before and after meals, and before bed. Some people check their blood glucose levels at each of these times every day, and some check them on different days. The best strategy is to establish a plan with your diabetes team that works best for you. They can help you decide how often to monitor your blood glucose and when to call with problems or concerns.

If you monitor and notice your readings regularly going out of range, you can call your doctor or nurse for guidance; this will help lower your risk of developing complications of diabetes, such as damage to the eyes, kidneys, and nerves. Also, monitoring is helpful if you have a break in your usual routine, such as a family reunion (more food than usual), travel across time zones (delayed meals), or have an illness. Monitoring gives you the information you need to make the right adjustments and will help you keep your blood glucose from going too high or too low. It may seem tedious sometimes, but it's essential for the best control of your diabetes.

151.
What is the HbA$_{1c}$ test?

The HbA$_{1c}$ (hemoglobin A$_{1c}$) blood test measures your average blood glucose over the three months preceding the test. It measures how much glucose is attached to hemoglobin, the specialized protein in your red blood cells that transports oxygen through your bloodstream. Hemoglobin picks up glucose that is floating around in your bloodstream. The more glucose in your blood, the more glucose the hemoglobin will pick up. By measuring the percentage of

Q   A

hemoglobin in the blood that is bound to glucose, your doctor can get a good estimate of your average glucose level over the preceding two to three months, which is how long a red blood cell stays in your blood before it is recycled.

Although the normal results for the HbA$_{1c}$ test range from 4% to 6%, the treatment goal for most people with diabetes is 6.5% to 7%. This allows for a certain percentage of blood glucose readings to be above and below the target range. Improved blood glucose, as documented by a decrease in HbA$_{1c}$ values, has been shown to prevent the microvascular complications of diabetes. For instance, if you lower your HbA$_{1c}$ by just 1%, you can decrease the possibility of damage to your eyes by at least 30%.

You can use HbA$_{1c}$ results to monitor the overall improvement in your blood glucose levels when you make a change such as adding exercise to your routine. An elevated HbA$_{1c}$ result can signal a need for a change in your treatment plan.

152.
Can't the HbA$_{1c}$ test take the place of blood glucose monitoring?

No. The HbA$_{1c}$ test will only give you and your diabetes team an idea of your average blood glucose level over the two to three months preceding the test. It doesn't give any specific information as to the degree or timing of blood glucose ups and downs. Home blood glucose monitoring can do that, allowing you to adjust your diabetes care with the help of your diabetes team as needed to correct blood glucose levels.

If you check your blood glucose meal to meal and day to day, you will be able to see patterns that might be occurring without your knowledge, and that could indicate a problem. For example, a high fasting blood glucose (before breakfast) could tell you that you had too much food the night before or that it rebounded after a low during the night. It could also be an early warning sign of an infection. In the absence of these possibilities, and if it is persistent, it could mean you need more insulin or diabetes medication in the evening.

Similarly, a persistent elevation of blood glucose in the afternoon before supper may prompt you to look at your daytime food intake and activity level to see what changes are necessary to correct the problem.

153.
How do I monitor?

Blood glucose monitoring can be done with a variety of devices; the most commonly used is a blood glucose meter. Checking your blood glucose level using a meter requires you to obtain a small drop of blood, which you then apply to a strip or cartridge connected to the meter. The meter calculates the level of glucose in the blood sample and gives you a digital readout of the blood glucose value. There are all kinds of meters on the market, but they are not all the same. They vary in cost, and they also vary in their suitability to different people's needs. For instance, one new device is worn like a wristwatch and periodically samples blood glucose levels, as frequently as every 10 minutes if you program it to do so. This device is available by prescription only and is intended to supplement, not replace, conventional blood glucose monitoring.

For some people, a very simple meter that just reads the blood glucose value is best; this requires the user to enter the time and blood glucose value into a logbook. Others might prefer a meter that automatically records the time and blood glucose in the meter's memory. Some meters can calculate averages at various times of day, and some even have the capacity to upload stored readings to a computer and provide graphs of your glucose readings. The meter that is right for you depends on your individual needs. Talk with your doctor or nurse about which meter is best for your needs.

154.
How often should I monitor my blood glucose?

Ask your diabetes team how frequently they think you should check your blood glucose. In general, people who have diabetes that can be controlled with pills or diet usually check their blood glucose level once or twice a day. However, they may check it more or less often depending on how well controlled they are, how they feel, or what activities are occurring that affect blood glucose.

Q A

People who use insulin need to check their blood glucose two to five times a day to see what their blood glucose is and make any necessary adjustments in their food intake and/or insulin dose. They should check it before exercise, after exercise, when they have symptoms of high or low blood glucose, and before bed. Safety also dictates that people who use insulin check their blood glucose before driving. A low blood glucose level may prompt you to take more food or less insulin, depending on your particular diabetes care plan. On the other hand, high blood glucose may prompt you to eat less food or take more insulin. Your doctor will give you directions about making these adjustments.

Regardless of treatment, when a person with diabetes becomes ill—for example, with intestinal flu—it is recommended they check blood glucose levels more frequently. Even if you are unable to eat, your blood glucose may go up higher than usual because the body releases glucose stores into the bloodstream to cope with illness. Thus, you may still need to take some portion of your usual medication to help your blood glucose come down, but you will have to check your blood glucose level first and then a few hours later to decide what you need to do. Always try to drink more water when your blood glucose is high or when you are ill, and check your blood glucose more often when circumstances are unusual.

155.
Why do I need to check my blood glucose more when I'm sick?

Checking blood glucose more frequently when you are sick is important for several reasons. For instance, your blood glucose may fluctuate more widely when ill. Or your illness may interfere with or mask the usual symptoms of high or low blood glucose. Checking your blood glucose will tell you if your blood glucose is rising or falling. Once you know this, you can make care adjustments, such as drinking more fluids or taking more or less medication as instructed by your diabetes team.

If you have stomach flu accompanied by nausea and diarrhea, you might not be able to eat. Since you are not eating, you may think that you do not need to take your diabetes medicine. However, when you are

Q A

ill your body releases hormones that cause blood glucose levels to rise. This is a protective response for people that do not have diabetes. For people with diabetes, your blood glucose can get too high and make you even sicker. By checking your blood glucose more often, you will know whether more medication is needed. In any case, drink extra fluids to avoid dehydration. If your stomach is upset, suck on ice chips or eat some sugar-free gelatin. As soon as possible, take an aid for your diarrhea to help prevent dehydration. Check your blood glucose as frequently as your diabetes team suggests and, if warranted, call them for further instruction.

156.
Does it hurt to get a blood sample?

The early meters required a large drop of blood, and the skin prick required to get it cut fairly deep and was painful for most people, even when they pricked the sides of their fingers, which have fewer nerve endings than the tip. As technology evolved, new methods for measuring blood glucose were developed. Some of the newest meters require a blood sample only about the size of the head of a pin. This smaller blood sample can be obtained from a much shallower skin prick with little or no pain. Another welcome development was the advent of "alternate-site" monitoring. Many newer meters can use a blood sample obtained from a finger or, alternatively, from the forearm or even the thigh, both of which have many fewer nerve endings than a fingertip. Many people find that getting a blood sample from either of these two sites quite painless. Another new device attaches to the wrist and allows most glucose samples to be assessed through the skin without blood even being drawn and with little or no discomfort.

157.
How often can I use the same lancet for pricking my finger?

Lancets are designed and labeled to be used once, then thrown away. While this is the ideal way to use them, there may be circumstances where you need to use your lancets more than one time each. If you decide to use a lancet more than one time, keep in mind the following recommendations:

Q A

■ Use a new lancet every 24 hours, regardless of how many times you have used it that day. Change the lancet if it appears or feels dull, looks deformed, or has touched any surface other than your skin. Also, keep the lancet clean and covered between uses.

■ Do not wipe the lancet with alcohol (or anything else), since that could remove the silicone coating that makes the poke less painful.

■ Always store your lancets in a clean, closed container.

■ Finally, make sure you wash your hands thoroughly before lancing your finger, and watch for signs of skin inflammation or infection at the lance site.

Dispose of all lancets in an appropriate container, such as a red plastic sharps holder, to avoid injury and contamination to other individuals. Check your clinic, community, or state guidelines for instructions on how to dispose of sharps safely.

158.
I have difficulty getting enough blood from my finger. What can I do to help this problem?

There are several things you can do to make it easier to get a drop of blood for a blood glucose test. First, wash your hands in warm water before testing to increase the blood flow to your fingertips. Next, let your hand or arm drop down by your side for a minute before poking your finger. This will also increase the blood flow to your finger. After lancing, gently massage or "milk" your finger until a blood droplet forms.

It's best not to use the same site for drawing blood each time. Instead, rotate to different fingers each time so you don't develop calluses over a particular area. And use the side of your finger rather than the tip; the side has fewer nerve endings, so you should feel the prick less.

Check to see if your lancing device has the ability to adjust the depth of puncture. If it does, adjust the device to allow for a slightly deeper puncture if you are having difficulty obtaining blood (check your instruction manual for information on how to do this). Also, some meters today are designed to require much smaller amounts of blood than some of the older meters. Your diabetes health-care team can

Q A

help you decide whether you might benefit from a meter that takes less blood than the one you might be using. You can also call the company that made your meter for questions and help with their equipment. The number to call is usually printed on the back of the meter.

159.
My fingers hurt from testing my blood. What can I do?

It is worth the time and effort to find a lancing product that minimizes the discomfort of puncturing your skin. Lancing devices are made of two main components: the lancet, which is a pointed piece of surgical steel encased in plastic that is used for puncturing your skin, and the lancing device, which pushes the lancet into your skin and then retracts it. Most lancing devices have a feature that allows you to dial in the penetration depth. Generally, children and adults with sensitive fingers prefer a shallower puncture; adults with callused fingers may need a deeper puncture to get an adequate blood sample.

The lancing device that comes packaged with your meter may not be the best one for you. If you find you can't get enough blood or it hurts too much, there are plenty of other devices to try. Also, the spring in your lancing device may weaken after a while, which makes it more difficult to draw blood. If the device came with your meter, sometimes the manufacturer may replace it free of charge.

Choosing the right lancet is as important as using the right lancing device. Lancets vary by gauge, that is, the width of the metal point that punctures your finger. A higher gauge indicates a smaller point. So a 30-gauge lancet makes a smaller hole than a 23-gauge lancet. Although a higher-gauge lancet may hurt less, you may not get enough blood when you puncture your skin. Trying a lancet with a lower gauge may allow you to get a larger drop of blood so you won't have to prick your finger more than once for one test.

Some test strips have been approved for use sites other than your fingertips, such as your forearm or thigh. These alternative sites may cause less discomfort, but they cannot be used if you are experiencing a low blood glucose reaction or when your blood glu-

Q A

cose is rapidly changing. In these cases, fingerstick results will be give you a more accurate result because blood flow to the fingers is faster and more direct than it is to these other sites.

160.
What about testing my urine for glucose?

Urine is generated as the kidneys filter blood for waste products. When blood glucose levels rise above approximately 180 mg/dl, the kidney will excrete some of the extra glucose into the urine; this urine is then stored in the bladder until the bladder is full.

Before the advent of home blood glucose monitoring in the 1980's, persons with diabetes used a home urine test for glucose. However, this is not as nearly as helpful as testing your blood. Because urine is stored in the bladder over time, urine testing cannot determine what the blood glucose level is at a specific time. For instance, a positive morning urine test could mean you had a blood glucose level over 180 mg/dl after you went to bed, but you would not know if it was still elevated at dawn. A second urination might determine that a more recent collection of urine contained no glucose, but it could not tell you how much lower than 180 mg/dl your blood glucose might be. Thus, a negative urine test for sugar does not mean blood glucose is normal, just that it wasn't recently over 180 mg/dl.

There still are some situations where urine testing is useful. An example would be a very frail older adult with heart disease who cannot or will not perform blood testing and in whom blood glucose levels under 180 mg/dl are generally satisfactory. Urine testing, where a persistent finding of more than trace glucose would indicate significant hyperglycemia, can then prompt blood testing by a helper or aide.

161.
What about checking my urine for ketones?

Checking urine for ketones is still done when a person with Type 1 diabetes is ill and concerned about his or her diabetes spiraling out of control. If a person with diabetes has too little insulin circulating to move glucose from the bloodstream into cells, then fat will be broken down as an alternative fuel source

Q A

(despite the fact that glucose is present in the bloodstream). Ketones are chemicals that are released into the bloodstream when fat is used this way for energy. During the process of burning fat, certain messenger proteins (hormones such as glucagon, adrenaline, and cortisol) are released and cause sugar stores to enter the bloodstream, raising blood glucose even higher.

If left untreated, this situation can progress to a medical emergency. The body tries to get rid of its excess blood glucose by "spilling" it into the urine, resulting in frequent urination and dehydration. As more and more ketones are released, the blood becomes acidic. This condition is called ketoacidosis and usually results in nausea, abdominal pain, shortness of breath, and clouded thinking. Ketoacidosis is a serious condition and should be managed by a doctor. If a person with Type 1 diabetes checks his urine for ketones early in the illness, he can make adjustments to avoid ketoacidosis by getting sufficient fluids and insulin. In Type 2 diabetes, ketoacidosis is quite rare since there is usually some insulin circulating in the blood, so urine testing of ketones is not usually ordered for people with Type 2 diabetes. However, people with Type 2 diabetes who have persistent high blood glucose can still become very ill and dehydrated, so blood glucose testing is critical.

162.
I've been checking my blood glucose, but I don't know what the numbers mean.

The glucose levels in your blood are constantly fluctuating. Glucose moves in and out of your bloodstream based on where and when your body needs it. So when blood glucose values are described, they are usually described in a range that allows for these fluctuations. People who do not have diabetes should have a premeal blood glucose level that is less than 110 mg/dl. For people with diabetes, the target goal is 90 mg/dl to 130 mg/dl before a meal. (If you use a whole-blood-calibrated meter such as the OneTouch Basic or OneTouch Profile, the target range is 80 to 120 mg/dl before a meal). The target level two hours after a meal is less than 180 mg/dl.

Q A

Looking at your blood glucose patterns gives you feedback that can help you make decisions about your diabetes care. For example, you may find that your blood glucose readings are within the target range before supper but above range before breakfast. Perhaps all of your readings two hours after lunch are within range, but your readings after dinner on weekends fluctuate depending on whether you ate out or at home. By looking at these patterns, you can see what is working for you (in this case, your food choices at lunch), decide if you need a change in medication (based on your higher-than-target readings before breakfast), or choose restaurants more carefully (as indicated by your weekend fluctuations).

The goal of monitoring is not to ensure that every blood glucose reading is within your target range. A more reasonable goal is to have most of your readings fall within target range, to understand and make decisions based on the patterns you observe, and to aim for an HbA_{1c} value of 6.5% to 7%. Regular monitoring is a tool that gives you the information you need to make adjustments in your diabetes care.

163.
I stopped checking my blood glucose because the high numbers scare me. What else can I do?

Blood glucose monitoring is a tool designed to help you self-manage your diabetes. If the high numbers upset you, by all means take a break from monitoring, but seek help from your health-care provider. The first step is to find out the reasons for your high blood glucose readings. Do you need a change or adjustment in medication? Do you need to take another look at your food choices and eating habits? Did you stop exercising? Do you have an infection? Any or all of these factors can be raising your blood glucose levels. Once the reasons have been identified, you can develop a new treatment plan and begin monitoring your blood glucose again.

It can be very frustrating to try your hardest, make the healthiest choices, and still see elevated or widely fluctuating readings. The good news is that your health-care team can help you to reevaluate your treatment plan, analyze the situation, and modify your treatment goals based on your lifestyle.

Q A

164.
What do I do when my blood glucose is high?

Don't panic, high blood glucose is treatable. Ask your diabetes team what they suggest you do if your blood glucose rises and when you should call for further direction. Every person's case should be treated individually. Many people with diabetes will find that their blood glucose will become high (over 200 mg/dl) when they eat extra food, are under stress, or don't get their usual amount of exercise. It may come down in an hour or so.

The first thing to do is drink a tall glass of water to dilute the blood and avoid dehydration, which often comes with high blood glucose. If you are feeling well and your blood glucose is under 300 mg/dl, a walk may help bring your blood glucose down. Avoid drinking any fluids that contain calories; water or diet caffeine-free sodas are good choices. In approximately one hour, check your blood glucose again to find out if your blood glucose is still rising or coming down.

If your blood glucose is over 300 mg/dl and still rising, your body may be starting to release hormones in an attempt to get more blood glucose to the muscles. This may further worsen your blood glucose level; insulin is needed to lower the blood glucose. Your diabetes team can tell you how much extra diabetes medicine or insulin to take.

If your blood glucose is over 400 mg/dl, you should get medical direction. Having blood glucose at this level can cause you to become dehydrated and ill if it isn't brought down. As long as you are feeling all right, call your physician. If you are feeling ill and don't think you can give yourself the care you need, treat this as an emergency and have someone take you to the nearest emergency room. The health-care team there will assess your condition and give you the fluids and insulin you require.

165.
What do I do when my blood glucose is low?

Low blood glucose (also called hypoglycemia) is a blood glucose value under 60 mg/dl (although in some clinical settings, it may be defined at a higher level). The symptoms of low blood glucose can

Q A

include shakiness, sweating, irritable mood, numbness around the mouth, nausea, blurred vision, and weakness. When your blood glucose is low, follow "the rule of 15's." This means you should ingest 15 grams of liquid carbohydrate such as four ounces of juice or a 10-ounce glass of milk. Then wait 15 minutes and check your blood glucose. If it's still low, repeat the rule of 15's until your blood glucose is in the normal range. If a liquid source of glucose is not handy, take three glucose tablets, six LifeSavers, or another sweet food containing 15 grams of sugar. If a meal is not to take place for some hours and your blood glucose falls below 50 mg/dl, eat a healthy snack (such as crackers and peanut butter or a slice of turkey on a piece of bread) to ensure you do not have another low episode before your next meal.

If you are about to eat a meal, skip the rule of 15's and drink some juice or six ounces of regular soda pop and eat your meal. Note the low blood glucose episode in your logbook. Watch your logbook carefully for a pattern of low blood glucose that could be avoided by changing your menu or diabetes treatment.

166.
How long do I have to keep checking my blood glucose?

You should monitor your blood glucose levels for as long as you want to control your blood glucose and avoid episodes of high and low blood glucose. Generally, people plan on monitoring their blood glucose for the rest of their lives. It is part of taking care of yourself when you have diabetes.

There are certain situations where a person can "take a break" from blood glucose testing. This can be done when you have a pattern of excellent control, are not ill or under stress, and have the recommendation of your diabetes team. One example: You are an adult who has had a normal HbA_{1c} test result since you started taking diabetes pills and following a prescribed menu plan. You have run out of strips and are waiting for the new order to come in the mail. You can skip your usual testing for a few days until your new supply of test strips arrives. However, it would be wise for you in this example to keep a couple of spare strips on hand in case you develop symptoms of high or low blood glucose or you get sick.

Q A

167.
Do I have to use my fingers to check my blood glucose level?

Recent technology is allowing people to use "alternate sites" (such as their forearms) to obtain a sample of blood for glucose testing. This is less painful for most people, but some have difficulty getting an adequate sample from alternate sites. Also, newer lancing devices make fingertip testing less painful.

If you are concerned that your blood glucose level may be low, it is recommended that you test your finger instead of using an alternate site. Blood flow to the fingers is faster than it is to alternate sites and it will reflect blood glucose changes more readily. Similarly, if you have had a history of low blood glucose without the usual symptoms ("hypoglycemic unawareness"), finger-stick testing is recommended to ensure you have the most current information about your blood glucose. Anytime an alternate-site sample gives a blood glucose reading that does not seem to be within your usual pattern, obtain a finger-stick sample.

168.
Can someone check my blood glucose for me?

Yes. You or your diabetes educator can teach anyone you like to check your blood glucose. This is very handy when you are ill and want or need the assistance of another person to check your blood glucose. This is an especially good idea if you are prone to severe high or low blood glucose levels and are too ill to realize that you need to get a test done and get treatment for your blood glucose level. Be sure that the person understands how to do the test, what the different levels mean, and when to call for help. If you have lost consciousness, your helper should be instructed to call 911 before trying to test your blood glucose. For people prone to severe low blood glucose episodes, a family member should be taught how to administer an emergency glucagon injection when you cannot swallow juice.

Sometimes a person with diabetes has very concerned and caring family members who will want do all of the blood glucose testing for him. In general, it is still best to do your own blood glucose testing when you are able. Playing an active role in your diabetes

Q A

management will give you a better idea of what foods and what activities have the greatest impact on your blood glucose. Further, knowing your blood glucose patterns through testing can give you the information you need to alter your food habits, activities, or medicines to maintain blood glucose levels in a better range. Another consideration when you let other people take over these tasks is that you may be putting more burden on them than is fair. If you think you are not getting enough help from family members or you think they are more involved than you want, it is a good idea to bring them to your diabetes healthcare appointments and discuss the sharing of your diabetes care with everyone concerned.

169.
Why do I have to keep a record of my blood glucose readings?

Keeping a record of your blood glucose levels helps you and your diabetes team to determine your blood glucose fluctuations and to adjust your diabetes program for better control of your blood glucose. The most helpful type of record allows you to record your blood glucose level, the time of day, and whether the blood glucose reading was taken before or after eating. This information is needed to best understand your diabetes. For example, suppose Mrs. Jones brings a pad of paper listing blood glucose values ranging from 57 mg/dl to 282 mg/dl, but not the times of day the readings were taken. Her diabetes team wouldn't know how to adjust her program to help her avoid the highs and lows. If her numbers are noted with times and meals indicated, it would be possible to see what her most typical reading is before breakfast and how it varies throughout the day. Her care plan could then be adjusted to help improve her range of blood glucose values.

Keeping track of your blood glucose levels also gives you a chance to record the foods or activities that led to wider ranges of blood glucose. For instance, if you had a higher than usual fasting blood glucose reading, you can note that you went out for dinner or ordered a pizza that might have led to the higher blood glucose. If you have a pattern of high morning blood glucose readings even if you ate according to the plan each night, then you need to consider a

Q A

change in your evening diabetes care plan. Similarly, if you have consistently high blood glucose before supper, you may need to change your daytime medication dose, reduce the amount of your daytime carbohydrates, increase your afternoon activity level, or all three. Record keeping will help you and your diabetes team address the appropriate issues more efficiently.

170.
Why does my doctor want to see my blood glucose records?

Your doctor wants you to be able to achieve blood glucose levels as close to normal as possible so you will have the least risk of developing complications of diabetes. By reviewing your blood glucose records, your doctor can see if your care plan needs adjusting to improve your control.

Your doctor also wants to compare your blood glucose levels at home to those obtained in the clinic from the hemoglobin A_{1c} (HbA_{1c}) test. If your blood glucose levels at home seem to fall in the target ranges but your HbA_{1c} result is too high, then your doctor can suggest that you get some blood glucose readings at other times of day to search for hidden high blood glucose levels.

Your doctor might also think that your care plan is fine based on an excellent HbA_{1c} result. On the other hand, your doctor may learn from examining your logbook and talking with you about your daily life that you are having frequent episodes of low blood glucose. Your diabetes care program should be designed to give you the best possible quality of life while minimizing your risk of diabetes complications. Tracking your blood glucose readings, bringing your logbook to appointments, and sharing your concerns with the diabetes team members will help you strike the best possible balance.

171.
Can test strips be used more than once?

Currently, all the test strips on the market are single-use strips (no more than one test per test strip). However, there are glucose meters that are loaded with a cartridge or barrel of multiple strips so that several tests can be done before the set of strips needs to be changed. Also, there are new devices being developed

Q A

that do not need test strips; such devices may become available in the future.

172.
Why do test strips cost so much?

A number of factors contribute to their high cost. In part, test strips are costly because the companies that developed these products have done so at great expense and need to recoup these costs. The manufacturer's research and development costs can be quite high. Sometimes the research and development period stretches over a period of a decade or more, but the products that research yields are usually superior to the products they replace. Typically, the prices of these products decrease with time as products are mass-produced. In the area of glucose monitoring equipment, new technology is replacing older technology at such a rapid pace that that there is barely enough time for some products to be on the market long enough for their costs to drop before they are discontinued and replaced by superior and more costly products.

Your diabetes educator can discuss options that might minimize your costs without compromising your overall diabetes management.

173.
How do I know if my blood glucose meter is reading correctly?

Most blood glucose meters come with control solution. The control solution has a set concentration of sugar. If the meter is working properly, when this control solution is placed on a test strip, the meter should give a reading within the control solution range. If it is not reading correctly, follow the instructions in the owner's manual or call the company. The company's customer service number is usually noted on the back of your blood glucose meter.

Be sure to follow the recommendations for keeping blood glucose test strips in good condition. In general, all brands should be protected from extreme temperatures and high humidity. Protect them from extreme weather conditions. Do not leave them in a car parked in the hot sun, for example. The extreme heat can damage the strips and give you false readings. Also, the meter itself and its batteries may not function properly if left in extreme conditions. For example, a meter packed in a suitcase and placed in

142

the very cold temperatures of a jet's baggage compartment may not be able to work properly until it returns to normal temperature (and be sure to test it with the control solution before using it again). When you travel, carry your blood glucose monitoring supplies and medication with you; do not expose them to damaging temperatures.

174.
What do I do if my meter is broken?

If your meter is not functioning properly, read the owner's manual to try to determine the problem. The display on the meter often gives an error code that indicates what the problem is. Frequently, it is a simple problem that is easily fixed by the user.

One common problem is not applying an adequate blood sample. Another is trying to apply blood to the test strip before the meter prompts you. When this happens, the meter "thinks" that the strip has already been used and shows an error code on the display screen instead of reading out your blood glucose value. This can be frustrating, but following the directions precisely avoids this problem. Review the owner's manual before concluding that the machine is broken and not usable.

If your meter is in fact broken, the manufacturer is often willing to replace it free of charge. If you filled out and returned the warranty card when you purchased the meter, it may still be under warranty. Even if it is not under warranty, the company may replace the meter for little or no cost. Call the company's customer service number noted on the back of the meter to discuss the problem. If you decide to get a new meter, find out about other meters that have become available; you may want to upgrade. Discuss this with your diabetes educator.

175.
At what blood glucose level should I call my doctor?

If your blood glucose level drops so low that you have trouble treating it yourself, you should call your doctor. A blood glucose level under 50 mg/dl does not allow the brain to function properly and needs to be treated quickly. Repeat episodes of low blood glucose are especially dangerous. If your blood glucose falls

Q A

too low more than once in 24 hours, you may not even feel symptoms the second time. Always carry a source of glucose with you to treat the first symptom of low blood glucose and talk to your diabetes team about this problem.

If your blood glucose levels are consistently high, say over 250 mg/dl, call to get instructions to bring it down. When blood glucose levels are above 400 mg/dl, you can become very ill and you should get advice immediately. If you feel ill, go to a local emergency room since you may need intravenous fluids, medicine, and correction of a hidden health problem that is contributing to your high blood glucose.

If your blood glucose is high or low but you feel fine, call your physician or clinic and get advice. Also, ask your diabetes team when they think you should call.

176.
I travel a lot and have learned from experience that test strips don't give accurate readings of my blood glucose level after I've left them in a hot car. I've seen advertisements for meters that operate over wide temperature ranges. Do these ranges apply just to the meter or are the strips temperature-resistant as well?

For accurate results, strips must be stored according to the manufacturer's guidelines. Although there are some variations, manufacturers agree that strips must be stored in the container (either the vial or foil wrapping) in which they came in a cool, dry place. Most strips can tolerate temperatures up to 86°F, but they should not be refrigerated or frozen.

Because meters and strips work as a unit and are carried as a unit, the storage requirements of the strips are your limiting factors. The operating temperature range listed for some meters indicates temperatures at which the meter was tested and was still found to be reliable. However, you still can't go beyond the temperature limits of the strips.

You might consider purchasing one of the travel organizers for people with diabetes. Some cases have separate compartments for keeping supplies cool or at room temperature.

5
Nutrition

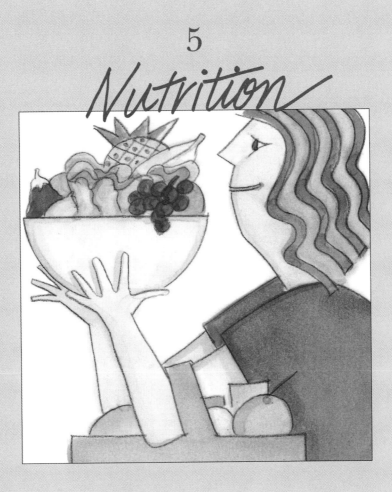

Basics

177. When I was first diagnosed with diabetes, my doctor put me on a special diabetic diet. Don't I still need to follow this diet to help control my diabetes?

178. I am newly diagnosed with diabetes. What is the first thing I should do?

179. I found out I have diabetes just a week ago, and I am waiting to meet with a dietitian next week. What should I do until I see the dietitian?

180. If you have Type 2 diabetes, what lifestyle strategies are important for you?

181. Why is it important to pay attention to what you eat when you have diabetes?

182. If you take insulin, what is the first priority for insulin and meal planning?

183. What diet is best for someone with diabetes? I hear a lot of different claims for both high-carbohydrate diets and low-carbohydrate diets. I don't know which one is best for my health.

184. How much carbohydrate do I need each day?

185. How does insulin use the carbohydrate I eat?

186. Does a bolus dose of insulin counter carbohydrates in the food we eat?

187. Can someone tell me what fruits are "good" for me and what fruits are "bad"?

188. I have heard talk about "free foods," but don't understand what "free" means. Can you please clarify?

189. Can people with diabetes eat sweets?

190. How many grams of sugar should I limit myself to each day?

191. Are there any proven strategies that can assist with making and maintaining lifestyle strategies?

Family Affairs

192. All that sugar-free food I have to buy for diabetes is so expensive, and no one else in the family eats it. What else can I do?

193. I am looking for quick and easy meals for a family member with diabetes. Most cookbooks I've looked at have been very bland and dull! Can you help?

194. I do not have diabetes, but my wife does. What can I do to encourage my wife to be more disciplined at meals?

195. I have heard that genetics plays a strong role in diabetes. What can my family do to avoid getting diabetes?

196. I want to be sure my child doesn't get diabetes. I've read that drinking milk puts a child at risk for getting Type 1 diabetes. Should I give my child soy milk instead?

197. It is very difficult for me to say "no" when my four-year-old asks me for cookies and ice cream when we are at a mall. He was diagnosed with diabetes only two months ago. What should I do?

198. My mother is older and has Type 2 diabetes. She doesn't always eat well, so I thought I would buy her some of those canned liquid supplements. Do I need to buy the kind especially for people with diabetes?

Carbohydrates

199. I am a little confused. How much carbohydrate can a person have per day? I thought that all I had to do was not eat sugar, yet my blood glucose is too high.

200. Are some carbohydrate foods better than others?

201. What is a carbohydrate serving?

202. How many carbohydrate servings should people with diabetes eat at a meal?

203. I've been reading about carbohydrate counting for diabetes, but I don't take insulin. Can I still try this?

204. My friend actually adjusts his insulin dose to match the amount of carbohydrate he wants to eat at a meal. I take insulin, too, but I've never heard of doing this. Should he be doing this?

205. I know that my triglyceride levels are high. How much carbohydrate should I consume so I can bring my triglyceride levels down?

206. I have heard that people with diabetes are carbohydrate sensitive. Is this true? I have always though of myself as being carbohydrate sensitive, so I severely limit carbohydrate intake to lose weight.

207. Why must I watch my portions of "no-sugar added" foods? Aren't they free foods?

208. I saw a snack bar with "extended-release carbohydrate" on the ingredient list. What does this do?

209. What is all the talk about the glycemic index?

210. Which foods have a low glycemic index?

211. Why did my dietitian suggest I include potatoes in my meal plan when they have a high glycemic index?

Fat

212. How does fat affect blood glucose levels? Does fat add glucose to the blood?

213. Does it matter which type of fats I eat or just the amount I eat?

214. What are the types of fat and which type is the better one to use?

215. What exactly are monounsaturated and polyunsaturated fats, and why do people with diabetes hear so much about them?

216. What are saturated fatty acids?

217. I've been hearing a lot about *trans* fatty acids lately. What are they? Are they bad for me?

218. My doctor told me I should eat more foods high in omega-3 fatty acids, but I'm not really sure what they are or what foods contain them.

219. How much omega-3 fatty acids do you need to stay healthy?

220. What are fat replacers?

221. I have heard a lot about plant stanol and plant sterol ester margarines lately. Are they good for people with diabetes?

222. How can I reduce my overall fat intake?

Fiber

223. What is "fiber"? Aren't foods high in fiber also high in carbohydrates?

224. What are soluble and insoluble fiber? Where do I find them?

225. I am trying to adjust my diet by introducing more vegetables and fruits with "juicing." Is this a good way to add more healthy foods?

226. Will eating foods containing fiber improve blood glucose levels?

227. How can I increase my dietary fiber intake?

228. I have cut starches almost completely out of my diet to keep my blood glucose levels low. I eat lots of high-fiber vegetables but stay away from breads, pasta, rice, and potato. This diet has been very hard to sustain. Any advice?

229. What is a resistant starch? Is it similar to fiber?

Protein

230. Does eating protein increase blood glucose levels?

231. Should people with diabetes eat a low-carbohydrate, high-protein diet?

232. My doctor suggests that I eat a diet extremely low in protein because I have protein in my urine. Where do I start?

233. Does eating protein cause renal (kidney) disease?

234. Will eating protein with a sweet or dessert slow the absorption of this "fast-acting carbohydrate"?

235. Should I always eat protein with my carbohydrates when I snack, or is it okay to eat the carbohydrate alone?

236. I'm trying to "bulk up" by lifting weights. Shouldn't I also be eating more protein in my diet to help me build more muscle?

Sweeteners

237. Can I eat sugar?

238. Is it safe to eat products that contain the sweetener aspartame?

239. What about saccharin, acesulfame-K, and sucralose? Are they safe?

240. How much diet soda can I safely drink during the day?

241. What are sugar alcohols? Do they affect my blood glucose in any way?

Vitamins and Minerals

242. Don't I need a special vitamin supplement for my diabetes? My drugstore carries some that are geared toward people with diabetes.

243. Are there some vitamin or mineral supplements that have been shown to be particularly helpful?

244. Should people with diabetes take antioxidant supplements?

245. What is alpha-lipoic acid? Is it something I should be taking for my diabetes?

246. What are the American Diabetes Association recommendations for people with diabetes regarding vitamin and mineral supplements?

247. How much calcium should I be consuming in a day? Should I take calcium supplements?

248. How can I be sure I am absorbing enough iron from the food that I eat?

249. Will taking chromium picolinate supplements improve blood glucose levels?

250. What about claims that chromium picolinate can burn body fat?

Blood Pressure

251. What can you do to lower blood pressure?

252. What are some tips for lowering sodium intake?

Alcohol

253. What effect does alcohol have on blood glucose levels?

254. Does the type of alcohol one drinks make a difference?

255. When a drug label says "avoid alcohol," does that mean "absolutely no alcohol," or is it all right for me to have a cold beer after mowing the lawn?

256. Are there other risks and benefits of alcohol consumption?

Physical Activity

257. I am looking for foods I can carry with me to treat possible hypoglycemic reactions when I am out walking. Any recommendations?

258. What insulin or carbohydrate adjustments should you make for exercise?

259. Wouldn't it be a good idea for a person to load up on carbohydrates before going out for a long run?

Common Concerns

260. What is the best way to treat a low blood glucose level?

261. Whenever I have a low blood glucose, I usually treat it with a candy bar. But then I find that my blood sugar level doesn't rise fast enough and I have to eat more. What's going on?

262. I have been told to drink water when my blood glucose is elevated. How does this help? Or does it?

263. Why are blood glucose levels often high in the morning even if you didn't eat at bedtime?

264. I have Type 1 diabetes. What should I do if I get the flu and can't eat?

265. I take insulin three times a day, and my blood glucose is under pretty good control. My dietitian wants me to take snacks between meals, but I usually don't feel hungry. Can I get by without having to eat all these snacks?

266. Sometimes when I have a meal, I only want to have a salad, but if I use two units of insulin, I will have low blood glucose within the next hour. Any suggestions?

267. Will becoming a vegetarian help my diabetes control?

268. I have always had a sweet tooth and can't seem to break the habit. I crave sugar, especially chocolate. Any ideas on how to break a bad habit?

269. This is my first holiday season with diabetes. Any suggestions?

270. I've read that caffeine can raise blood glucose levels. Does this mean I should stop drinking my morning coffee?

271. My doctor just diagnosed me with gastroparesis. He said to eat six small meals per day. What does this mean?

272. I saw an advertisement for an all-natural pill that can lower my blood sugars—some kind of ancient remedy. Does this really work?

Q A
Basics

177.

When I was first diagnosed with diabetes, my doctor put me on a special diabetic diet. Don't I still need to follow this diet to help control my diabetes?

Would you believe that there is no such thing as a "diabetic diet"?

Nutrition guidelines for people with diabetes have really come a long way. Back in the days before insulin was discovered, people were literally put on starvation diets, which contained relatively no carbohydrate. After the discovery of insulin, things changed for the better; carbohydrate was added back in, but in controlled and measured amounts.

Up until about 20 years ago, health-care professionals required their patients with diabetes to follow fairly rigid dietary guidelines. You might remember this if you've had diabetes for a while. Perhaps your doctor or dietitian gave you a printed meal plan restricting you to 1,800 calories a day, for example, with instructions to follow it carefully. What you may remember most is that you couldn't eat sugar or foods that contained sugar. After all, eating sugar would sharply raise your blood glucose (or so we thought).

Fortunately, times have changed. Gone are the days of strict meal plans and the avoidance of favorite foods. Eating foods that contain sugar is permissible (in moderation, of course). Unfortunately, not all health-care professionals are relaying this message to their patients, and even today, people with diabetes are still being told that eating sugar is taboo and that they must see a dietitian for a "diabetic diet."

You should see a registered dietitian, but not for a diabetic diet! Rather, meet with a dietitian to work out an individualized eating plan that is right for you. This means that the eating plan should be based on your food preferences, your weight goals, your lipid goals, and of course, your blood glucose goals. The meal plan may have to change as your life circumstances change—if you gain or lose weight or if your diabetes changes, for example.

Q   A

178.
I am newly diagnosed with diabetes. What is the first thing I should do?

First, you should seek out a diabetes team to help you learn about diabetes. A diabetes team will consist of various health-care professionals in addition to your physician: for instance, a nurse, a registered dietitian, an exercise physiologist, a mental health professional, and a podiatrist. Diabetes is not a do-it-yourself disorder, and it is best managed with diabetes self-management education input from all the team members. Everyone will have important information for you, so learn the facts. As Dr. Elliott Joslin once said, diabetes is a disorder that "deserves the best effort of the doctor and the patient from start to finish."

179.
I found out I have diabetes just a week ago, and I am waiting to meet with a dietitian next week. What should I do until I see the dietitian?

These simple tips should work fine until you can meet with a dietitian:
- Eat your meals at the same time each day.
- Avoid eating excessive amounts of any foods.
- Do not skip meals.
- Coffee, tea, diet drinks, and water can be taken anytime.
- When you're thirsty, drink water, not juice.
- Eat the same foods as the rest of your family, providing they are healthy eaters.
- Keep a written record of what you eat at each meal and bring this along to your appointment. This will help the dietitian develop nutrition strategies and education tailored specifically to your needs.

180.
If you have Type 2 diabetes, what lifestyle strategies are important for you?

Nutrition recommendations for a healthy lifestyle for the general public also apply to people with diabetes, whether Type 1 or Type 2 diabetes. However, if you have Type 2 diabetes, you want to focus on food and physical activity choices that will help keep your blood glucose in your target goal range. It is often

Q A

helpful to begin by learning what foods are carbohydrates, average portion sizes, and the number of carbohydrate servings you should select for meals and, if appropriate, snacks. At the same time, you will want to limit the size of your meat and fat portions. Being careful about portion size is the first step in reducing calories. Doing this may or may not lead to small amounts of weight loss, but even if weight is not lost it can lead to improvement in blood glucose control. Remember, what is important is reaching your blood glucose and blood fat (cholesterol and triglycerides) goals.

Along with following your meal plan, regular physical activity is helpful. The goal is to do physical activity for 30 minutes nearly every day of the week. Regular physical activity can improve blood glucose control, decrease insulin resistance, and reduce your risk factors for heart and blood vessel disease.

Type 2 diabetes is a progressive disease, which means that you will probably need to combine medication with your meal plan eventually. Over time, many persons will require insulin along with their meal plan to achieve good blood glucose control. Some people may mistakenly think this means that they have done something wrong. This is not the case. Type 2 diabetes is caused by both insulin resistance and insulin deficiency, and as diabetes progresses, the insulin-producing beta cells of the pancreas progressively fail, and insulin deficiency becomes more and more the problem. The best way known today to keep your beta cells working longer is to keep your blood glucose levels as near to normal as you can. Do your best with lifestyle, but when necessary add appropriate medicines; at the same time continue following your meal plan and doing regular physical activity. The medicines will work better when you also pay attention to lifestyle.

181.
Why is it important to pay attention to what you eat when you have diabetes?

Balancing what you eat with the insulin your body makes or with the insulin you take by injection is essential to achieve and maintain target blood glucose goals. It is important that blood glucose levels be

Q A

as close to a nondiabetic range as is safely possible to prevent or reduce the risk for complications. For some people with Type 2 diabetes, just following a meal plan will be sufficient to improve and maintain control of blood glucose levels. For other people with Type 2 diabetes, medicine may need to be combined with a meal plan to control blood glucose levels. And for some, insulin may need to be integrated into the overall management plan. But for everyone who has diabetes, following a meal plan helps with glucose control and can help improve cholesterol and blood pressure levels as well.

Improving health through healthy food choices and physical activity is an important goal of diabetes nutrition therapy. Many studies have tried to identify the role of a single nutrient, food, or food group in preventing chronic disease or for the promotion of health. However, it appears not to be a single nutrient or food that is important, but instead there are health benefits from food patterns that include mixtures of food. For example, the American Diabetes Association and the American Heart Association recommend five or more servings per day of a variety of fruits and vegetables; six or more servings per day of grain products, including whole grains; daily servings of fat-free or low-fat dairy products; two or three servings of fish per week; legumes, poultry, and lean meats.

To make permanent changes in your eating habits, you need to find ways to fit the foods you enjoy into your everyday life. A meal plan is your personalized guide to what you need to eat each day to meet your diabetes and health goals. If you don't have a meal plan, you need to have one developed for you. Usually this is done with a registered dietitian. The key is to make reasonable changes that you can stick to over the long term.

182.
If you take insulin, what is the first priority for insulin and meal planning?

Nutrition recommendations for a healthy lifestyle for the general public also apply to persons with diabetes. What differs for individuals who require insulin is the importance of integrating an insulin regimen into your lifestyle. Today, there are many insulin

Q A

options available, and if your health-care team is aware of your preferred meal schedule and the kinds and amounts of food you like to eat, an appropriate insulin regimen can usually be developed. Therefore, your first priority is to be sure your health-care team, especially your dietitian, is aware of your lifestyle.

To determine your basic insulin doses, it is important that you eat fairly consistently for a period of weeks. Then by using your food and blood glucose records, adjustments can be made in your insulin doses to help you meet your target blood glucose goals. Once you and your dietitian determine the amount of rapid-acting insulin you require to cover the usual amount of carbohydrate you eat for meals, an insulin-to-carbohydrate ratio can be calculated. This is the amount of rapid-acting insulin you need to cover one carbohydrate serving (15 grams of carbohydrate) at breakfast, lunch, or dinner. If you plan to eat more or less than you usually do for a meal, you can adjust your dose of rapid-acting insulin based on the amount of carbohydrate servings you are planning to eat. This type of approach will give you more flexibility in your food choices and the amount that you can eat.

183.
What diet is best for someone with diabetes? I hear a lot of different claims for both high-carbohydrate diets and low-carbohydrate diets. I don't know which one is best for my health.

The U.S. Dietary Guidelines for Americans (with and without diabetes) as well as the American Diabetes Association and the American Dietetic Association have established healthy eating guidelines from evidence-based research. The healthiest distribution of calories is 50% to 60% of calories from carbohydrate, 10% to 20% of calories from protein, and 20% to 30% of calories from fat. If a person has cardiac or cholesterol issues, the fat may be lower; if a person has kidney problems, the protein may be lower; if a person has high triglyceride levels, the carbohydrate may be lower. It is really the job of the registered dietitian to assess and evaluate each person and individualize the distribution.

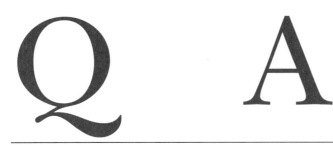

184.
How much carbohydrate do I need each day?

The amount of carbohydrate a person needs on a daily basis is very individualized, and depends on a number of factors: height and weight, desired weight, age, activity level, type and amount of medications used for diabetes management, hemoglobin A_{1c} level, lipid profile (cholesterol and triglycerides), cultural factors, personal preference, and lifestyle.

In other words, there is no one right amount of carbohydrate for everyone. However, we generally recommend that at least half of your total caloric intake come from carbohydrate. In case this sounds like a lot to you, remember that carbohydrate is the major fuel source for the body. An inadequate carbohydrate intake can lead to some serious health problems and can adversely affect your diabetes control. On the other hand, too much carbohydrate can do the same. The key is learning how much carbohydrate you need to stay healthy and manage your diabetes.

The best person to help you figure out how much carbohydrate you need is a registered dietitian. She or he can work with you to develop an eating plan and specify a carbohydrate goal for meals and snacks based on the various factors mentioned above. This meal planning method is called *carbohydrate counting*.

To get you started until you meet with a dietitian, use the following guidelines:

	DAILY CALORIES	DAILY CARBOHYDRATE
Women	1600–2200	220–300 grams
Men	2300–2800	315–385 grams

Remember that these are just general guidelines. Some people will need more or less carbohydrate. Also, keep in mind that your carbohydrate intake should be spread fairly evenly throughout the day for good blood glucose control. Aim to keep the amount of carbohydrate fairly consistent from meal to meal. And don't forget to monitor your blood glucose levels.

185.
How does insulin use the carbohydrate I eat?

Think of your body using insulin in two ways: There is background insulin, which is a slow, constant infu-

Q A

sion of insulin to keep your blood glucose stable overnight and between meals. If you inject insulin, this is your *basal* dose of long-acting insulin.

Then there is the *bolus* dose, which is the short burst of insulin the pancreas secretes to cover a meal. If you inject insulin, rapid-acting insulins such as Humalog or Novolog or short-acting (Regular) insulin can be matched to the number of carbohydrate grams in the food you are about to eat. Your physician and registered dietitian can help you fine-tune this method, called carbohydrate counting, to keep your blood glucose level in a desirable range.

186.
Does a bolus dose of insulin counter carbohydrates in the food we eat?

Yes. A bolus dose is the amount of insulin given to cover incoming food and also to correct a high blood glucose. Rapid-acting and short-acting insulins like Humalog, Novolog, or Regular can be matched to the carbohydrate grams in the food you are about to eat. A basal dose is your "background" insulin. This is insulin that is released slowly into the bloodstream to mimic the pancreas's slow, constant secretion of insulin to help keep blood sugar stable between meals and overnight. This insulin also helps cover small snacks.

187.
Can someone tell me what fruits are "good" for me and what fruits are "bad"?

Fortunately, there are no longer "good" and "bad" foods—and that includes fruit choices. All foods that contain carbohydrate affect your blood glucose similarly in equal amounts. One serving of strawberries is equal to 1¼ cups and will have the same effect as one serving of 12–15 grapes. Both of these fruits have about 15 grams of carbohydrate per serving. The serving size is not the same for all fruits, so it is important to be aware of the correct portion size for each fruit so you can be flexible with your fruit choices and not affect your blood glucose level adversely.

Q A

188.
I have heard talk about "free foods," but don't understand what "free" means. Can you please clarify?

A free food is a food so few in calories per serving that it will have little impact on your blood glucose. Foods containing less than 20 calories per serving are considered free foods. Although these can be consumed without worry, free foods should be limited to no more than 3–4 servings per day. Free foods include salad greens and raw vegetables such as celery, onion, peppers, and mushrooms, as well as sugar-free drinks, condiments, and seasonings. A good, basic list of free foods and serving sizes can be found in the American Diabetes Association's booklet *Exchange Lists for Meal Planning.*

189.
Can people with diabetes eat sweets?

In nearly 20 studies, beginning with the first study in 1976, researchers have reported that when the same number of calories from sugars such as sucrose (table sugar) is substituted for the same number of calories from starches, the effect on blood glucose and insulin levels will be the same. For years, people with diabetes were told not to eat added sugars and to restrict naturally occurring sugars because they were small molecules and therefore would be rapidly digested and quickly enter the blood stream, thus causing blood glucose levels to go higher than after eating starch foods. When research studies were finally done to see if this was true, it was found that sugars do not cause blood glucose levels to increase more rapidly and higher than equal amounts of starch.

However, the advice to be careful of sugars was good advice, even if the advice was given for the wrong reason. Often, foods that contain sugars are high in total carbohydrate, as well as fat and calories. So when people with diabetes were careful to avoid sugars, it may have helped control their blood glucose levels. For example, if people with diabetes drink a can of regular soda containing the equivalent of 11 teaspoons of sugar, it is very likely to raise blood glucose levels. However, if people with diabetes substitute a cookie containing 15 grams of carbohydrate

Q A

for a slice of bread containing 15 grams of carbohydrate, the effect on blood glucose levels should be quite similar. Or if they put a teaspoon of sugar (4 grams of carbohydrate) on their cereal, it is unlikely to affect their blood glucose level.

So, people with diabetes can eat sweets. However, the sweet should be substituted for another carbohydrate in their meal plan. If it is added to that meal plan it would need to be covered with additional insulin or some other glucose-lowering medicine. And remember, as for the general population, sweets should be eaten in the context of a healthful diet.

190.
How many grams of sugar should I limit myself to each day?

If you've had diabetes for a while, chances are you've been told at some time or another that you shouldn't eat sugar. And in a way, it makes sense, right? If you eat sugar, it will raise your blood glucose.

Well, not so fast. That's what we used to think. Fortunately, thanks to great research done about 20 years ago, we've learned a lot. Even if you've never had a biology course in school, you mostly likely know that carbohydrate is what turns into blood glucose, or glucose. What are sources of carbohydrate in the diet?

Starches, for one—think of cereals, pasta, bread, rice, potato...

What else? Sugar! Whether it's plain old table sugar (sucrose), fruit sugar (fructose), or even milk sugar (lactose), sugar is a carbohydrate, too! Sugar isn't bad. We know that fruit and milk, for example, are healthful foods. The sugars in these foods are natural. Furthermore, eating sugar does not raise your blood glucose any more than eating starch. What's important is not the source of the carbohydrate, but rather the amount. If you eat 15 grams of carbohydrate from a piece of bread, or 15 grams of carbohydrate from a chocolate chip cookie, you can expect that the effect on your blood glucose from these two foods will be pretty much the same.

The question really is not how much sugar should you limit yourself to each day, it's how much carbohydrate you should consume each day. The best person to help you figure this out is a registered dietitian.

159

Q A

She'll work out an eating plan tailored to meet your particular nutrient needs and fit your lifestyle and food preferences.

So you can eat foods that contain sugar, as long as you count them as your carbohydrate choices in your eating plan. Even the American Diabetes Association states that moderate amounts of sugar can be part of a well-balanced diet for people with diabetes. Remember, though, that foods high in sugar—cakes, cookies, ice cream—tend to be high in calories and fat, and they don't contain many other nutrients, such as fiber, vitamins, and minerals. Overall nutrition is still important. In addition, because foods high in sugar are obviously high in carbohydrate, you may be surprised how small a serving size really is (ice cream servings are based on ½ cup servings—who eats just a ½ cup?). So, everything in moderation. But the next time your family goes out for an ice cream cone on a hot summer night, feel free to join in (just make sure to count that carbohydrate!).

191.
Are there any proven strategies that can assist with making and maintaining lifestyle strategies?

In spite of all that's known about the importance of healthy eating and regular physical activity, changing lifestyle habits isn't easy for most people. Adopting healthy habits is a long-term proposition, and success can easily be thwarted by a short-term approach. That's why it's important to create built-in support for your efforts. Many people have found the following strategies to be effective aids to long-term success.

Recognize your meal plan as a tool for good health. It is not a "diet." Rather, it is a guide that will allow you to take charge of your eating habits and your health.

Seek support from your family and friends. Having family members eat the same healthy foods that you do and having them join you in regular physical activity such as walking, bike riding, and swimming can help reinforce your efforts over time.

Focus on personal motivation. You may start making changes because your family wants you to, or because your doctor told you to, but to be successful you need to make changes because it is important for

Q   A

you, and because you want to be in charge of your health.

Focus on positive changes in health risks. For example, higher energy levels, improved blood glucose and cholesterol levels, and reduced blood pressure are more important than what the scale says.

Get and stay physically active. Physical activity is the strongest predictor of long-term adherence to healthy meal planning.

And finally, good food, good health, good taste. Healthy food can and does taste good!

Family Affairs

192.
All that sugar-free food I have to buy for diabetes is so expensive, and no one else in the family eats it. What else can I do?

The foods that you eat don't need to be different from what the rest of the family eats. Often, "no sugar added" or "sugar free" foods such as ice cream, cookies, and candy have about the same carbohydrate content as the regular foods they are replacing and have similar impact on blood glucose. Learning to count grams of carbohydrate (carbohydrate counting) is the easiest way to learn how to fit in any food (within the context of healthy eating) and yet maintain good blood glucose control. By knowing how much carbohydrate to aim for at meals and snacks, you can "spend" your carbohydrate grams on regular foods and not feel different from the rest of the family.

193.
I am looking for quick and easy meals for a family member with diabetes. Most cookbooks I've looked at have been very bland and dull! Can you help?

People with diabetes do not have to eat bland and dull meals, although this is the general perception. Meals for a family member with diabetes should not be any different than meals for a family member without diabetes—assuming that the family eats in a healthy way. People with diabetes do not need to eat special foods. A visit with a registered dietitian is in

Q A

order to help you identify any misconceptions and learn about all of the newest nutrition guidelines for people with diabetes.

194.
I do not have diabetes, but my wife does. What can I do to encourage my wife to be more disciplined at meals?

Family and friends want to ensure that their loved ones remain healthy, and they are often quick to point out what they perceive as dietary indiscretions. Although these people want to be supportive, the person with diabetes is receiving a negative message, and mealtimes become a daily chore rather than a source of enjoyment. Some quick tips:

■ Become more flexible. It is not necessary for your wife to follow an inflexible diet.

■ Let go. No one is going to be able to do everything expected all of the time.

■ Be realistic. Labeling food as "good" and "bad" often creates guilt and stress.

■ Remain neutral. Do not blindly attribute poor control to dietary indiscretions, as this may not be the case.

■ Set a good example. Maintain the same healthy diet as your spouse.

195.
I have heard that genetics plays a strong role in diabetes. What can my family do to avoid getting diabetes?

Since family members of individuals who have diabetes are at increased risk for developing diabetes, it is very important that the whole family develop a healthy lifestyle. In the past, it was often assumed that only older adults developed diabetes, but the sad news is that more and more younger adults and even children are developing diabetes. The bottom line is that all individuals, especially family members of individuals with Type 2 diabetes, should be encouraged to participate in regular physical activity. Both moderate and vigorous exercise decrease the risk of prediabetes and Type 2 diabetes.

Prediabetes is the condition where blood glucose levels are not in the normal range but are not yet in a

Q & A

diabetic range. Genetic factors do play a powerful role in determining who is likely to develop Type 2 diabetes. However, lifestyle habits can also help determine who does or does not develop diabetes. Studies have reported on associations between lifestyle factors and diabetes, and they have identified strategies that people can use to help ward off diabetes: (1) sustaining a weight loss of 5% to 10% of body weight; (2) participating in regular, moderate-intensity physical activities, such as brisk walking, as well as participating in more vigorous exercise; (3) eating a lower-fat diet (especially one lower in saturated fat); high-fat diets over time can contribute to weight gain, which increases the risk for diabetes; and (4) increasing intake of whole grains and dietary fiber.

In the Diabetes Prevention Program, a research study done in the United States, lifestyle changes that included a reduced fat and calorie intake, regular physical activity (30 minutes a day or 150 minutes a week), and an education program that included regular participant contact led to a weight loss of 5% to 7% of starting weight and dramatically reduced the risk of developing diabetes.

**196.
I want to be sure my child doesn't get diabetes. I've read that drinking milk puts a child at risk for getting Type 1 diabetes. Should I give my child soy milk instead?**

Several years ago, some inconclusive studies indicated that children with a strong risk for developing Type 1 diabetes were more likely to develop diabetes if they drank cow's milk at a very early age. One study showed that children who had a sibling with Type 1 diabetes were more than five times as likely to develop diabetes if they drank three or more glasses of milk each day. Further evidence indicated that children who were not breastfed or only breastfed for a short amount of time were at higher risk of getting diabetes than children who were breastfed for longer periods of time.

These studies suggested that early exposure to cow's milk may cause the body to launch an immune response to the body's own insulin, potentially because of some of the proteins that are found in cow's milk. The body ends up "attacking" its own beta

163

Q A

cells (insulin-producing cells) in the pancreas, hence leading to Type 1 diabetes.

However, many factors are potentially involved in identifying who gets Type 1 diabetes. The "milk theory" is still just that; researchers don't know enough at this point to recommend avoiding cow's milk. And to throw more confusion into the mix, new studies show that children and adults who drink milk may be at lower risk for developing Type 2 diabetes!

A woman who has an infant at risk for diabetes should try to breastfeed her baby as long as possible, and probably limit how much cow's milk the baby drinks after weaning. Feeding your child soy milk is an option, as long as the soy milk is fortified with calcium and vitamin D. If your child does not like soy milk, speak with your child's pediatrician or dietitian to discuss how to obtain other sources of calcium and vitamin D in his or her diet.

197.
It is very difficult for me to say "no" when my four-year-old asks me for cookies and ice cream when we are at a mall. He was diagnosed with diabetes only two months ago. What should I do?

You would say "no" to a your child in the same way you would say "no" to a child who did not have diabetes. There is no difference in their food choices. We all want our children to eat healthfully, and children eat best when their parents are neither overly permissive nor overly restrictive. Children learn their food behaviors at a very early age, and they may try to manipulate their parents around food issues (particularly when the child has taken premeal insulin). There is nothing wrong with a child having a cookie or ice cream, even a child with diabetes. However, as parents, we cannot give into our children's every request for food. If it is snack time anyway, a cookie or a scoop of ice cream would be all right, but if the child has just eaten a meal or snack, why not buy the treat for your child to eat at the next snack or meal. This is not a diabetes issue; it is an eating behavior issue. Establishing a smooth pattern of eating for any child is a healthier way to eat, and the child will learn that he cannot "panhandle" for food.

Q A

198.
My mother is older and has Type 2 diabetes. She doesn't always eat well, so I thought I would buy her some of those canned liquid supplements. Do I need to buy the kind especially for people with diabetes?

Liquid supplements, such as Ensure and Sustacal, have been available for many years, primarily to help people who were hospitalized or just not eating well improve their nutritional status.

Today, there are even more supplements to choose from, and they're not necessarily just for "sick people" anymore, or so advertisements would have you believe. Now, supplements are available for just about everyone—children, busy parents, and older adults. There are even specialized supplements for people with heart disease, renal disease, or diabetes. The next time you're in your local pharmacy or grocery store, scan the shelves; you may be amazed at the variety of choices! The pharmaceutical companies who manufacture the supplements market them aggressively to everyone (you might have seen the ads on television claiming that we don't eat a balanced diet, or that we're too busy to eat right).

Most of these liquid supplements contain approximately 240 calories for eight ounces, along with varying amounts of fat and protein. They generally contain little fiber, are soy based, and often loaded with different kinds of sugars, including sucrose and corn syrup. In addition, they don't contain the numerous nutrients that whole foods contain and that are needed for good health. They don't come cheap, either; a typical 8 ounce can costs $1.40 or more, depending on the formula.

Supplements do have their place, though. If someone is not eating well due to illness, recent surgery, or chewing or swallowing problems, they can be very useful. The supplements intended for people with diabetes are very similar to the "traditional" supplements (Ensure, Sustacal), except that they contain a small amount of fiber, and a blend of complex and simple carbohydrates. However, the total carbohydrate is pretty much the same. In fact, it's not absolutely nec-

Q A

essary for someone with diabetes to use only the diabetes supplements; the others are appropriate, as well. Remember, too, that these are supplements and are not intended to be the sole source of nutrition for anyone. It's still important to eat regular foods, and the last thing you want is for the supplements to fill you up so much that you can't eat your meals!

Finally, if you or someone close to you is not eating well, it's very important to speak with your doctor or dietitian to find out why. A poor appetite can be the result of many conditions, including illness, poorly controlled diabetes, and depression, to name a few. It's best to get to the root of the problem before starting supplements of any kind.

Carbohydrates

199.
I am a little confused. How much carbohydrate can a person have per day? I thought that all I had to do was not eat sugar, yet my blood glucose is too high.

It is not sugar per se, but rather carbohydrate, that affects blood glucose levels, and sugar is just a type of carbohydrate. I suggest that you make an appointment with a registered dietitian (R.D.) who specializes in diabetes. Look for the additional credential of "Certified Diabetes Educator" (C.D.E.). An R.D. can work with you to develop a meal plan, which is a guideline indicating the amount of carbohydrate to aim for at meals and snacks. This is very individualized, so it is impossible to give you a definite number without knowing a lot about you. To determine your carbohydrate allowance, an R.D. would take into account your weight, height, age, type of diabetes, diabetes medications, other medical issues, lifestyle, favorite foods, and ask for your overall input. This way, a "designer" meal plan can be developed that you would be willing and able to use day to day.

200.
Are some carbohydrate foods better choices than others?

There is an awful lot of confusing news about carbohydrates these days. Some health professionals may

Q A

suggest that all carbohydrates should be restricted because they stimulate insulin release. Other health professionals may suggest that particular types of carbohydrates are better than others. So how do you know what is important?

First of all, remember that foods containing carbohydrate are important for a healthy diet. Researchers consistently report that eating carbohydrate foods such as whole grains, fruits, vegetables, and low-fat milk decreases the risk of many chronic diseases, including Type 2 diabetes. Taking a supplement to replace the nutrients found in these foods is not an alternative because nobody knows for certain what it is in these foods that decreases risk. If you have diabetes, you deserve the right to eat healthfully, and eating healthfully includes eating healthy carbohydrate foods.

Second, remember that it is the glucose from carbohydrate foods that provides energy for your body and allows you to do all the activities you enjoy. However, to use glucose, your body needs the right amount of insulin to be available. And even though protein and fat do not add glucose to the blood, they also require insulin for the body to use them correctly. In fact, gram for gram, protein stimulates as much insulin as carbohydrate does, and in people with Type 2 diabetes it may even stimulate more insulin than carbohydrate does. To control your blood glucose levels, it is important to balance the food you eat, including carbohydrate, protein, and fat, with the right amount of insulin.

What is important, then, with regard to carbohydrates? Many research studies have shown that if people with either Type 1 or Type 2 diabetes choose either a variety of starchy foods or a variety of starchy foods and foods containing sugars, and in both cases the amount of carbohydrate is the same, the blood glucose response will also be similar. So the first priority for people with diabetes is to focus on the total amount of carbohydrate they eat.

201.
What is a carbohydrate serving?

A carbohydrate serving is generally considered to be the amount of food that contains 15 grams of carbo-

Q A

hydrate. These foods can be starches, starchy vegetables, fruits, milk, or sweets. Examples of 1 carbohydrate starch serving are 1 slice of bread, 1 small tortilla or pancake, or ½ English muffin, hot dog or hamburger bun, or bagel (1 oz); ½ cup dry cereal or ½ cup cooked cereal; 1 small baked potato or ½ cup mashed or boiled potato; ⅓ cup rice or pasta; ½ cup cooked beans, peas, or corn. Examples of one fruit serving are 1 small fresh fruit, 1 cup melon cubes, ½ cup unsweetened canned fruit, ½ cup fruit juice, or ¼ cup dried fruit. Examples of one milk serving are 1 cup (8 oz) fat-free or reduced-fat milk or 1 cup of fruited yogurt sweetened with a noncaloric sweetener, or 1 cup fat-free or low-fat plain soy milk. Examples of one sweet or dessert serving are 2 small cookies, a 2-inch square of unfrosted cake or brownie, ½ cup ice cream or light ice cream, or ½ cup sherbet. Raw vegetables like salads or relish (such as 1 cup raw vegetables or carrot or celery sticks) are considered to be "free foods." They have less than 20 calories or less than 5 grams of carbohydrate in a serving and will not have much of an effect on blood glucose levels. If you are tightly controlling your carbohydrate intake, 3 servings of a raw vegetable can be counted as 1 carbohydrate serving.

Food labels are very useful for determining carbohydrate servings. First, look at the serving size and make sure that this is the serving size you will be eating. Next, look at the section on the nutrition label where it lists the total grams of carbohydrate in that serving size. Divide that number by 15 and this is the number of carbohydrate servings. This is often not an even number, so use your judgment in deciding if it is, for example, 1, 1½, or 2 carbohydrate servings. Ignore the grams of sugar listed under total carbohydrate. The grams of sugar include both added and naturally occurring sugars and are included in the total grams of carbohydrate. In most cases, you can also ignore the grams of fiber. Technically, fiber is that portion of carbohydrate that is not absorbed, so there may be times when the amount of fiber should be subtracted from the total grams of carbohydrate. Again, if you are tightly controlling your intake of car-

Q A

bohydrate, and if there is more than 5 grams of fiber in a serving, you can subtract that from the total grams of carbohydrate and then divide that number by 15 to determine the number of carbohydrate servings. However, for most individuals the amount of fiber in foods will not have much of an effect in either raising or lowering blood glucose levels and does not need to be subtracted.

202.
How many carbohydrate servings should people with diabetes eat at a meal?

The number of carbohydrate servings you should eat for a meal or snack is influenced by two factors. First, and of most importance, is the number of carbohydrate servings you would like to eat for meals and snacks. Second, the approximate number of calories you need in a day also determines how many carbohydrate servings you need each day. For instance, if you look at a food label, the number of recommended grams of carbohydrate for 2,000 calories per day is listed. This number is 300 grams daily; divided by 15, this is 20 servings of carbohydrate in a day. This can be divided so that you have 6 carbohydrate servings at each meal and 2 for snacks. Often, adult women with Type 2 diabetes will start with 4–5 carbohydrate servings per meal and adult men with 5–6 carbohydrate servings per meal, and both can have 1–2 carbohydrate servings for snacks. If you don't want snacks, those carbohydrate servings can be added to your meals. Your dietitian will then ask you to keep food and blood glucose monitoring records to determine the effect this amount of carbohydrate has on your blood glucose levels. In addition, is this a comfortable and realistic amount of carbohydrate for you to eat? Are your blood glucose readings in your target goal range with this amount of carbohydrate, or are changes needed in the amount of medicine or insulin you take? It is a trial-and-error method, and the person with diabetes has to be the one who determines the comfortable number of carbohydrate servings per meal.

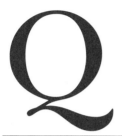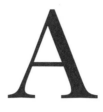

203.
I've been reading about carbohydrate counting for diabetes, but I don't take insulin. Can I still try this?

Absolutely! Carbohydrate counting is really just one other method of meal planning available to people with diabetes. If you've had diabetes for a while, you might be familiar with the traditional "exchange system," where you exchange one food for another within the same food group. This system, developed in 1950, is actually very efficient and well balanced, but many people with diabetes find it just too confusing, time-consuming, or inflexible.

Carbohydrate counting is an option that has gained popularity over the past decade. You can use this meal-planning method whether you control your diabetes with pills, insulin, or simply by diet and exercise. Carbohydrate counting is based on the fact that all dietary carbohydrate (meaning starches and sugars) is converted into blood glucose approximately two hours after eating. By eating a set amount of carbohydrate at each meal and snack during the day, blood glucose levels are more easily managed. When you start to use carbohydrate counting, you may be provided with a goal of carbohydrate (measured in grams) for each of your meals and snacks. For example, your dietitian may suggest you consume 60 grams of carbohydrate for breakfast, 45 grams for lunch, and another 45 grams for supper. Your carbohydrate goals are based on many factors, such as your daily schedule, weight goals, exercise routine, and food preferences. Another way to use carbohydrate counting is by using "choices": one carbohydrate choice equals 15 grams of carbohydrate. Either way is fine.

It's fairly easy to find carbohydrate information for most foods, unlike the exchange system. The Nutrition Facts section on a food label lists the number of carbohydrate grams per serving. You may also want to buy a food counts book that lists the number of carbohydrate grams for foods that don't have nutrition labels, such as fruits and restaurant foods, for example.

The best way to get started with carbohydrate counting is to set up an appointment with a registered dietitian. He or she will recommend an amount

Q A

of carbohydrate that is right for you and give you further instruction. You'll even learn how to fit in your favorite foods while still maintaining good blood glucose control. Now what could be better than that?

204.
My friend actually adjusts his insulin dose to match the amount of carbohydrate he wants to eat at a meal. I take insulin, too, but I've never heard of doing this. Should he be doing this?

Anyone with diabetes can determine the amount of carbohydrate in a meal; people who take insulin can take it one step further. If you take a fast-acting insulin before a meal, you can actually base your insulin dose on your current blood glucose level plus how much carbohydrate you want to consume. Does this sound suspicious? Read on.

Many people who take insulin were taught that the insulin dose should not change unless blood glucose levels were high. Meal planning, therefore, was based more on what the insulin dose was rather than what the person actually wanted to eat. Not surprisingly, people became frustrated with the rigidity of a "diabetic diet." Fortunately, times have changed for the better. You are the one who can make the decision as to what and how much you want to eat while still achieving and maintaining good diabetes control. Of course, nutrition and a balanced diet are still key.

Chances are, your friend is using something called an insulin-to-carbohydrate ratio. Everyone has a different "ratio" based on the total daily amount of insulin they take. For example, if you have a 1:15 ratio, this means you take one unit of fast-acting insulin for every 15 grams of carbohydrate you consume. This ratio allows you to decide how much carbohydrate you want to eat; you're no longer limited to a set amount of carbohydrate anymore, but be careful, as weight gain can be a side effect. While this sounds easy, and it actually is, there are a few things to consider: You need to be very certain of how much you're eating and how much carbohydrate is in what you're eating. Also, using a ratio means you must check blood glucose levels not only before you eat a meal, but two to three hours after, at least for a while, until you can be

Q A

sure your ratio is correct. In addition, your friend might be using a sensitivity, or correction, factor that is really just a supplemental insulin dose to take before a meal if blood glucose levels are too high.

If this level of carbohydrate counting is something you'd like to try, speak to your health-care team to find out if it's right for you. Be prepared for more frequent blood glucose monitoring, portion control, careful label reading, and diligent record keeping.

The homework that's involved can ultimately give you much more dietary flexibility and improved blood glucose control.

205.
I know that my triglyceride levels are high. How much carbohydrate should I consume so I can bring my triglyceride levels down?

A dietitian can prescribe an eating plan tailored just for you to help you reduce your triglyceride levels. Usually, the carbohydrate in your daily intake is reduced to 45% to 50% of your total calories. Your "healthy fat" (monounsaturated) may then be increased to make up for your reduction of carbohydrate. Here are some tips in order of effectiveness:
- Reduce or eliminate alcohol intake
- Lose weight
- Reduce carbohydrate intake with the help of your registered dietitian (to 45% to 50% of total calories)
- Eat less fat, especially saturated fat
- Exercise regularly

206.
I have heard that people with diabetes are carbohydrate sensitive. Is this true? I have always thought of myself as being carbohydrate sensitive, so I severely limit carbohydrate to lose weight.

Some people with Type 2 diabetes are thought to be more sensitive to carbohydrates than others, but carbohydrates per se do not cause weight gain. Eating excess calories from any food, particularly fat, is what causes weight gain, together with a sedentary lifestyle. The reason you lose weight when you strictly limit carbohydrates is that you are eating fewer calories.

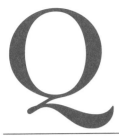 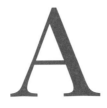

207.
Why must I watch my portions of "no-sugar added" foods. Aren't they free foods?

Go to any supermarket and you'll find an abundance of both "no-sugar-added" and "sugar-free" foods, including ice creams, cookies, candies, and jellies. Chances are you've tried some of these foods, and perhaps even thought that you could eat as much or as many as you like. After all, these are "sugar-free," right?

Well, it's not as simple as that. Sugar is just one kind of carbohydrate found in food. The other major carbohydrate in food is starch. The term "sugar-free" typically means that no sucrose (plain old table sugar) has been added to the food. However, the food manufacturer often will replace sucrose with other forms of sweeteners, including fructose, polydextrose and maltodextrin, as well as a group of sweeteners called sugar alcohols (sorbitol, mannitol). All of these sweeteners are simply different forms of carbohydrate. And remember: all carbohydrate (except for fiber) turns into blood glucose.

Even foods that are sweetened with artificial sweeteners, such as aspartame or sucralose, often still contain other forms of carbohydrate.

This means that eating sugar-free or no-sugar-added foods can affect your blood glucose just as much as eating the "regular" version of a food.

Before you become too overwhelmed or confused with trying to decipher all this, don't forget that an easy way to determine how to fit any food into your eating plan is to read the Nutrition Facts Label. Make sure you look at the Total Carbohydrate listing on the label and not the sugar listing. The sugar listing might read "0 grams" but chances are, there will still be a significant amount of carbohydrate in the food that you'll need to consider. Your dietitian can help you learn how to read the Nutrition Facts Label if you think you need more help with this.

Remember, "sugar-free" does not mean "carbohydrate-free."

Q A

208.

I saw a snack bar with "extended-release carbohydrate" on the ingredient list. What does this do?

Currently, there are a few snack bars on the market that contain something called "extended-release carbohydrate". The carbohydrate in this case is uncooked cornstarch. While that may not sound too tasty, there are several studies out now that have shown that consuming uncooked cornstarch at nighttime can reduce the frequency of hypoglycemia overnight and in the morning. (These studies were done with children and adolescents). In fact, one of the companies that make these snack bars reports that hypoglycemia is reduced by up to 75% for up to nine hours after consuming their extended-release snack bar. They also recommend these bars for other times when hypoglycemia can occur, such as during exercise.

What's so unique about uncooked cornstarch, you may be wondering? Think back to basic digestion. Remember that carbohydrate is converted into glucose in the small intestine and then absorbed from there into the bloodstream. This generally takes one to two hours after eating. (Protein and fat are not so readily converted to glucose, and they are much slower acting). However, uncooked cornstarch, while definitely still a carbohydrate, is more slowly digested and absorbed. In fact, it takes up to six hours for this to happen! Oh, and yes, the cornstarch does get a little help from the protein and fat in the bar to help slow things down a bit.

Should you try these bars? It might be worth it if you tend to experience hypoglycemia either overnight or during exercise. However, you have other options, too, such as decreasing your medication or insulin, for example, or eating "regular" snacks beforehand, such as peanut butter and crackers, or nuts and fruits. Extended-release bars are convenient, but they do cost more. Also, don't forget that these bars contain between 15 and 30 grams of carbohydrate and that they need to be included as part of your daily carbohydrate allotment.

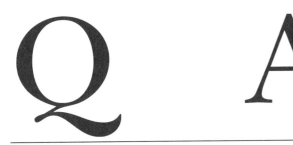

209.
What is all the talk about the glycemic index?

Research has shown that when carbohydrate foods are eaten separately and in 50-gram serving sizes, some foods raise the blood glucose level more than others. This difference in how much carbohydrate in foods raises blood glucose is referred to as the "glycemic index" of carbohydrate. Interestingly, foods containing sugars, either natural or added, tend to have a lower glycemic index than starches.

The important question is whether your HbA_{1c} level would improve if you chose only foods with a low glycemic index. Fourteen studies have compared diets with foods with a low glycemic index to diets with foods with a high glycemic index for at least four weeks. Two studies showed improvements in HbA_{1c}, while eight studies reported no differences in HbA_{1c} levels. Six studies showed improvement in fructosamine test results (a short-term measure of overall glucose control), while six studies showed no difference. (Not all studies measured both tests.) You can see that the results do not convincingly suggest that low-glycemic index diets over longer periods of time improve overall glucose control.

The bottom line is that some people may benefit from choosing low-glycemic index foods, and some may not. By testing your blood glucose before and after eating meals, you may be able to determine whether some foods will raise your blood glucose level more than others. If you do this, be sure to keep the total carbohydrate amount in the meals the same and your blood glucose in a normal range before the meal. This information may lead you to choose smaller portions of foods that raise your blood glucose more than others or to cover the food with the right amount of medication (insulin).

210.
Which foods have a low glycemic index?

Whole grains, such as barley, oatmeal, and rice; most fruits and vegetables; dried beans and peas; peanuts; low-fat yogurt and milk; and soy milk, to name a few. However, beware that some not-so-nutritious foods have a low glycemic index as well, including Snickers

Q   A

bars, potato chips, and pound cake. These foods still need to be limited in your diet.

You might be wondering about foods that have a higher glycemic index, such as potatoes, raisins, or cornflakes. Have these suddenly become foods to avoid?

Certainly not. Remember that all foods can fit into your meal plan. The key is to balance foods that have a low glycemic index with those that have a higher glycemic index. Experts recommend trying to include at least one food with a low glycemic index at each meal.

Speaking of experts, not all agree with the practicality of using the glycemic index. It works well in controlled environments such as a research study, but it can be difficult to apply in the everyday world. A number of factors can affect the glycemic index of a food, such as how much protein and fat you consume with that food, or how that food is cooked, or even the physical state of that food (whole versus chopped, for example). And what if you don't want to bother with choosing your foods off a scale?

That's all right. The lesson behind the glycemic index, whether you choose to use it exactly or use it in theory, is that whole-grain, high-fiber, unrefined foods eaten in their natural state are the best foods for us. Isn't that what we've been recommending all along?

211.
Why did my dietitian suggest I include potatoes in my meal plan when they have a high glycemic index?

The whole concept of the glycemic index is something new in the area of nutrition and diabetes. The glycemic index is a way of ranking foods based on how those foods affect blood glucose levels: A food with a low glycemic index will lead to a smaller rise in blood glucose after digestion than a food with a medium or high glycemic index, which will cause a higher rise in blood glucose.

The issue that many researchers and nutritionists struggle with is that this system seems too "black or white." In other words, many view foods as being

Q A

either good or bad. On the one hand, foods with a low glycemic index are, for the most part, quite healthful and nutritious. No one will argue that peaches, whole-wheat pasta, or lentil soup are bad for you. Yet, if you scrutinize the list closely, you will see wedged in there some foods that don't win any awards for nutrition: Chocolate bars? M&M's? Potato chips? Very few dietitians will promote these as part of good eating plan.

Along those lines, take a look at foods that have a high glycemic index. Yes, you'll see doughnuts, French fries, and honey. But what about Grape-Nuts Flakes, or baked potatoes, or dates? These foods offer a lot of nutritional benefits, including vitamins, minerals, and even fiber. There is no need to eliminate these foods from your diet.

If you're still not convinced, or if you're concerned that your blood glucose will go sky-high after eating a baked potato, try these tips:

■ Eat a food with a low glycemic index along with the food that has a higher glycemic index. Eat vegetables or lima beans, for example, along with that potato.

■ Include a small amount of healthful fat at your meal, which can help to blunt the rise in blood glucose after eating.

■ Eat foods in their whole state whenever possible. For example, eat the potato whole rather than mashing it.

■ Don't forget to eat the skin of the potato, which is where most of the fiber hides out.

■ Check your blood glucose level about two hours after your meal to see how that meal affected your blood glucose.

■ One last important point: All carbohydrate foods, whether they have a high or low glycemic index, will have an effect on blood glucose. Just because a food has a low glycemic index does not mean you can go overboard with the amount you consume. Portion size still matters, and eating too much of any food will lead to a higher blood glucose level.

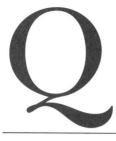 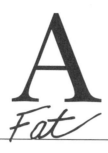

Fat

212.
How does fat affect blood glucose levels? Does fat add glucose to the blood?

Fat does not directly contribute glucose to the blood. Glycerol, which is a very small part of the fat molecule, can be converted to glucose, but this glucose is probably stored in the liver. The fatty acids from food are primarily stored in the fat cells to be released when needed for energy. However, some research has shown that large amounts of dietary fat can cause insulin resistance. This might have the effect of raising blood glucose levels, but again this is not very well studied.

As you can see, what affects blood glucose levels is not as simple as the information often given to people with diabetes. The main point to remember, from the standpoint of what is important on a day-to-day basis, is that it is the total amount of available carbohydrate from foods eaten that will determine what happens to blood glucose levels after eating. The glucose from carbohydrate is the body's primary source of energy. And your body must have enough insulin available to use or store carbohydrate for energy, just as it must have enough insulin to metabolize protein and fat. It is the balance between foods eaten and insulin that keeps your blood glucose levels normal.

213.
Does it matter which type of fats I eat or just the amount I eat?

The type of fat is most significant, for all people. However, the amount is also important. Fats are often categorized as either "good fats" or "bad fats," referring to the form the fat is in at room temperature: saturated (solid) or unsaturated (liquid). Eating a lot of saturated fat causes blood cholesterol levels to rise, more so than eating a lot of foods containing cholesterol (animal foods) that are not also high in fat (white meat chicken/turkey, fish, skim dairy products). Remember, too, that fat, whether "good" or "bad," contains 9 calories per gram versus 4 calories per gram for carbohydrate and protein. So quantity as well as quality is essential.

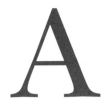

214.

What are the types of fat and which type is the better one to use?

Liquid fats (oils) are better than solid fats. Monounsaturated fats such as olive, canola, and peanut oils can lower blood cholesterol and increase HDL cholesterol if the diet is low in saturated fat. Polyunsaturated fats such as corn oil, safflower oil, sunflower oil, sesame oil, and soybean oil are found to only lower blood cholesterol when the diet is low in saturated fat. Omega-3 fats are polyunsaturated fat found in fish such as mackerel, salmon, tuna, sardines, bluefish, walnuts, and flaxseed oil and may reduce the risk of heart disease. Omega-3 fats help prevent clotting and stickiness on artery walls, but they are most beneficial when obtained from foods and not supplements. Saturated fat, mostly from fatty animal and dairy products, is the main culprit in raising blood cholesterol levels. *Trans* fats are oils that have been changed from a liquid into a more solid fat. Although making fats more solid allows for a longer shelf life, *trans* fats raise your blood cholesterol levels just like saturated fats.

215.

What exactly are monounsaturated and polyunsaturated fats, and why do people with diabetes hear so much about them?

Monounsaturated fats and polyunsaturated fats are long chains of carbons connected by bonds. Monounsaturated fats have one (mono) double bond while polyunsaturated fats have many (poly) double bonds. Saturated fats have no double bonds and are therefore completely "saturated" with hydrogen atoms along the entire carbon chain. Monounsaturated and polyunsaturated fats do not raise cholesterol levels and when eaten in very large amounts (which is not recommended) may actually lower cholesterol levels. Therefore, they are often thought of as being good fats, especially the monounsaturated fats.

Sources of polyunsaturated fats are cottonseed oil, corn oil, safflower oil, sunflower oil, soybean oil, and walnuts. Sources of monounsaturated fats are canola oil, olive oil, peanut oil, olives, avocados, and most nuts. Monounsaturated fats are also found in many of the foods that contain saturated fat, so that when

Q A

individuals cut back on saturated fats, they also reduce their intake of monounsaturated fats. That means to increase intake of monounsaturated fat, people have to use more oils and eat more nuts. The problem with this is that these food products are also high in calories, so if you are trying to increase your intake of monounsaturated fats, you need to also monitor your total calorie intake and your weight.

Some studies suggest that total fat, regardless of the type, contributes to insulin resistance. Saturated fats do cause insulin resistance, but the effect of monounsaturated and polyunsaturated fats on insulin resistance is unclear at this time.

216.
What are saturated fatty acids?

All fats are composed of fatty acids, which can come from either plant-based or animal-based foods and are the building blocks of fat. There are three types of fatty acids: saturated, monounsaturated, and polyunsaturated. They differ primarily in the number of carbons in a molecule and the amount of hydrogen they contain. Saturated fats contain the most hydrogen; that is, they are "saturated" with hydrogen at every possible point along the carbon chain. Monounsaturated and polyunsaturated fatty acids contain the least amount of hydrogen. A food is classified based on the type of fatty acids it contains in the largest amount. One quick way to tell the difference in fats is to see if they are liquid or solid at room temperature. Saturated fats are solid at room temperature and monounsaturated and polyunsaturated fatty acids are liquid at room temperature.

Saturated fats raise blood total and LDL cholesterol levels. When substituted for saturated fats, monounsaturated and polyunsaturated fats do not raise cholesterol levels and may even help lower blood cholesterol levels. It is recommended that all adults with diabetes have an LDL cholesterol level less than 100 mg/dl. To help achieve this goal, it is recommended that foods with a high content of saturated fatty acids be limited to less than 10% of total calories per day for all persons, and for persons with LDL cholesterol equal to or higher than 100 mg/dl to less than 7% of total calories. However, percentage of calories from a nutrient is not very helpful advice for choosing

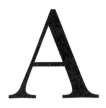

foods because on the food label, it lists grams of fat per serving. The goal is to keep saturated fat intake to less than 15 grams per day for someone on a lower-calorie diet and to less than 20 grams a day for someone eating about 2,000 calories a day. Knowing this you can look at food labels and try and find foods with 5 or less grams of saturated fat in a serving.

Although saturated fats are found mainly in animal foods, there are some vegetable fats that also contain saturated fats. Some common food sources of saturated fats are meats, cheese, butter, hardened shortenings, milk-fat dairy products, lard, coconut oil, palm oil, and palm kernel oil.

217.
I've been hearing a lot about *trans* fatty acids lately. What are they? Are they bad for me?

All fats and oils are made up of fatty acids. Fatty acids are classified as being either saturated, monounsaturated, or polyunsaturated. A saturated fat is a solid fat at room temperature; picture a stick of butter or a can of vegetable shortening. Saturated fats can raise your blood cholesterol levels. On the other hand, polyunsaturated and monounsaturated fats are liquid at room temperature; corn oil and olive oil, for example. These are known as the "heart healthy" fats, since they can help lower your blood cholesterol level if it is high.

Trans fats are formed when unsaturated fats such as vegetable oils undergo the process of hydrogenation where hydrogen atoms are added to fill the empty slots on the carbon chain, thus "saturating" it. Hydrogenation is used to extend the shelf life of some products. *Trans* fats are found in solid margarines and in food prepared or fried in hydrogenated vegetable oils. They also occur naturally in some meats and dairy products. Other foods that have been hydrogenated and therefore contain *trans* fats include store-bought cookies and crackers, cake mixes, potato chips and fast-food French fries, to name a few.

Similar to saturated fats, *trans* fats raise LDL cholesterol levels, but they have the added disadvantage of lowering HDL cholesterol (the good cholesterol). The good news is that only about 3% of total calories on average are from *trans* fats compared to 11% to 12% from saturated fats. Although it is important to

Q A

try to avoid *trans* fats whenever possible, cutting back on saturated fats is likely to be more beneficial in terms of lowering cholesterol because more saturated fats are eaten than *trans* fats.

218.
My doctor told me I should eat more foods high in omega-3 fatty acids, but I'm not really sure what they are or what foods contain them.

Your doctor is right! We all should aim to include more omega-3 fatty acids in our diets. Omega-3 fatty acids, or omega-3's for short, are a type of polyunsaturated fatty acid found in abundance in fish, especially fatty fish (omega-3's are sometimes called "fish oils"). Omega-3's get their name from the fact that the first double bond is found at the third carbon, whereas other polyunsaturated fats are omega-6 fatty acids because they have their first double bond at the sixth carbon. These fats are found in cold-water or oily fish such as salmon, mackerel, perch, cod, tuna, sole, and some plant sources such as flaxseed and flaxseed oil, canola oil, soybean oil, and nuts. Increasing intake of the omega-3 fatty acids has been shown to be beneficial to people with diabetes. Nutrition researchers have known for several decades that omega-3's can play a big role in the prevention of heart disease. More specifically, eating a diet rich in omega-3's can help in the following ways:
- Lower blood triglyceride (fat) levels
- Lower your chances of developing blood clots by thinning the blood
- Lower blood pressure
- Regulate heart rhythm

The coronary heart disease rate is low in countries where fatty fish is eaten often, even if the total fat intake is high. This is why it is recommended to eat two or more servings of fish per week.

219.
How much omega-3 fatty acids do you need to stay healthy?

Well, here's where experts are divided. But all agree that most of us don't consume enough, and that we should try to eat at least two fish meals each week. The fish that contain the highest levels of omega-3s

Q A

are salmon, mackerel, sardines, trout, tuna, herring, and swordfish.

Don't like fish? Don't despair. Omega-3 fatty acids are also found in plant foods, such as flaxseed and flaxseed oil, walnuts and walnut oil, canola oil, and soybean oil.

What about just popping a capsule of fish oil? You may have seen these supplements in your drugstore. Unless your physician advises otherwise, avoid doing this. Fish oil capsules contain a concentrated amount of omega-3 fatty acids that can be potentially dangerous, especially if you're taking other medications. Besides, getting your omega-3s from food sources rather than a pill will give you so many other nutritional benefits: less saturated fat, more protein, more vitamins, more minerals, and even fiber. You can't get all that in a pill!

220.
What are fat replacers?

Food fat can be decreased by eating less high-fat food or by substituting lower-fat or fat-free food for high-fat food. To help accomplish this, food companies can either decrease the amount of fat in foods or they may use fat replacers or substitutes, which are ingredients that mimic the properties of fat with fewer calories. You may see some of the following fat replacer ingredients on the ingredient list on the food labels of light or reduced-calorie foods: maltodextrin, hydrolyzed corn starch, sugar beet fiber or powder, cellulose gel, xanthan gum, microparticulated egg white, milk protein.

Used wisely as a part of a plan of healthy eating, foods containing fat replacers can help you reduce the fat and calories you eat while allowing you to eat foods you like. But fat replacers are not the complete answer. These foods still have calories, and it can be easy to overeat with these foods just as it is easy to overeat with regular foods.

Some people think that as long as a food is low fat they can eat as much as they want, but this is not true. A food labeled "low in saturated fat" or "cholesterol-free" can be loaded with *trans* fat. But beginning January 1, 2006, food companies are required to add the amount of *trans* fat in a particular food to the Nutrition Facts label of the product.

Q A

Without the Nutrition Facts label, how would you know if a food contains *trans* fat? Read the ingredient list and look for the words "hydrogenated," "partially hydrogenated," or "fractionated." The closer to the top of the list these words are, the more *trans* fat the food contains.

To minimize your intake of *trans* fats, limit the number of processed foods you eat (fatty snack foods, fast foods), choose lower-fat dairy foods (skim or low fat milk), eat less red meat, and choose a margarine that contains no *trans* fatty acids (this will be stated right on the container). You can't totally avoid consuming *trans* fats, but you can definitely consume less.

221.

I have heard a lot about plant stanol and plant sterol ester margarines lately. Are they good for people with diabetes?

Plant sterol and plant stanol esters, naturally occurring substances in plants, block the absorption of food cholesterol from the intestine. Plant stanols and plant sterols in the amount of about 2 grams per day have been shown to lower total and LDL cholesterol. The new margarines on the market (for example, Benecol, Take Control) contain these ingredients. In the future they may also be found in salad dressings. Two to three servings of plant stanols or plant sterols per day can be substituted for similar foods such as butter or regular margarine as part of an overall plan to improve your cholesterol.

222.

How can I reduce my overall fat intake?

The most important thing to pay attention to is the total amount of saturated fat and calories. The following are some tips to help lower the fat in your diet:

■ Eat smaller and fewer meat servings. Most adults should try to limit total meat intake to about 6 ounces after cooking per day. Some women need 4–5 ounces a day. People on meal plans of more than 2,000 calories may be able to have up to 8 ounces of meat a day.

■ Choose leaner meats such as lean beef, pork, fish, or poultry. If you eat luncheon meats, look for those with 3 or fewer grams of fat per ounce.

Q A

- Restrict your high-fat meat servings to no more than two or three times per week. Regular luncheon meats, other processed meats, frankfurters, wieners, sausage, bacon, and prime cuts of meat are all high-fat meats.
- Cook using low-fat cooking methods such as baking, broiling, or roasting. When frying or sautéing foods, use nonfat cooking spray or a small amount of vegetable oil.
- Chill gravies, soups, and stews until the fat hardens. Remove the fat layer, reheat, and serve.
- Drink skim or 1% milk.
- Use plain nonfat yogurt (2 tablespoons = less than 20 calories) instead of sour cream (2 tablespoons = 50 calories) or mayonnaise (2 tablespoons = 200 calories) as a condiment or in recipes for dips and salad dressing.
- Choose cheeses that have 5 or fewer grams of fat per ounce.
- Use a soft margarine or one made with a stanol or sterol ester instead of butter, but be careful of amounts. The calories in margarine and butter are the same, but because butter is primarily a saturated fat, margarine is recommended. Look for margarine that lists a liquid fat such as corn, safflower, or soybean oil as the first ingredient. A soft or tub margarine is a better choice than solid or stick margarine.
- Choose low-fat or fat-free salad dressings. One tablespoon of a low-fat or fat-free salad dressing generally has less than 20 calories and is considered a "free food"; two or three tablespoons is one fat serving. One tablespoon of a regular dressing is one fat serving.
- Try some of the many light or low-fat sour creams, mayonnaise, and salad dressings on the market.

Fiber

223.
What is "fiber"? Aren't foods high in fiber also high in carbohydrates?

Fiber is a carbohydrate. It comes from plant foods (not animal products), cannot be digested by the human digestive system, and does not provide calories. Fiber is what gives plants their structure and is found in vegetables, fruits, and grains. Fiber gives bulk and helps push food through the digestive tract. Soluble fiber has also

Q   A

been shown to have beneficial effects on cholesterol levels. So it is actually beneficial to eat high-fiber foods since you often do not have to count the fiber grams as part of the number of carbohydrate grams. If one serving of a food contains five or more grams of fiber, the fiber should be subtracted from the total carbohydrate listed on the Nutrition Facts label, because the carbohydrate portion that is fiber is not absorbed.

224.
What are soluble and insoluble fiber? Where do I find them?

The two types of fiber are called soluble and insoluble. Soluble fiber dissolves in water to form a gel and is found in citrus fruits, apples, strawberries, vegetables, oats and rice bran, barley, dried beans, and peas. Soluble fiber has been shown to have a cholesterol-lowering effect and, in large amounts, may even delay the rise of blood glucose after a meal. Insoluble fiber is known as roughage. It is the part of a plant that gives it its structure, and is called insoluble because it doesn't dissolve in water. Insoluble fiber is found in wheat and corn bran, whole grains, nuts, fruits, and vegetables, particularly root vegetables. Insoluble fiber adds bulk to the diet, giving a feeling of fullness. It helps to prevent constipation, keeping the digestive tract healthy.

225.
I am trying to adjust my diet by introducing more vegetables and fruits with "juicing." Is this a good way to add more healthy foods?

It's always a good idea to introduce more fruits and vegetables into your diet. However, juices probably are not the best choice. A piece of fruit or a vegetable in a raw or cooked state is more healthy for you because it contains fiber as some of its carbohydrate. The problem with juicers is that you usually end up throwing out the fiber, the part that gives you the most benefit. Any vegetable or fruit in a liquid form is absorbed more quickly and disappears more quickly, not the most beneficial for blood glucose and a feeling of satisfied fullness.

226.
Will eating foods containing fiber improve blood glucose levels?

The short answer is yes, if you eat an awful lot of it.
   The average dietary fiber intake is 19 grams a day

Q A

for men and 13 to 16 grams a day for women. For health, it is recommended that all Americans try to increase this amount to 25 to 35 grams a day. Eating five or more servings of fruits and vegetables and three or more servings of whole grains from cereals, bread, and legumes in a day can help meet this goal.

Studies in people with Type 1 and Type 2 diabetes have shown that eating 50 grams of fiber a day compared to more usual amounts (20 to 24 grams) can improve blood glucose levels. However, it seems that very large amounts of fiber need to be eaten to see beneficial effects. It is not known today if people with diabetes can eat that much fiber every day and if eating that amount of fiber would be acceptable to most people.

Does this mean you shouldn't bother trying to increase your fiber intake? Certainly not! Any increase in fiber has benefits. Insoluble fiber helps ensure that your digestive track runs smoothly by preventing constipation and diverticulosis. It may also help prevent against colon cancer. Foods rich in insoluble fiber include bran cereals, whole wheat bread, and vegetables. The other kind of fiber, soluble fiber, forms a gummy gel in your intestinal tract and, like insoluble fiber, has a laxative effect. However, this kind of fiber can also bind up excess cholesterol, ultimately helping you to lower your blood cholesterol level if it is high. People with elevated cholesterol levels were more likely to see a benefit than individuals with normal cholesterol levels. However, as with blood glucose, it also takes a lot of dietary fiber to have beneficial effects on cholesterol. Foods high in soluble fiber include oat bran and oatmeal, dried beans and peas, and some fruits and vegetables.

The American Diabetes Association recommends that people with diabetes, just as people in the general population, eat foods containing fiber as an important part of a healthy diet. Foods that are high in fiber are often good sources of important vitamins and minerals but it is not known, and probably unlikely, that people with diabetes will eat enough fiber to improve their blood glucose levels.

The best way to determine how fiber affects your individual blood glucose level is to gradually increase your intake by about 3–5 grams every few days and

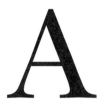

monitor your blood glucose. Be sure to include foods high in soluble fiber in your eating plan every day, since this kind of fiber is most likely to improve blood glucose levels. Last but not least, don't forget to increase your fluid intake as you increase your fiber intake to prevent any chance of becoming constipated.

227.
How can I increase my dietary fiber intake?

Fiber is found in a broad range of plant foods, which give you a wide variety to choose from. The following table lists carbohydrate foods that are good sources of fiber.

FOOD	SERVING SIZE	AVERAGE GRAMS OF FIBER
Starch		
Breads: whole wheat, whole grain, or crackers	1 slice or 1 oz	2
Cereals: dry or cooked	varies	3
Bran cereals	⅓–½ cup	8
Starchy vegetables: potatoes, brown rice, green peas	½ cup	3
Legumes: peas, beans, lentils	⅓ cup	4–5
Grains: kasha, couscous, bulgur, wild rice	½ cup	2
Fruit		
Fresh, frozen, or canned	½ cup	2
Fresh	1 small	2
Vegetables		
Cooked, canned, or frozen	½–¾ cup	2
Raw	1–2 cups	3

Here are some tips to help you increase your fiber intake and to meet the guidelines for a healthy diet:

Q A

Switch from white bread to whole-grain varieties. Choose products made from stone ground flour, 100% whole wheat, or other whole-grain flours, which should be the first ingredient listed on the label. "Brown-colored" breads contain little or no whole grain, just molasses for coloring. If the ingredients list says "wheat flour," it usually refers to bleached or white flour.

Select whole fresh fruit and vegetables instead of juices. Eat the skin of cleaned fruit (such as apples), the membranes (such as oranges), and seeds (such as strawberries). Eat more raw and slightly cooked vegetables such as corn, peas, beans, legumes, and potatoes with skin. The stems and leaves of salad greens and broccoli are also fibrous. Don't throw away good fiber sources. Add dry beans and peas to soups, stews, and casseroles. Use legumes as main dishes, along with whole wheat pasta.

Choose high-fiber, low-fat snacks. Snack on vegetables, fruits, air-popped popcorn, and cereals, rather than cakes, cookies, and chocolate.

Start adding up your servings each day. It won't take long to see a healthy increase in your daily intake of fiber.

228.
I have cut starches almost completely out of my diet to keep my blood glucose levels low. I eat lots of high-fiber vegetables but stay away from breads, pasta, rice, and potatoes. This diet has been very hard to sustain. Any advice?

High-fiber foods are always good choices because they make you feel more satisfied and full, without extra calories. Since fiber is not digested or absorbed, it does not provide calories or affect your blood glucose. But there is no reason that you can't eat starchy foods if you choose; it's the quantity that you eat that is important. If you overeat carbohydrate foods, you will probably raise your blood glucose. It does not matter where the carbohydrate comes from, as far as your blood glucose is concerned, but the total number of carbohydrate grams you eat at each meal that makes the difference. Allow yourself some flexibility in food choices. You are missing out on some perfectly healthy foods by eliminating so many starchy foods.

189

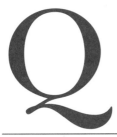 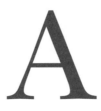

229.
What is a resistant starch? Is it similar to fiber?

Resistant starch is a type of starch that is resistant to (not easily broken down by) digestive enzymes, so it is absorbed much more slowly in the bloodstream than other starches. It is similar to fiber but found in different food sources, such as uncooked cornstarch. Foods containing naturally occurring resistant starch (cornstarch) or foods with added resistant starch might help lower blood glucose levels after eating, prevent low blood glucose levels (hypoglycemia), and reduce high blood glucose levels (hyperglycemia). Resistant starch is used in some diabetes snack bars designed to improve blood glucose control and reduce the risk of nighttime hypoglycemia. Studies have suggested that diabetes snack bars may have a positive effect on blood glucose control, but the studies are not conclusive. The research available has been of questionable quality, and it has not been established that bedtime snacks with resistant starch are more effective in preventing hypoglycemia than other types of carbohydrate. The best advice to prevent hypoglycemia during the night is to consistently choose a carbohydrate snack at bedtime that you enjoy the taste of, to test blood glucose levels, and then—if necessary—to adjust your medication.

Protein

230.
Does eating protein increase blood glucose levels?

Indirectly, protein may contribute glucose to the blood, but when and how much is determined by how much insulin you have and your glucose needs. Protein is composed of about half essential and half nonessential amino acids. Essential amino acids are used to repair or make new body tissues such as muscle; that is why they're called essential. In the liver, the nonessential amino acids can be changed into glucose, but this glucose does not enter the general blood circulation. People with diabetes are often told that about 50% of protein eaten changes into glucose and enters the blood 3 to 4 hours later. Where this assumption came from is unknown, because as early

Q   A

as 1936 it was reported that no glucose entered into the blood stream during the 10 hours after eating a very large portion of protein (lean meat). In 1984, it was shown again that no glucose entered the blood stream during the 8 hours after 50 grams of protein (again, lean meat) was eaten. And again in 2001, it was shown that some protein does change into glucose in the liver; however, the glucose does not enter the general circulation and the fate of the glucose is unknown at this time. It is speculated that this glucose is stored in the liver as glycogen, as is some carbohydrate, and when needed the liver releases glucose from this glycogen into the circulation. At this point, whether the glucose came originally from protein or carbohydrate would not be known.

To be metabolized, however, protein does require as much insulin as does carbohydrate. In fact, in some people with Type 2 diabetes, protein may require more insulin than carbohydrate. If the amount of insulin available is inadequate, it may be possible that blood glucose levels may increase after eating protein. This last possibility has not been well studied.

231.
Should people with diabetes eat a low-carbohydrate, high-protein diet?

Aside from the concern about how high protein diets might affect your kidneys, are there advantages from these diets that outweigh their risks? Weight loss and improved blood glucose control are claims made for the high-protein, low-carbohydrate diets. Although the authors of the popular books on this subject all use a slightly different tactic—you need a gimmick to set you apart from the "pack"—the basic idea is the same. Eating a high-carbohydrate diet makes people fat because carbohydrates increase blood glucose levels, causing a greater release of insulin and higher insulin levels cause carbohydrates to be easily stored as fat. By eating a high-protein diet, weight is lost, insulin levels decrease, and blood glucose levels improve. However, the research to back these claims is missing. There is no good evidence to suggest that eating starchy foods and sugar is the cause of obesity or insulin resistance. What research there is suggests that eating carbohydrates actually improves insulin sensitivity, not decreases it. In fact, it is obesity that is associated with insulin resistance. Increased physical activity, reduced fat and calorie intake, and small amounts of weight loss—not changes in the percentage of protein or carbohydrate—have been shown to improve insulin sensitivity.

The advantage of high-protein, low-carbohydrate diets is that when you eliminate a whole category of foods, such as carbohydrates, you decrease calories and weight is lost. Few people can eat endless amounts of animal protein and fat for weeks on end and they therefore end up eating less and less; that's the good news. The bad news and the major disadvantage is that you have eliminated many foods that are important for a healthy diet, such as whole grains, fruits, vegetables, and low-fat milk. When these diets are analyzed, they come up seriously short of fiber and essential nutrients such as vitamin C, D, folic acid, and especially calcium. Taking a supplement to replace missing nutrients is not the answer either, because all of the essential nutrients in foods have not yet been identified and thus cannot be replaced. These diets are also high in cholesterol and fat and increase your risk of heart disease, gout, and kidney stones. People with diabetes deserve to eat healthfully. These diets have not been shown to be of benefit for the general public, and certainly not for people with diabetes.

Popularity is not credibility. There is little research published in reputable medical journals showing that people maintain weight loss better from these diets than from other low-calorie diets. High-protein diets are based on personal experiences and testimonials. Long-term studies are needed to prove these diets are safe and to determine how much protein should be consumed and for how long people can stay on these diets.

232.
My doctor suggests that I eat a diet extremely low in protein because I have protein in my urine. Where do I start?

You need to get your doctor to give you a referral to a trained registered dietitian (R.D.) who can explain the best way to fit this modification into your eating

Q A

plan. Look for somebody who is also a certified diabetes educator (C.D.E.). Here are some tips to get you started:

■ Your body needs protein, but most people eat much more than they need.

■ Decrease your portions of animal products; all animal and dairy products contain protein. Animal and dairy products are also high in fat, so eating less will be more heart-healthy.

■ Eat two or three meatless meals each week; vegetable protein may be easier on your kidneys. Try dried beans, peas, lentils, tofu, soy products, nuts, seeds, and grains.

■ Eat a fruit with each meal to fill you up; fruit does not contain protein.

It is important to eat the right amount and type of protein. If you eat too little, you can lose protein from cells and tissue such as muscle. If you eat too much protein, it may harm your kidneys. A prudent treatment approach includes having a protein intake no greater than what your body actually needs (0.8 g protein/kg body weight). A registered dietitian can create an individualized meal plan with the amount of protein that is just right for you, while keeping your weight considerations in mind.

233.
Does eating protein cause renal (kidney) disease?

People with diabetes often ask if eating a high-protein diet, in particular, will cause renal disease. The answer to this is not a simple yes or no. For people who get 20% or less of their calories from protein, the answer is no. In seven studies, protein intake for people who developed renal disease was identical to the protein intake for people who did not develop renal disease. In all of these studies protein intake was in the range of usual intake, which is between 15% and 20% of total calories. However, if you eat a high-protein diet—that is, if more than 20% of your calories comes from protein—the answer is not so clear. In one study of 2,500 persons with Type 1 diabetes, those who reported protein intakes greater than 20% of their calories had average albumin excretion rates in the range of microalbuminuria (small amounts of albumin, a protein, in the urine;

Q A

albumin in the urine is a measure of deteriorating kidney function). In those who had macroalbuminuria (overt kidney disease) 32% got more than 20% of their calories from protein. This study only shows an association between high-protein diets and renal disease and does not prove cause and effect, but it does suggest that a high protein intake may have detrimental effects on kidney function. The bottom line is that protein intake in the usual range does not appear to cause renal disease, but the answer regarding high-protein diets is not clear. It seems prudent, though, to avoid diets with greater than 20% of the calories from protein until we know the answer to this question.

234.
Will eating protein with a sweet or dessert slow the absorption of this "fast-acting carbohydrate"?

There really are not any "fast-acting carbohydrates," despite the fact that this is a commonly used term. If you look at research studies, almost all carbohydrates are absorbed from the small intestine into the bloodstream in the form of glucose at very similar rates, although a small amount of other sugars (fructose and lactose) also enters the bloodstream. The small difference in absorption between carbohydrates does not have much of an effect on blood glucose levels. When we talk about carbohydrates, the terms we should use are starch, sugars, and fiber. There are no clear definitions of what a "complex carbohydrate" is and all sugars are basically "simple."

We should also note that very few foods contain only protein. Most foods that are commonly called protein also contain fat. Even lean meat will have about the same number of calories from fat as it does from protein. Common "protein foods" such as meat, poultry, fish, eggs, cheese, or nuts also contain fat. Other common "protein foods" such as cooked dried peas, beans, or lentils, and even milk, also contain carbohydrate.

However, regardless of whether these foods are called protein or meats and meat substitutes, eating them with carbohydrates does not slow the absorption of glucose from carbohydrate. There are a number of research studies in which a standard amount of

194

Q A

carbohydrate is eaten with different amounts of protein. In all of these studies, regardless of the source of the carbohydrate or the amount of protein, the glucose response and peak is similar: The blood glucose level peaks about 45 to 90 minutes following the meal. And if adequate insulin is available, blood glucose levels return to premeal values in 4 to 5 hours. If less is eaten, the return to the premeal blood glucose level may occur sooner, but there are no studies that show you can lengthen the time of this response beyond 4 to 5 hours.

That was the long answer. The short answer is no, eating protein with a carbohydrate does not change the peak blood glucose response.

**235.
Should I always eat protein with my carbohydrates when I snack, or is it okay to eat the carbohydrate alone?**

Eating a snack with carbohydrate and protein together is not necessary. The first consideration is to keep your snack about 15–20 grams of carbohydrate or the amount your dietitian has prescribed for you. Eating a carbohydrate on its own works well for most people. However, if you plan to have a very active day, eating a carbohydrate with added fat such as the fat in a tablespoon of peanut butter, a cheese stick, or some nuts may help the snack stay with you longer. It is usually the fat in the protein choice that can delay the absorption of carbohydrates from your intestine into your bloodstream and not the protein, as we once thought.

**236.
I'm trying to "bulk up" by lifting weights. Shouldn't I also be eating more protein in my diet to help me build more muscle?**

No. It's really a common misconception that just because you want to be more muscular, you should eat more protein. Before you choke down a glass full of egg yolks or polish off a pound of hamburger, read on.

Protein is an essential nutrient needed to (among other things) build muscle tissue. The Recommended Dietary Allowance (RDA) for protein is 0.8 grams per kilogram of body weight each day. Believe it or not, weight lifters do just fine with the same amount of protein than someone who has never picked up a dumbbell in his life! This is because a regular weight lifter uses dietary protein more efficiently to help build muscle mass. Only endurance athletes require slightly more protein (approximately 1.0 to 1.2 grams per kilogram of body weight daily).

Cramming more protein into your diet really doesn't do any good. Unlike carbohydrate and fat, protein cannot be stored in the body. The excess protein that you ingest merely gets stored—as fat. Too much protein can be harmful and can lead to kidney damage and possible leaching of calcium from the bones, which means an increased risk for osteoporosis. There's even some evidence that consuming a high-protein diet can increase the risk for some types of cancer. Keep in mind, too, that eating protein foods that are high in saturated fat, such as red meats and cheeses, can also increase your risk of heart disease.

Too much protein can also affect blood glucose. We usually think that only carbohydrate-containing foods raise blood glucose levels. But taking in more protein than is recommended can also affect your blood glucose.

You may have heard people talk about getting extra protein by taking protein supplements. These supplements, usually in the form of a powder, can be found in all different varieties at health-food stores, health clubs, and of course, on the Internet. The protein in these powders is usually derived from either milk, eggs, or soybeans. The directions on the container indicate that a serving, or a "scoop," of the powder contains approximately 21 grams of protein. This is equivalent to eating three ounces of chicken breast, for example. You have the option of mixing the powder into water, milk, or juice. The directions also tell you that the goal is to consume several servings of the supplement each day. When you do the math, you'll end up consuming at least 60 grams of protein from the powder alone—and that doesn't include the protein from food that you eat. People typically consume at least 100 grams of protein from food every day; add the amount from three servings

Q A

of the protein supplement, and you'll get almost 200 grams of protein in one day! This is much more than what is recommended and what is considered to be healthy.

Finally, it's highly unlikely that you're consuming too little protein. The typical American diet provides about 100 grams of protein per day, which is actually twice the RDA for protein.

Sweeteners

237.
Can I eat sugar?

Yes. Remember that the focus nowadays is on total carbohydrate intake, not sugar intake. If you choose to eat a food that contains sugar as one of your carbohydrate choices, go ahead. Just be sure not to constantly sacrifice nutritious foods for sugary, empty-calorie foods. The dietary guidelines for people with diabetes are the same as for people without diabetes. Good nutrition is key for everyone, yet all foods can fit, in moderation.

If you want sweetness without the calories and without affecting your blood glucose level, try using one of the artificial sweeteners on the market.

238.
Is it safe to eat products that contain the sweetener aspartame?

People with diabetes, as well as the general public, periodically receive e-mail messages linking aspartame to fibromyalgia, lupus, multiple sclerosis (MS), Alzheimer disease, diabetes, Gulf War syndrome, and seizures. These messages, and others like them, continue to be passed around on the Internet even though there is no scientific evidence for the concern. Many organizations—including the Multiple Sclerosis Foundation, the Arthritis Foundation, the American Diabetes Association, and the American Dietetic Association—have issued statements refuting the claims that have circulated. However, people with diabetes become concerned, and rightly so, whenever they hear or read these messages.

So what is the evidence for aspartame's safety? Repeated studies in peer-reviewed journals show no adverse effects of aspartame in relation to seizures;

Q A

cognitive/behavioral/neuropsychiatric/neurophysiologic function; brain/intestinal/liver hormones or enzymes; brain tumors; cancer; birth defects; weight loss; Parkinson disease; allergic responses; blood pressure; or carbohydrate or lipid metabolism. As you can see from this lengthy list, the safety and possibility of side effects have been studied and reviewed extensively.

In 2001, the journal *Regulatory Toxicology and Pharmacology* published an evaluation of aspartame's use and safety since its approval. This evaluation, which cited extensive scientific research investigating various allegations, reported that no relationship had been found between aspartame and adverse effects and that, even in amounts many times what people typically consume, aspartame is safe.

For example, 12 ounces of a typical diet soda contains about 200 mg of aspartame. Healthy men have consumed up to 10,000 mg of aspartame without exhibiting any side effects. Aspartame does contain methanol, an ingredient many of the reports seem to be concerned with. However, many fruits and vegetables also contain methanol. In fact, there is more methanol in a glass of tomato juice than in a diet soda. The body treats methanol the same whether it comes from fruit or from aspartame.

All non-nutritive sweeteners—aspartame included—must undergo rigorous testing and must be judged safe for the public to consume before the Food and Drug Administration (FDA) approves them for marketing. Furthermore, the FDA establishes an Acceptable Daily Intake (ADI) for many food additives, including nonnutritive sweeteners. The ADI defines the amount considered very safe even if consumed on a daily basis over a person's lifetime. In the case of aspartame the ADI is 50 mg per kilogram of body weight, which is 1% of the level that has been tested and shown to be safe. To reach this level, an adult would need to consume 15 diet sodas or 86 packets of Equal per day and for every day of a lifetime and a 50-pound child would need to consume 7 diet sodas or 32 packets of Equal every day.

Q A

239.
What about saccharin, acesulfame-K, and sucralose? Are they safe?

All sugar substitutes are often referred to as non-nutritive sweeteners or low-calorie or noncaloric sweeteners, because they contribute few or no calories. They are intensely sweet, so only very small amounts are needed to sweeten food products. Saccharin, acesulfame-K, sucralose, and neotame are sugar substitutes approved by the Food and Drug Administration (FDA) for sale in the United States. Just as for aspartame, the FDA sets an ADI for these non-nutritive sweeteners, which includes a very generous safety factor.

Although saccharin has been used for over 80 years, in the 1970's it was designated by the FDA as a possible cancer-causing agent and packages of saccharin were required to carry a warning label. This happened because a study showed a probability of causing cancer in rats that had a daily saccharin intake equal to about 800 cans of diet soda. Further research found no evidence to suggest that saccharin caused cancer in humans if used in food products, and in late 2000 Congress voted to repeal the requirement for the warning label.

Acesulfame-K is a man-made sweetener and is marketed under the brand names Sunett and SweetOne. It has been reviewed and determined to be safe by regulatory authorities in more than 20 countries. Its safety is supported by more than 90 studies conducted over 15 years. Unlike aspartame, it is heat-stable and can be used in cooking and baking.

Sucralose is the first sugar substitute made from sugar and is marketed as Splenda. It has no calories and can be used virtually anywhere sugar can be used, including cooking. It can be used in baking as well, but it works best in recipes developed specifically for its use. Extensive studies have been conducted and evaluated to show and support that sucralose is safe for humans to use.

The newest non-nutritive sweetener approved by the FDA is neotame. It is similar to aspartame in that it is composed of two amino acids, aspartic acid and phenylalanine. Neotame can be used alone or in combination with other nonnutritive or nutritive sweeteners in foods and beverages.

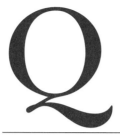 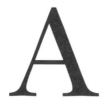

240.
How much diet soda can I safely drink during the day?

The majority of diet sodas available in stores these days contain aspartame, also known as NutraSweet and Equal. Aspartame is a noncaloric sweetener (others include saccharin, acesulfame-K, sucralose, and neotame) available for use in foods and as a tabletop sweetener. Comprised of two amino acids, aspartic acid and phenylalanine, aspartame breaks down during digestion and is then used in normal body processes.

Aspartame is approximately 200 times sweeter than regular sugar, and it has no effect on blood glucose levels, making this an acceptable sugar alternative for people who have diabetes.

In addition to diet sodas, aspartame can be found in many low-calorie foods, such as chewing gum, candy, dessert mixes, gelatins, yogurt, and even some medications.

The question of safety always arises when anything considered "artificial" is added to food products, and it's no different with aspartame. This sweetener has been tested for three decades in no less than 200 clinical studies, all of which have produced similar results—that aspartame is safe for human consumption. Both the American Medical Association and the American Diabetes Association have reviewed the studies on aspartame and concluded that it is safe to use. Furthermore, the Food and Drug Administration (FDA) has set an Acceptable Daily Intake (ADI) for aspartame, which indicates the amount of the sweetener that can be safely consumed on a daily basis over one's lifetime without causing adverse effects. This ADI is expressed as an amount per body weight. The ADI for aspartame is 50 milligrams per kilogram of body weight per day.

Here's an example to give you an idea, then, of how much diet soda you can drink daily without exceeding the ADI for aspartame: A 150-pound person would have to consume twenty 12-ounce cans of diet soda each day to reach the ADI.

That's a lot of diet soda! However, if you drink more than this amount of diet soda daily, chances are that you're still within safety limits set by the FDA. The

Q A

ADI amount is a conservative amount and has an automatic safety level built in. In fact, the ADI is just 1% of the level that has been tested and shown to be safe. Nevertheless, if you're at all concerned about the amount of aspartame in your diet, decrease the amount of diet soda and other aspartame-containing foods you consume. Remember that water is always the best choice!

The only people who should not consume aspartame are those who have phenylketonuria, a rare genetic disorder (about one in 15,000 babies born in the United States inherits this disorder). People who have this disorder cannot metabolize phenylalanine, one of the ingredients in aspartame, which can cause health problems, including mental retardation. In the United States and many other countries, routine screening for this disorder is required for all newborns. Foods that contain aspartame, including diet soda, must carry a warning label with these words: "Phenylketonurics: Contains Phenylalanine."

241.
What are sugar alcohols? Do they affect my blood glucose in any way?

Sugar alcohols, sometimes called polyols, are sweeteners that are naturally found in plant foods such as berries and fruits. (By the way, these substances do not contain alcohol!) They are typically used by food manufacturers for their sweetening ability. When used as a replacement for regular sugar, sugar alcohols provide between one-third to one-half fewer calories than sugar. In addition, sugar alcohols have little affect on blood glucose levels, since they don't require insulin to be metabolized.

You can identify a sugar alcohol by scanning the ingredient list on the Nutrition Facts Label. Typical sugar alcohols include sorbitol, mannitol, xylitol, isomalt, lactitol, maltitol, and hydrogenated starch hydrolysates (HSH). Foods that contain these ingredients are generally the "no sugar added" and "sugar free" versions of ice creams, cookies, and candies, but you'll also find sugar alcohols in cough drops, toothpaste, and some mouthwashes.

Before you jump on the sugar alcohol bandwagon and assume you can eat a whole box of sugar-free cookies, remember to check the label for total carbohydrate content. You may be surprised to see that, yes, even these sugar-free foods can have a considerable amount of carbohydrate. For example, a regular ice cream bar (1 serving) contains 15 grams of carbohydrate and 160 calories and is one carbohydrate serving. An ice cream bar (1 serving) sweetened with a sugar alcohol contains 13 grams of carbohydrate and 120 calories and is also one carbohydrate serving. As you can see, either ice cream bar is 1 carbohydrate serving. So why are sugar alcohols used, then?

Well, food manufacturers use them for a couple of reasons, one being to help market "special" foods to people with diabetes. Another reason is that sugar alcohols contain fewer calories than regular sugar—about 2 calories per gram instead of 4 calories per gram.

The downside of these sugar alcohols is that, when eaten in excess, they can cause some unpleasant gastrointestinal side effects such as gassiness, cramping, and diarrhea. Some people are very sensitive to even very small amounts of sugar alcohols in foods. A warning concerning excess consumption and the laxative effects is only required on the food label for certain foods and when used in large amounts.

In addition, many foods that contain ingredients such as sorbitol and mannitol can be high in overall calories and total fat. When eaten in excess, these foods could lead to both higher blood glucose levels and weight gain.

Sugar alcohols must be listed in grams on the Nutrition Facts panel for all sugar-free and no-sugar-added foods, just under the Total Carbohydrate section.

Vitamins and Minerals

242.
Don't I need a special vitamin supplement for my diabetes? My drugstore carries some that are geared toward people with diabetes.

There are so many varieties of nutrition and vitamin supplements on the market these days that you may

Q A

feel you need a medical degree to figure it all out. It certainly becomes confusing, especially when you see special supplements aimed at people who have diabetes. Should you spend the extra few dollars on these in hopes of helping to manage your diabetes?

First off, realize that nutritional supplements are big business. Almost half of all Americans take a multivitamin, and of these, 80% take them for good health. Yet, on the flip side, many people don't take supplements, either because they don't know what to take or because they prefer to get their nutrition in food form.

Second, there is some evidence that people with diabetes need higher levels of the antioxidant nutrients, such as vitamin C and vitamin E, for example. Antioxidants help to counteract the effects of free radicals, which are by-products of cell metabolism. The chief danger of free radicals is the damage they can do when they react with important cell components. The body has several enzyme systems that scavenge free radicals, but the principal antioxidants come from vitamins in the diet. Studies have shown that some of the complications of diabetes (retinopathy and neuropathy) may occur due to damage from free radicals.

Third, people with diabetes are more prone to developing heart disease. High levels of homocysteine, an amino acid, have been linked to heart disease in Type 2 diabetes and to kidney disease. The B vitamins can help to lower levels of homocysteine, and therefore help reduce the risk of these two complications as well.

Many of the "diabetes" vitamin supplements contain higher doses of the above nutrients, plus some other nutrients that are also thought to play a role in reducing diabetes complications. However, it's important not to "megadose" on any one nutrient. Remember that nutrients, while natural, can have harmful effects in large amounts. Also, popping pills does not substitute for a nutritious diet. You still need to aim for at least 3–5 servings of fruits and vegetables every day.

While there's still a lot to learn about nutrient requirements for people with diabetes, most experts in the field agree that you don't need to spend more

Q   A

money for a diabetes vitamin supplement. The store brand is usually just fine, or choose a brand name that you trust. If you're not sure, speak with a dietitian or the pharmacist at your drugstore. And look for supplements that have expiration dates and display the USP (United States Pharmacopeia) symbol on the bottle. Last but not least, speak with your physician or dietitian before taking any kind of nutrition supplement (vitamins included), and always be sure to inform your health-care team at each visit of any supplements you take.

**243.
Are there some vitamin or mineral supplements that have been shown to be particularly helpful?**

Folate and calcium are two micronutrients that people with diabetes may need to take as supplements. The role of folate in preventing birth defects is widely accepted, and as a result many wheat and grain products in the United States are fortified with folate. Folate supplementation is especially important for any women considering becoming pregnant; 400 micrograms of folic acid from fortified foods and/or as a supplement is recommended for all women of childbearing age for the prevention of neural tube defects and other congenital abnormalities. Another role for folate is under investigation. An association between elevated levels of homocysteine and coronary heart disease has been shown to exist, and it has been speculated that folate supplementation may lower homocysteine levels. Stay tuned as the results from research trials are reported. The good news is that there are very few health concerns from folate supplementation.

A daily intake of 1,000 to 1,500 milligrams of calcium, especially in older persons with diabetes, is recommended. Women with Type 1 diabetes are at increased risk for an early onset of osteoporosis, and older women with Type 2 diabetes are at increased risk of bone fractures compared with women who do not have diabetes. In one study, older women with diabetes were 80% to 90% more likely to have a hip or shoulder fracture. Men with diabetes are also at risk for osteoporosis and fractures. The reason is not completely clear, but it may be because insulin is

Q A

needed for the development of strong bones. Foods, juices, and supplements can all be good sources of calcium. If you use calcium supplements, take them with meals to improve absorption. In addition, the body can absorb only a certain amount of calcium, so no more than 500 to 600 milligrams of calcium should be taken at a time.

Besides calcium, the National Osteoporosis Foundation recommends 400–800 IU per day of vitamin D. Ninety percent of our vitamin D supply comes from the skin, which synthesizes it when exposed to sunlight. Therefore, vitamin D deficiencies can occur in people who spend most of their time indoors. Vitamin D is added to most milk, but if people do not drink milk and are not exposed to the sun, they may need to take a supplement.

244.
Should people with diabetes take antioxidant supplements?

The evidence here is mixed. The Institute of Medicine of the National Academies assembles authorities in nutrition and medicine to determine what nutrients and how much are necessary for good health and to prevent disease. After reviewing all the evidence, they concluded that megadoses of antioxidants—vitamin C, vitamin E, selenium, beta-carotene, and other carotenoids—have not been proven to protect against heart and blood vessel diseases, diabetes, or various forms of cancer. In fact, they concluded the opposite may be true, that high dosages of antioxidants may lead to health problems, including diarrhea, bleeding, and toxic reactions.

Large population studies that looked at associations between nutrients and prevention of health problems did show a positive relationship between good health and antioxidant intake. However, large intervention studies in which supplements of antioxidants were compared to placebos failed to show any benefit from taking supplements, and in some cases suggested adverse effects. For example, two studies of cigarette smokers at high risk for the development of lung cancer found an unexplained increase in lung cancer in those taking beta-carotene.

Other studies have looked specifically at vitamin E and potential benefits. Of interest is the Heart Out-

205

Q A

comes Prevention Evaluation (HOPE) trial, which included 9,541 persons, 38% of whom had diabetes. Supplementation with 400 IU of vitamin E per day for four to six years failed to show either a decrease or an increase in the number of heart attacks, strokes, and deaths. Some researchers hypothesized that the primary function of antioxidants may be to prevent the formation of lesions that lead to athero-sclerosis and that for the people in this study, who were already at high risk for cardiovascular disease, vitamin E supplementation may have been a case of too little too late.

In any case, the American Diabetes Association does not advise routine supplementation with antioxidants because of their uncertainty regarding long-term benefit and safety.

245.
What is alpha-lipoic acid? Is it something I should be taking for my diabetes?

Alpha-lipoic acid is sometimes nicknamed the "universal antioxidant" because it can help fight off many different kinds of free radicals, by-products of metabolism that can cause cellular damage in the body. This vitamin-like antioxidant is produced in the body and is more powerful than vitamins C, E, and beta-carotene.

Because it is made in the body, alpha-lipoic acid is not considered an essential nutrient. However, many researchers feel that this substance plays important roles in maintaining good health.

Alpha-lipoic acid has shown some promise in the management of diabetes. It's currently used in Europe to treat and prevent diabetes-related complications, cataracts, and macular degeneration, and even to reduce insulin doses. In particular, diabetic neuropathy (nerve damage) has been shown to be relieved by taking alpha-lipoic acid. A few studies indicate that when people with neuropathy were given 600 milligrams of alpha-lipoic acid each day, symptoms of this painful condition were greatly reduced. A four-year clinical trial in the United States and in Europe is currently under way to determine if alpha-lipoic acid can be effective in treating neuropathy.

Q   A

This antioxidant may also help reduce blood glucose levels, based on some research with people with Type 2 diabetes. Again, it's still too soon to say for certain if it works well or not.

In case you're wondering, alpha-lipoic acid is found in some foods, but in very small amounts. To reap any benefit from this substance, it needs to be consumed in capsule form.

As you may have gathered, it's still a little early to routinely recommend alpha-lipoic acid as part of a diabetes treatment plan. However, if you have diabetic neuropathy, it's worthwhile to discuss taking this with your physician. The supplement is relatively inexpensive, and there are no known major side effects. If you do decide to try this, as with any supplement, be sure to inform your health-care team and be diligent about monitoring your blood glucose levels.

246.
What are the American Diabetes Association recommendations for people with diabetes regarding vitamin and mineral supplements?

After reviewing all the research, the American Diabetes Association nutrition technical review concluded that there is no clear evidence that people with diabetes will benefit from vitamin or mineral supplements if they do not have underlying deficiencies. The problem is that it is difficult to test and know if individuals are deficient in vitamins and minerals, but if a deficiency can be determined, supplementation can be beneficial. There are two exceptions: Folate is recommended for the prevention of birth defects and calcium for the prevention of bone disease.

It is important that everyone, including people with diabetes, get their daily vitamin and mineral requirements from a healthy diet. A healthy diet is one that includes at a minimum five servings a day from fruits and vegetables, three servings of whole grains, and one to two glasses of low-fat milk or its equivalent. There are, however, some groups within the population who might benefit from supplementation with a multivitamin supplement. These are elderly individuals, pregnant or lactating women, strict vegetarians, and people on calorie-restricted diets.

Q   A

247.

How much calcium should I be consuming in a day? Should I take calcium supplements?

Here is a rough guide to the amount of calcium people need:
- Ages 11–24: 1,200–1,500 mg/day
- Healthy adults: 1,000 mg/day
- Pregnant or lactating women: 1,200 mg/day
- Postmenopausal women (not on hormone replacement therapy): 1,500 mg/day
- Men over 65: 1,500 mg/day

If you are not reaching your calcium needs, consult your physician as to the best supplement to take. People who are prone to kidney stones or who have a family history of kidney problems should consult a doctor before taking any calcium supplement.

248.

How can I be sure I am absorbing enough iron from the food that I eat?

Iron in animal foods (poultry, lean beef, fish, pork, liver) is more easily absorbed than iron in plant foods (dried beans and peas, vegetables, and fruits). For best absorption, these foods should be eaten together. To absorb more iron from the food you eat, here are some tips:
- Cook foods in iron cookware. The longer it is cooked, the more iron the food will absorb.
- Eat foods that are high in vitamin C together with iron-containing plant foods such as potatoes, tomatoes, strawberries, and cantaloupe for better iron absorption.
- Iron absorption from food may be blocked when you drink coffee or tea with meals. Instead, drink your coffee and tea between meals.

249.

Will taking chromium picolinate supplements improve blood glucose levels?

Recently, two randomized, placebo-controlled studies of Chinese persons with diabetes reported beneficial effects on glucose using very large amounts (1,000 micrograms) of chromium picolinate. Unfortunately, in these studies the chromium status of the participants was not evaluated either at the beginning or at

Q A

the end of the studies. Therefore, it is not known if the study population was or was not deficient in chromium. In the United States, the group that set the Dietary Reference Intake recommendations could not find enough evidence to set a requirement for chromium, but they did determine that an adequate intake is 35 micrograms for men under 50 and 30 micrograms for men over 50. For women, an adequate intake was determined to be 25 micrograms for those under 50 and 20 micrograms for those over 50. These are very small amounts, easily attainable through a normal diet. Since chromium is quite widely distributed in a variety of foods, it is unlikely that persons living in the United States are chromium deficient.

Prior to these studies, three well-designed studies in persons with diabetes compared chromium to a placebo and found no benefit from chromium. Recently, the Office of Dietary Supplements, National Institutes of Health, reviewed all the randomized clinical trials of chromium done in subjects with and without Type 2 diabetes to determine the effect of dietary chromium supplements on blood glucose control. They concluded that data from randomized controlled trials show no effect of chromium on glucose or insulin levels in persons without diabetes and that the data from similar trials in persons with diabetes was inconclusive. They summarized data from 15 trials and 618 participants and reported that only the study done in subjects with diabetes in China found that chromium reduced average blood glucose levels. However, even though chromium supplementation is unlikely to be beneficial, few adverse effects have been reported with excess intake of chromium. As a result, the Dietary Reference Intake committee could not establish an upper level that would be safe (called a tolerable upper intake level).

250.
What about claims that chromium picolinate can burn body fat?

You've heard the saying, "If it sounds too good to be true, it probably is." Once again, there is no reliable evidence that shows taking chromium picolinate can help with weight loss or help build muscle.

Q A
Blood Pressure

251.
What can you do to lower blood pressure?

Reducing sodium intake and moderate weight loss are proven strategies for lowering blood pressure. For some reason, people with diabetes appear to be more "sodium sensitive" than people who don't have diabetes. As a result, persons with diabetes and either normal or high blood pressure may experience a more positive response to lowering sodium intake than the general public will. The goal should be to reduce sodium intake to 2,400 mg sodium per day. In addition, a modest amount of weight loss beneficially affects blood pressure.

Perhaps you have heard or read about the DASH diet. The Dietary Approaches to Stop Hypertension (DASH) study revealed that a diet low in total fat, saturated fat, and cholesterol and that includes fruits and vegetables (five to nine servings per day) and low-fat dairy products (two to four servings per day) can effectively lower blood pressure, even without weight loss. Reducing sodium intake lowered blood pressure levels further.

252.
What are some tips for lowering sodium intake?

Table salt is composed of two minerals: sodium and chloride. About one-third of the sodium in our diets comes straight from the saltshaker, so cutting down on table salt is a good way to cut down on sodium. However, two-thirds of the sodium in our diet comes from other sources, primarily processed foods, so cutting back on these can also reduce your sodium intake.

Although some sodium is necessary for the body to function, we consume far more than we need. The body requires only about 220 milligrams of sodium per day, or the equivalent of one-tenth a teaspoon of salt. (One teaspoon of salt contains 2,300 milligrams of sodium). We could easily get all the sodium we need, even if we never added salt in processing or cooking food. The average daily intake of sodium is 4,000 to 5,000 milligrams, or two to three teaspoons of salt. The following are some tips for reducing salt in your diet:

Q A

- Add little or no salt to foods at the table. Leave the saltshaker in the cupboard, and pass the pepper!
- Taste foods before deciding if they really need salt.
- Cook without adding salt. When cooking pastas, vegetables, and cereals you can skip the salt without losing the flavor. In some recipes, you can leave out the salt altogether or you can use half the salt called for. However, many recipes for baked foods, especially those with yeast, require salt for the recipe to work.
- Read food labels and look for foods with 400 milligrams or less sodium per serving and 800 milligrams or less sodium per convenience dinner or entrée.
- Avoid high-sodium foods such as ham, bacon, sausage, and cold cuts.
- Rinse canned foods with fresh water to reduce the sodium content. For example, rinsing the contents of a can of tuna for one minute will wash away three-fourths of the sodium. Almost half the sodium can be removed from canned vegetables by rinsing for one minute and heating the vegetables in water instead of the canning liquid.
- Use herbs and spices instead of salt. Begin by using no more than one or two herbs or spices at one time. As a general rule, use ¼ teaspoon of dried herbs or 3 to 4 teaspoons of the fresh herb for every 4 servings of food. Add herbs or seasonings to soups or stews during the last hour of cooking to retain flavor. In cold dressings, dips, or marinades, add herbs and spices several hours before serving to blend the flavors.
- Limit your use of salt-based condiments such as soy sauce, steak sauce, catsup, and Worcestershire sauce, or use low-salt varieties.
- Substitute onion or garlic powders for onion or garlic salts.
- Choose low-sodium or lower-salt crackers, snacks, and soups.
- Limit your use of fast foods. If you have a meal of fast foods, be especially careful of your food choices containing sodium for the rest of the day.

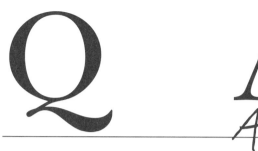

Alcohol

253.
What effect does alcohol have on blood glucose levels?

The effect of alcohol on blood glucose levels depends on how much an individual drinks, if the alcohol is consumed with or without food, if alcohol use is chronic and excessive, and if an individual uses insulin or certain glucose-lowering drugs. Research in people with either Type 1 or Type 2 diabetes who drank moderate amounts of alcohol (two drinks or less) with food showed no effect from alcohol on blood glucose or insulin levels. However, in persons who use insulin, drinking alcohol without food has been shown to cause hypoglycemia (low blood glucose levels), and this risk of hypoglycemia can continue for 12 hours or more. Alcohol can lower blood glucose levels because it does not get changed into glucose when being metabolized. So if individuals drink without food, there is no new source of glucose available and hypoglycemia can result.

For those who choose to drink alcoholic beverages, adult men should limit their consumption to two drinks per day, and adult women to one drink per day. When moderate amounts are consumed with food, blood glucose levels are not affected. For people who use insulin or oral blood-glucose-lowering drugs that stimulate insulin release, alcohol should be consumed with food to reduce the risk of hypoglycemia. The same precautions that apply to the general population regarding alcohol use also apply to persons with diabetes. Pregnant women and people with medical problems such as pancreatitis, advanced neuropathy, or alcohol abuse shouldn't drink at all.

254.
Does the type of alcohol one drinks make a difference?

Before you use alcohol of any type, discuss with your doctor how alcohol may interact with any drugs you are using. The type of alcoholic beverage you drink does not make a difference. All alcoholic beverages begin as carbohydrates (grains or fruit). By the process of fermentation, the glucose is converted to alcohol. Generally, different drinks contain alcohol in different concentrations. One drink of alcohol is usually defined as 5 ounces of wine, 1.5 ounces of distilled spirits (hard liquor), or 12 ounces of beer. Each of these contains about ½ ounce or about 15 grams of alcohol. Light beer is usually recommended because it has less carbohydrate than regular beer. Alcoholic beverages should be considered an addition to your meal plan and no food should be omitted.

Alcohol appears in the blood within five minutes after drinking. Food in the stomach will slow the rate of alcohol absorption by delaying stomach emptying. Dry wines and light beer may be better choices since they are lower in carbohydrate. However, alcohol itself is high in calories and is usually planned into the meal plan as the equivalent of two fat exchanges (calorie-wise). In general, alcohol should be consumed only when diabetes is well controlled and with the advice of your physician.

255.
When a drug label says "avoid alcohol," does that mean "absolutely no alcohol," or is it all right for me to have a cold beer after mowing the lawn?

As with any drug interaction, the overall effect depends on several variables. Drug interactions with alcohol can be categorized into five main types:

1. Enhancing or multiplying the effect of central nervous system depressants. Usually a result of combining alcohol with other sedative or depressant agents—including diazepam (brand name Valium) and other benzodiazepines, chloral hydrate (Noctec, Aquachloral), over-the-counter sleeping aids, barbiturates, muscle relaxants, and some drugs used to treat anxiety—this interaction can cause altered coordination and impaired judgment.

2. Accumulating a toxic chemical called acetaldehyde because of altered alcohol metabolism. This may result in flushing, increased breathing and heart rate, and even death. Specific drugs leading to this toxic interaction with alcohol include disulfiram (Antabuse), some injectable cephalosporin antibiotics, the antimicrobial furazolidone (Furoxone), and the more commonly prescribed antibiotic metronidazole (Flagyl). People taking metronidazole should avoid drinking alcohol until at least 48 hours after their last dose.

3. Increasing the concentration of alcohol in the blood when a drug inhibits an enzyme in the stom-

ach responsible for helping to break down alcohol. The degree and severity of this interaction depends on the amount of alcohol-metabolizing enzyme in the gut and the dose or concentration of the inhibitor. This interaction, which can lead to acute intoxication, is reported with over-the-counter agents used for heartburn or dyspepsia, such as cimetidine (Tagamet), famotidine (Pepcid), and ranitidine (Zantac).

4. Increasing the amount of certain enzymes within the liver that metabolize other drugs, especially with chronic or daily alcohol ingestion, particularly heavy intake. The most significant interaction causes acetaminophen (Tylenol) to be toxic to the liver at smaller doses than usual. Acetaminophen should be limited to no more than 2 grams per day in people who drink alcohol regularly.

5. Increasing the rate of absorption of alcohol because of a drug that promotes stomach emptying. This can lead to acute intoxication. Taking alcohol with metoclopramide (Reglan), an agent frequently used to treat slow stomach-emptying, or gastroparesis, in people who have diabetes, may lead to a sharper than usual rise in blood levels of alcohol.

So whether to have that cold beer after mowing the lawn depends on which medicines you might be taking and how much alcohol you drink on a regular basis. Of course, it would be ill advised to drink beer—with or without another depressant drug— before going out to mow the lawn or handling heavy equipment or machinery. It is always best to ask your physician or pharmacist about the likelihood of a severe adverse effect resulting from the use of alcohol and alcohol-containing products with any drug you are taking.

People who have diabetes must also consider the effects of alcohol on blood glucose and their overall health. On average, people with diabetes should not exceed one drink per day for women or two drinks per day for men and should always drink alcohol with a meal rather than on an empty stomach to avoid the risk of hypoglycemia. Furthermore, the calories in the alcohol-containing beverage should be considered in the overall count for the meal.

Q A

256.
Are there other risks and benefits of alcohol consumption?

Heavy and excessive alcohol consumption is a leading, avoidable cause of death in the United States. Furthermore, chronic alcohol consumption (three or more drinks per day) can lead to deterioration in both short- and long-term blood glucose control.

However, some benefits from alcohol have also been reported. In persons without diabetes, light-to-moderate amounts of alcohol are associated with decreased risks of Type 2 diabetes and stroke and improved insulin sensitivity. In adults with diabetes, light-to-moderate amounts are associated with decreased risk of coronary heart disease, which may be because alcohol can raise HDL cholesterol (the good cholesterol) and improve insulin sensitivity.

Light-to-moderate amounts of alcohol also do not raise triglyceride or blood pressure levels, but excessive intakes of alcohol can cause elevated blood pressure and possibly high triglyceride levels.

If you don't drink, you probably shouldn't start. Regular exercise can have the same potential benefit as moderate amounts of alcohol, and for many people, exercise will be more appropriate. If you do choose to have an alcoholic beverage, watch the amount. And enjoy!

Physical Activity

257.
I am looking for foods I can carry with me to treat possible hypoglycemic reactions when I am out walking. Any recommendations?

The general rule for treating a low blood glucose is to consume about 15 grams of carbohydrate and recheck blood glucose levels in 15 minutes. Some easy-to-carry treatment foods that contain 15 grams of carbohydrate include a 4-ounce "kid size" juice box, 8 LifeSavers, 9 small gumdrops, 10 small jelly beans, or 6 large jelly beans. However, 3–4 glucose tablets work as well as any of these and provide fewer calories. Remember, never use a treatment food that has fat in it, such as chocolate. The fat can delay the food from

Q A

emptying from your stomach and may work too slowly.

258.
What insulin or carbohydrate adjustments should you make for exercise?

For people who take insulin (and perhaps for individuals who use medicines that stimulate the release of insulin), exercise can increase risks for both hypoglycemia (low blood glucose levels) and, occasionally, hyperglycemia (high blood glucose levels). The most common risk is for hypoglycemia, but the most common time for hypoglycemia to occur is after, not during, exercise. This is because when you exercise your body uses stored glucose (glycogen) when you exercise, and glucose stores must be replaced after exercise, thus lowering blood glucose level. Furthermore, your body is more sensitive to the actions of insulin after exercise. However, hypoglycemia can occur during exercise if your blood glucose level started to drop before you began. This illustrates one of the problems of blood glucose testing: It only tells you what your blood glucose level is at the moment of testing and not, for example, what it was an hour before.

Hyperglycemia can be the result of high-intensity exercise. High-intensity exercise, just like illness, can be stressful, and stress hormones can raise blood glucose levels. We need energy for this type of exercise, but not knowing how much is needed, our bodies will release excessive amounts of glucose from glycogen stores. You can't do much about this situation except wait for your blood glucose level to drop again, but you can take some precautions to prevent hypoglycemia.

To prevent low blood glucose, you can reduce your insulin dose for the time of exercise or you can eat extra carbohydrate. For planned exercise, reducing your insulin dose may be preferred. However, carbohydrate-containing foods should always be readily available during and after exercise. The amount of carbohydrate you should plan on needing should be based on your blood glucose levels before and after exercise, previous exercise experiences,

Q A

and your insulin regimen. In general, exercise of moderate intensity requires about 8–13 grams of carbohydrate per hour above your usual (non-exercise) requirements. During high-intensity exercise, this requirement is doubled. This need for additional carbohydrate is the basis for the recommendation to eat 15–30 extra grams of carbohydrate either before or after an hour of exercise, depending on the intensity of the exercise and your blood glucose level at the start of exercise.

259.
Wouldn't it be a good idea for a person to load up on carbohydrates before going out for a long run?

Carbohydrate loading is a strategy used by endurance athletes to increase the body's reserve of muscle glycogen and thus improve their performance. Glycogen is the body's storage form of glucose. When carbohydrates are eaten, the body changes much of them into glucose. The glucose that is not needed immediately is stored as glycogen for later use. Unfortunately, people with diabetes have an impaired ability to store and mobilize carbohydrate in the right amounts at the right times. This means that carbohydrate loading is not an option for people with diabetes. Instead, extra calories need to be consumed during exercise, based on one's current blood glucose level, insulin action, the intensity of the exercise, and how long the exercise will last.

Common Concerns

260.
What is the best way to treat a low blood glucose level?

You may have heard the 15:15 rule: If blood glucose levels are lower than 50 mg/dl you should immediately ingest 15 grams of carbohydrate, wait 15 minutes, and test again, and, if necessary, treat again with 15 grams of carbohydrate. (However, blood glucose levels between 60 mg/dl and 80 mg/dl also usually require treatment.) This is a good rule, but something should be added: Just testing in 15 minutes is not enough. Blood glucose levels begin to drop again

Q A

in about 60 minutes, so it is important to retest at that time, as treatment with additional carbohydrate may be needed.

Research studies suggest that glucose is the preferred treatment for hypoglycemia, although any form of carbohydrate that contains glucose may be used. There really is no "fast-acting carbohydrate" that will be absorbed faster than another carbohydrate (glucose would be the only possibility). When blood glucose levels are low, the gastric tract will speed up gastric emptying and any form of carbohydrate—liquid or solid—will be absorbed as rapidly as is possible.

Treatment of low blood glucose (hypoglycemia) with 10 grams of glucose has been shown to raise plasma glucose levels from approximately 60 mg/dl to approximately 100 mg/dl over 30 minutes, with plasma glucose levels starting to fall again after 60 minutes. Treatment with 20 grams of glucose raised plasma glucose from about 60 mg/dl to about 120 mg/dl over 45 minutes, with plasma glucose again starting to fall in 60 minutes. In short, 15–20 grams of carbohydrate can be an effective, but temporary treatment for hypoglycemia. Adding protein to the treatment of hypoglycemia has been advised in the past as a way of slowing the absorption of glucose, but the practice has not been shown to be helpful. In a study in which either 15 grams or carbohydrate or 15 grams of carbohydrate plus 14 grams of protein were used to treat blood glucose levels of 50 mg/dl, both treatments were equally effective, and adding the protein did not prevent blood glucose levels from dropping again in about 60 minutes. The researchers concluded that adding protein to the treatment of hypoglycemia only added unnecessary and often unwanted calories.

The bottom line: Although glucose is recommended as the optimal treatment for low blood glucose, use whatever type or form of carbohydrate is convenient. Remember, all carbohydrates will eventually raise glucose levels, so just *treat*.

Q A

261.
Whenever I have a low blood glucose, I usually treat it with a candy bar. But then I find that my blood glucose level doesn't rise fast enough and I have to eat more. What's going on?

Low blood glucose, known as hypoglycemia, typically occurs when blood glucose levels drop below 70 mg/dl. At this point, it's very important to treat it to prevent it from dropping further and, of course, to raise the level.

Symptoms of hypoglycemia include shakiness, lightheadedness, sweating, irritability, and confusion, to name just a few. Sometimes, people with diabetes do not experience symptoms; they may feel fine, but unless they receive treatment, there's a real danger of their blood glucose dropping too low, with a resulting loss of consciousness.

The best way to treat low blood glucose is to take in some form of carbohydrate, usually in the form of sugar. Examples include glucose tablets, LifeSavers, fruit juice, regular soda, and honey. After checking your blood glucose level, eat 15 grams of carbohydrate. Recheck your blood glucose 10–15 minutes later to be sure it has risen above 70 mg/dl. If it has not, treat again with another 15 grams of carbohydrate. Any of the following is equal to about 15 grams of carbohydrate:

- 4 glucose tablets
- 1 tablespoon of honey
- 4 teaspoons of sugar
- 4 ounces of fruit juice
- 6 ounces of regular soda
- 8 LifeSavers

You will notice that candy bars are not on the list, nor is any kind of chocolate, for that matter. The reason has to do with the high fat content of chocolate. Fat slows down the digestion and absorption of carbohydrate from the intestinal tract to the bloodstream. Under normal circumstances, say after a meal, this is good—it means that your blood glucose won't "spike" so high after eating. But when you're experiencing a hypoglycemic episode, you need that carbohydrate to work fast. Candy bars and other high-fat foods are

219

Q A

therefore not recommended for treating low blood glucose.

Another reason that chocolate is not such a good choice to use as a treatment for low blood glucose is that it's quite high in calories. It's very common for people with diabetes to overtreat low blood glucose. If you constantly use chocolate for treatment, not only will your blood glucose not rise quickly enough, you may end up gaining weight in the process!

It's always a good idea to review the treatment of hypoglycemia with your health-care team and discuss your individual blood glucose goals.

262.
I have been told to drink water when my blood glucose level is elevated. How does this help? Or does it?

Drinking water doesn't actually help to lower your blood glucose. However, high blood glucose can cause dehydration. The body responds to a high blood glucose level by increasing urination, and "flushing out" the blood glucose into the urine. This, in turn, leads to dehydration. Therefore, it is important to drink water or noncaloric, decaffeinated drinks (6 to 8 cups per day) to make sure you stay well hydrated on a daily basis.

263.
Why are blood glucose levels often high in the morning even if you didn't eat at bedtime?

People with diabetes often mistakenly believe that blood glucose levels are high before breakfast because they ate too much either for dinner or before they went to bed the night before. First, let's review what happens to blood glucose levels after eating food or a meal. After eating, blood glucose levels reach a peak between 45 to 90 minutes and, if there is adequate insulin available, return to premeal blood glucose levels in four to five hours. No research is available to suggest there are ways to extend this time frame. Therefore, what you eat is used for energy or stored in four to five hours. (If you eat smaller amounts of food, this time can be shorter). What you eat the evening before can affect your blood glucose levels during the middle of the night but not the next morning.

Q   A

So why are blood glucose levels often higher in the morning than they were before bedtime? The answer has to do with the liver and the glucose stored there in the form of glycogen. Sometimes, blood glucose may be elevated in the morning because of the "dawn phenomenon," which simply means that in the early morning hours the liver releases glucose, presumably to prepare the body for daytime activity. This happens in everyone, but in people who do not have diabetes, their bodies make enough insulin so the glucose can be used and blood glucose levels are normal. But if you have diabetes, the beta cells of your pancreas may not be able to release enough insulin to keep your blood glucose level normal, and this results in above-normal blood glucose levels.

There may be another reason for elevated morning blood glucose levels in persons who take insulin or perhaps medicine that stimulates the release of insulin. If your blood glucose level drops too low during the night, your liver will sense this drop and respond by releasing glucose. This can happen because you ate nothing or not enough, or simply because too much insulin was available. Because your liver does not know exactly how much glucose to release, it will likely release more than is actually needed, thus leading to the elevation in morning glucose readings. This is called a rebound hyperglycemia or the Somogyi effect.

A less likely explanation is that your body simply may not sense that your blood glucose levels are already elevated, or that you have enough available glucose, and the liver just keeps on releasing glucose.

The bottom line is that it is more complicated than just blaming food at bedtime.

264.
I have Type 1 diabetes. What should I do if I get the flu and can't eat?

Colds, fever, flu, vomiting, and diarrhea—all common problems—can cause special problems for people with diabetes. If not handled appropriately, these types of short-term illness in individuals with Type 1 diabetes can quickly result in diabetic ketoacidosis, a life-threatening condition that requires prompt treatment. During illness, stress hormones increase, caus-

221

ing the liver to release extra glucose to give your body extra energy to cope with the illness, which in turn causes an increased need for insulin. For that reason, you must take your insulin, even if you can't eat because of nausea or vomiting.

When you're sick, it is essential that you test your blood glucose levels and your ketone level. If your blood glucose reading is higher than 240 mg/dl, it is especially important to test for ketones. The combination of a high blood glucose level and a moderate to high ketone level is a danger signal. It means you need more insulin. Call your health-care team if this happens.

It is also important to drink adequate amounts of fluid and to eat some carbohydrate, especially if your blood glucose level is less than 100 mg/dl. To prevent dehydration, begin by trying to drink a large glass of calorie-free liquid (water, diet soft drink, or tea) every hour. If you're nauseated or vomiting, take small sips of liquid—one or two tablespoons every 15 to 30 minutes. Fluids that contain sodium, such as broth, tomato juice, or sports drinks, are also helpful. To prevent starvation ketosis (ketones produced from breakdown of fat when glucose is unavailable for energy), you need about 150 to 200 grams of carbohydrate each day. This works best if you eat 45–50 grams of carbohydrate every three to four hours. If you can't tolerate regular food, eat liquid or soft carbohydrate foods, such as regular (not diet) soft drinks, juices, soups, and ice cream.

Call your health-care team immediately if you have any of the following symptoms:

■ You are vomiting and can't keep any liquids or carbohydrate down for more than three to four hours.

■ You have ketones in your urine or you test positive for ketones in your blood.

■ You begin to breathe rapidly or become drowsy. If you lose consciousness, someone must immediately call for assistance.

The bottom line: Never omit insulin. Remember that you may also need supplementary insulin. When the illness is over, return to your regular meal plan and insulin schedule. If you need help making insulin adjustments, call your physician or nurse educator for help.

Q A

265.
I take insulin three times a day, and my blood glucose is under pretty good control. My dietitian wants me to take snacks between meals, but I usually don't feel hungry. Can I get by without having to eat all these snacks?

The management of diabetes has come a long way since the discovery of insulin. For a long time, there were few kinds of insulin available, and for people who took insulin, this meant totally rearranging eating schedules to accommodate the "peak" times of these insulins. This also meant that people were often forced to eat between meals to prevent hypoglycemia.

Fortunately, with so many kinds of insulins available these days, rigid eating plans and strict schedules are a thing of the past. Eating plans can be much more individualized and tailored to your lifestyle and preferences.

The issue of snacking is often surrounded by controversy. On the one hand, you may be told to eat one to three snacks each day, and that otherwise you run a risk of having low blood glucose. On the other hand, if you don't feel hungry, or if your physician has recommended you lose weight, why eat more?

The best advice is to talk with your dietitian about your insulin regimen and your daily schedule. If your mealtimes are fairly close together, you may not need to eat a snack. If you take a longer-acting insulin that peaks midafternoon, see if the dose can be reduced to prevent having to eat at this time. You may even be able to decrease your shorter-acting insulin at mealtimes to prevent unnecessary snacking.

There are some instances where you may need (or want) to have a snack. For example, if you eat lunch at noon and supper not until, say, seven o'clock, you might be hungry. A small snack can ward off hunger pangs and prevent overeating at supper. Or if you exercise before supper, you may need to eat a snack to prevent low blood glucose during your workout. Finally, be sure to check your bedtime blood glucose level. You may need a small snack (even if you're not hungry), depending on the reading, to prevent your blood glucose from getting low overnight.

Q A

Remember, too, that a snack does not mean eating a large amount of food. A typical snack choice might be a piece of fresh fruit or 4–6 crackers, for example. Be sure to choose nutritious snacks and avoid "empty calorie" foods such as chips, cookies, or candy bars.

If your weight is a concern, but you find you need to take a snack or two during the day, your dietitian can help adjust your eating plan to reduce calories elsewhere, perhaps at one of your meals. And if you're snacking just to prevent frequent episodes of low blood glucose, speak to your physician or diabetes educator about reducing your insulin dose. Depending on your diabetes control, you may find that you can avoid having to snack altogether.

266.
Sometimes when I have a meal, I only want to have a salad, but if I use two units of insulin, I will have low blood glucose within the next hour. Any suggestions?

A registered dietitian can help you determine the ratio of insulin to carbohydrate that is right for you. This will allow you to calculate your insulin dosage at a meal based on your premeal blood glucose reading and the amount of carbohydrate you plan to eat at that meal. This will give you more flexibility to eat according to your appetite.

267.
Will becoming a vegetarian help my diabetes control?

A well-planned vegetarian diet can actually be a lot healthier than eating a meat-based diet. Studies show that vegetarians tend to have lower blood pressures, lower cholesterol levels, less heart disease, less cancer, and, overall, tend to be leaner than people who eat meat. So there's no reason for you not to follow a vegetarian meal plan, provided that it's well balanced and meets all your nutrient needs.

You may wonder how switching to vegetarian eating will affect your medication or insulin doses. Many people who take insulin end up needing less, and many people with Type 2 diabetes who manage their diabetes with pills can often decrease the dose or even get off the medication altogether. One main reason for this is that most people who become vegetari-

Q A

ans end up losing weight (as long as they also decrease their fat intake). Weight loss can help improve blood glucose control and can reduce medication requirements.

There are different kinds of vegetarian diets. Most people who become "vegetarian" tend to include some animal foods, usually from eggs and/or dairy products. These vegetarians are called "ovo-" or "lacto-ovo" vegetarians. Someone who totally avoids animal foods altogether is called a "vegan." Vegans need to be very careful to assure they receive adequate nutrition, especially protein and certain vitamins and minerals.

You can meet your nutritional needs with a vegetarian diet quite easily, but it does take some planning. It's a good idea to talk this over with a dietitian who is well-versed in planning vegetarian diets to make sure you're getting enough nutrients, especially protein, calcium, iron, and vitamin B_{12}. Your dietitian can also give you meal and snack suggestions. In addition, let your health-care team know if you make the switch; you may need guidance on how to reduce your insulin dose.

You'll need to monitor your blood glucose levels frequently when you change over to a vegetarian diet. This kind of food plan tends to be fairly high in carbohydrate, since many protein sources, such as dried beans and peas, will also contain carbohydrate. On the other hand, you'll likely be eating more fiber-rich foods, which may help to better control your blood glucose.

Finally, don't assume a vegetarian diet is always low in fat and saturated fat. If you're not careful, you can end up consuming more fat than you realize if you include cheeses, butter, and eggs in your eating plan on a regular basis. While a vegetarian eating plan can be heart-healthy, it still takes some effort to plan it appropriately.

268.
I have always had a sweet tooth and can't seem to break the habit. I crave sugar, especially chocolate. Any ideas on how to break a bad habit?

Nobody with diabetes is expected to give up all of his favorite foods. Within the context of a healthy

Q A

intake, you can select which foods you wish to spend your carbohydrate grams on. Remember, sugar is just a carbohydrate and is found naturally in some foods and added in other foods. Your main goal should be to eat healthy foods, but still allow yourself a treat once in a while. A registered dietitian can teach you how all foods can fit in a healthy meal plan.

269.
This is my first holiday season with diabetes. Any suggestions?

Holiday meals usually center around traditional holiday fare and old family favorites, which typically translates into calories, sugar, and fat. The true meaning of the holiday season often gets buried under the food table. However, food can still be enjoyed without putting on the pounds and wrecking your diabetes control. Here are some tips that will help:
■ Focus on conversation instead of standing next to the food table.
■ Avoid skipping meals or snacks in anticipation of a dinner party.
■ Don't be afraid to say "no, thanks" to food you really don't want.
■ Eat slowly and enjoy the flavor. You will end up eating less.
■ Use your carbohydrate "allowance" for treat foods.
■ Don't take a holiday from exercise.

270.
I've read that caffeine can raise blood glucose levels. Does this mean I should stop drinking my morning coffee?

No, but before you pour your sixth cup of coffee for the day, you might consider the possible effects of caffeine on your blood glucose levels. Caffeine, which is actually a drug, can enter the brain and cause hormonal changes. Some of these hormones (the "stress" hormones) cause a rise in blood pressure and also lead to higher blood glucose levels by stimulating the liver to release stored glucose. One of the stress hormones, epinephrine, is what causes your heart to pound and makes you feel jittery and nervous (think of how you feel when you've had too much coffee or diet cola).

Q A

One study published in the early 1990's did link higher blood glucose levels to an increased intake of caffeine—500 mg, to be exact. A cup of coffee contains about 100–150 mg of caffeine. Recently, though, another study was published that looked at the effect of caffeine on insulin sensitivity. The more "sensitive" to insulin you are, the more insulin will help to move glucose from your blood into your cells. This study found that caffeine decreased insulin sensitivity by 15% by stimulating epinephrine release. Blood pressure increased slightly, as well.

What does this mean? First, realize that this study looked at people who don't have diabetes. We don't know if the results would be the same in people with diabetes. Second, remember that this is just one study; you can't really make firm conclusions based on just one study. However, if you've been seeing some higher blood glucose readings, and/or if you find yourself taking more insulin or oral medicine to bring down blood glucose levels, and you consume a fair amount of caffeine (coffee, tea, diet colas), you might try cutting back on your caffeine intake to see how your blood glucose levels respond.

By the way, it's not a bad idea to decrease your caffeine intake anyway, especially if you have difficulty getting to sleep, are pregnant or lactating, have high blood pressure, or are at risk for osteoporosis.

271.
My doctor just diagnosed me with gastroparesis. He said to eat six small meals per day. What does this mean?

About 30% of persons with diabetes have this disorder. Gastroparesis is the complication that results when neuropathy strikes the nerves controlling your digestive tract. This abnormality interferes with the emptying of the stomach and absorption of food. This delay in stomach emptying does not match the peak action of insulin taken before meals and thus can cause wild swings in blood glucose levels. Symptoms of gastroparesis include nausea, vomiting, diarrhea, and constipation. Eating six small meals per day allows the stomach to empty more easily. Here are some other tips that can help:

Q A

- Eat a low-fat diet (fat slows down gastric emptying).
- Eat a low-fiber diet (indigestible fiber and skins from vegetables can collect in the stomach and form a ball called a bezoar).
- Try switching to liquids when you experience difficulty with gastric emptying.
- Stop smoking.
- Keeping blood sugar within the near-normal range is also very important to protect further nerve damage.

It is also a good idea to work with a dietitian to make sure you avoid foods that can contribute to delayed stomach emptying and to ensure you are getting all the nutrients you need in your meal plan.

**272.
I saw an advertisement for an all-natural pill that can lower my blood sugars—some kind of ancient remedy. Does this really work?**

These days, there's a natural "solution" for just about anything that ails you, ranging from colds to depression to obesity to…diabetes! The majority of these pills, or supplements, contain a mixture of various herbs and nutrient supplements. These supplements appeal to people because the thinking is, if it's natural, it's got to be safe, right? Not always!

Many of the supplements marketed to people with diabetes have been found to contain blood-glucose-lowering substances. But some have been contaminated with dirt or bug parts. And some don't contain any significant amount of the ingredients listed.

Supplements, by law, are not regulated by the Food and Drug Administration (FDA), although the FDA is imposing some standards for manufacturers of these supplements.

As far as ancient remedies go, it is true that many herbs do have blood-glucose-lowering effects. In fact, certain herbs such as fenugreek, gymnema sylvestre, and bitter melon, for example, have been used in various cultures for centuries to help treat diabetes. Other herbs, such as bilberry and ginkgo biloba, have been touted as helping to treat diabetes-related complications.

Do they work? Some do. The concern, though, is that knowledge is lacking as far as how much of these

Q A

supplements to take to lower blood glucose levels, or treat retinopathy, for example. And many of these herbs can have dangerous side effects if taken in large amounts, taken for an extended period of time, or if taken in conjunction with other medicines.

If you are truly interested in taking a supplement for your diabetes or any health-related condition, here are a few suggestions to heed:

■ Discuss the use of any supplement (herb, vitamin, or mineral) with your health-care team, especially if you take other medicines.

■ Avoid supplements if you are pregnant or lactating, unless advised otherwise by your health-care team. Also avoid giving supplements to children.

■ Become an informed consumer and learn more about the supplement you're interested in. Your physician may not know much about it, but share what you've learned with him or her.

■ Monitor your blood glucose levels carefully, and take note of any unusual symptoms or side effects; stop taking the supplement if these occur.

■ Use reputable, national brands of supplements, and shy away from foreign products, as these are more likely to be contaminated.

■ Follow directions on the container for dosage and frequency. If the amount seems excessive, avoid taking it or speak with your physician first.

Finally, remember that most supplements are not necessarily intended for long-term use. Evaluate your progress, if any, and stop taking the supplement if you don't see any beneficial effect.

6

Weight Loss

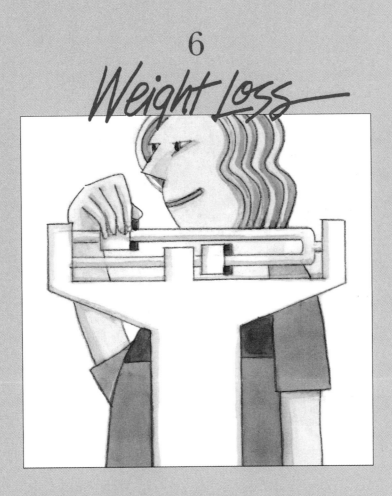

273. Will my blood glucose improve if I lose weight?

274. How much weight do I need to lose to lower my blood glucose levels?

275. How many pounds a week should I try to lose?

276. What is a realistic weight loss?

277. I cannot stop myself from overeating and have picked up considerable weight. I am really getting desperate. What can I do?

278. I switched from cooking with butter to cooking with olive oil, but I still haven't lost any weight. What am I doing wrong?

279. I seem to get better control of my blood glucose if I have food with fat in it. I am trying to lose weight by walking. Is this okay?

280. Which vegetables are best for losing weight?

281. I have heard the term "grazing" in connection with weight loss. What does this mean and how does it help with weight loss?

282. Why is it so hard to keep weight off once you lose it?

283. Are meal replacers helpful for weight loss?

284. How do weight-loss drugs work, and are they safe for people with diabetes?

285. Should people with diabetes consider gastric reduction surgery?

286. Can exercise help with weight loss?

287. Can exercise help maintain weight loss?

288. What kind of exercise will help me lose weight?

289. What's the difference between the "fat-burning" and "cardio-vascular training" ranges that I see listed on my treadmill?

290. I have Type 2 diabetes, am obese, and am thoroughly frustrated. I have tried every exercise and diet plan you can think of, not to mention health clubs, hypnosis, and various pills, but nothing has changed. What I need is the energy and stamina to exercise. Where do I get that?

291. My doctor told me to lose weight to control my blood glucose, so I started an exercise program three months ago. I have not lost as much weight as I expected from all my exercise (only five pounds), and I'm feeling very frustrated. What's going on?

292. I am about 150 pounds overweight, and I was recently diagnosed with Type 2 diabetes. My doctor told me to exercise to lose weight to help lower my blood glucose, but it's really hard for me to do most exercise. What can you suggest for someone in my situation?

293. My friend walks every day. After her latest visit to her doctor, she now tells me that she is fit. But it's obvious that she is overweight. Is it possible to be "fit and fat"?

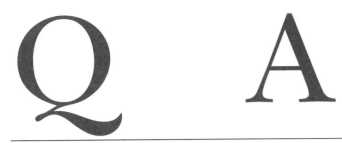

273.
Will my blood glucose improve if I lose weight?

If you need to lose weight, weight loss can indeed help your blood glucose control. Short-term studies have shown that people with Type 2 diabetes who lose weight not only improve their blood glucose, but their bodies become less resistant to their own insulin, and they often experience improvements in blood cholesterol and blood pressure levels as well. The difficulty with weight loss is in maintaining it. The reason it is difficult to maintain weight loss is that body weight is regulated by several different factors, including genetic factors that might predispose people to become obese. Environmental factors, such as the eating habits of one's family, can also make it difficult to lose weight and maintain that loss.

People who are most successful with losing and maintaining weight loss are those who participate in an intensive lifestyle program that involves education, individualized diet counseling, reduced intake of fat and calories, and regular physical activity. These changes for a healthier lifestyle are for life, not just until you reach your goal weight. With these changes in place, people can greatly enhance their success with long-term weight loss.

Talk with your doctor and dietitian to decide how much weight loss would be reasonable for you. And then ask for help in making a weight-loss plan that includes a healthy food plan, an exercise plan, and an individual or group support plan. A steady loss of 1 pound to 1½ pounds per week is a safe and healthy rate of weight loss.

274.
How much weight do I need to lose to lower my blood glucose levels?

If you are overweight, losing just 10% to 15% of your weight may be enough to bring your blood glucose levels down, possibly even to normal levels. This amount of weight loss may also lower your levels of cholesterol and triglycerides and improve your blood pressure. If you weigh 200 pounds, a 10% weight loss is 20 pounds; if you weigh 300 pounds, 10% would be 30 pounds.

233

Q   A

Talk to your doctor or dietitian for advice on how to lose weight. The best approach is to come up with a healthy eating plan that is rich in nutrients, but low in fat and calories, combined with an exercise plan. Most people do better if they have some form of support, either with an individual counselor or dietitian or from a support group such as Weight Watchers or Overeaters Anonymous. A loss of about 1 pound to 1½ pounds per week is a safe and healthy goal.

275.
How many pounds a week should I try to lose?

Slow and steady is the way to go when losing weight. Most people do best losing a maximum of 1½ to 2 pounds per week. If you starve yourself to lose more weight, you may not get enough nutrients. You may also be constantly hungry and irritable, and you may have trouble with your glucose control. And quick-loss diets don't teach you long-term healthy eating habits that will help you keep off the weight you lose.

Even with this slow weight loss, you'll reach your weight goal in a reasonable time. Suppose your goal is to lose 30 pounds, and you lose just one pound a week. You will still meet your goal in less than eight months. Talk to your doctor or dietitian about developing a healthy weight-loss plan that includes a varied low-fat and low-calorie diet, exercise, and support.

276.
What is a realistic weight loss?

If by "realistic" you mean "possible," there are many factors that may limit or inhibit the amount of weight you can lose. If, however, you mean "reasonable," meaning how much weight you can lose to have a positive effect on your diabetes control, every little bit helps. A loss of even 10–15 pounds will have a significant effect.

Most people can lose about 1% of their starting weight each week for 4–6 weeks before they hit a plateau, a temporary pause in weight loss. This can be a blow to motivation, but if they are patient, weight loss will resume for most people.

A second weight-loss plateau occurs weeks or months later and tends to be more permanent. This happens for two reasons. First, the caloric restriction necessary for any weight loss causes a decrease in the

Q A

activity of the thyroid hormones, the hormones that regulate the metabolic rate. Less activity results in a lower rate of metabolism; that is, your body uses calories more slowly. The second reason is that weight loss decreases the size of the body, and by doing so, lowers the amount of energy the body burns. When the body's energy expenditure decreases while caloric intake remains the same, weight loss will come to a halt.

At this point, most people will have lost 5% to 10% of their starting weight, which can be very beneficial to your health. This amount of weight loss can lower blood pressure, lower triglycerides, raise HDL ("good") cholesterol, and improve insulin sensitivity.

However, if you have had diabetes for a number of years, losing weight might not improve blood glucose levels, The reason for this is that the longer you have diabetes, the more likely you are to be deficient in insulin. Weight loss does help with insulin resistance but not with insulin deficiency. The remedy for insulin deficiency is medication, either glucose-lowering oral medicine or insulin, together with physical activity and nutrition therapy.

277.
I cannot stop myself from overeating and have picked up considerable weight. I am really getting desperate. What can I do?

Often, uncontrolled eating is a response to other issues in our life that are out of control; and food is often a comforting response to an emotional issue. Another possible cause is high blood glucose. When blood glucose is high, body cells don't get the "fuel" they need, and the body increases appetite in response to lack of food (fuel). Keeping food records and discussing them with your dietitian will help you determine whether your overeating is an emotional response or an appetite response from high blood glucose.

278.
I switched from cooking with butter to cooking with olive oil, but I still haven't lost any weight. What am I doing wrong?

Before you despair, congratulate yourself for lowering your saturated fat intake. Butter is one of the highest

Q A

saturated-fat foods there is, and we know that a diet high in saturated fat is a definite risk factor for heart disease, heart attack, stroke, and clogged arteries.

A saturated fat is one that is solid at room temperature—butter, lard, and shortening are just three examples. Saturated fat is also hidden in foods—whole milk, ice cream, and red meat, for instance. This kind of fat is not considered a "heart healthy" fat, as it can raise blood cholesterol levels, which in turn puts you at risk for having a heart attack or a stroke. It's important for everyone, especially people with diabetes who are already at an increased risk for heart disease, to limit their intake of saturated fat.

Olive oil is a prime example of a monounsaturated fat. Monounsaturated fats are always liquid at room temperature. Canola oil and peanut oil are two other examples of monounsaturated fat. Olives, peanuts, peanut butter, and avocado are also rich in this heart healthy fat.

Obviously, it makes sense to substitute as much saturated fat as you can for monounsaturated fat, especially when you are cooking.

However, there's still a catch. If you're trying to lose weight, calorie for calorie and serving for serving, there is no difference in calories between butter and olive oil. One tablespoon of either butter or olive oil contains approximately 100 calories and 11 grams of fat. The only difference is that most of the fat in the butter is saturated. Using too much of either type of fat can lead to weight gain, or at least make it difficult to lose weight.

To reduce calories when cooking, try putting your olive oil in a spray bottle and coating the pan lightly, rather than pouring oil directly into the pan. You might also consider sautéing without fat altogether—use chicken broth or vegetable broth, wine, or even water. Save the olive oil to drizzle lightly over your salad, or to dip your bread into (just a little).

279.
I seem to get better control of my blood glucose if I have food with fat in it. I am trying to lose weight by walking. Is this okay?

Your question raises a very good point. Which is more important: blood glucose control or weight loss?

Q A

Both are equally important, but keep in mind that if you lose weight, you may find that your blood glucose levels improve. Some fat is good, but I wouldn't suggest following a high-fat diet for blood glucose control, as this will certainly make weight loss difficult and may increase your risk for heart disease. A registered dietitian can work out a realistic eating plan that will help you lose weight *and* control your blood glucose.

280.
Which vegetables are best for losing weight?

With very few exceptions, vegetables contain fewer than 100 calories per half cup. So although vegetables do differ in calorie count, these differences aren't worth taking into account in a weight-loss plan. Vegetables contain hundreds of useful chemicals, and no one vegetable contains them all. So to get the best health benefit, eat a wide variety of vegetables. Dark-colored and brightly colored vegetables tend to be particularly high in nutrients.

The only exception to this rule is starchy vegetables like corn, beans, peas, and potatoes. These are still healthy for you; it's just wise to limit your portions of these types of vegetables if you are trying to lose weight.

281.
I have heard the term "grazing" in connection with weight loss. What does this mean and how does it help with weight loss?

Grazing in the context of weight loss means eating five or six small meals per day, spread out fairly evenly, with a fairly set number of calories per day. The idea is that by eating six mini-meals instead of the standard three main meals most people are used to, you can reduce your total calorie intake without feeling hungry. It can also prevent hunger before a main meal that may make you overeat. Of course, the key to weight loss is to eat fewer calories than you burn.

Five or six meals per day might sound overwhelming, but if you add one meal at a time until it becomes a habit, increasing the number of meals will not seem difficult.

Q   A

Obviously, a controlled, consistent plan is essential if you intend to graze. A registered dietitian (R.D.) who is also a certified diabetes educator (C.D.E.) can help you develop a plan that works and be there for you if you need advice as you proceed with your grazing regimen.

Remember that since you will be eating less food over the course of the day, your medication will probably need to be adjusted, so make sure that you involve your physician in your weight-loss plan before you start.

282.
Why is it so hard to keep weight off once you lose it?

When you lose weight, compensatory mechanisms take over to protect the body from "starvation." The center of this control appears to be in the hypothalamus, which is in the brain. Signals to areas in the hypothalamus, perhaps from the hormone leptin released from fat tissue when its fat content is decreased, increase appetite. The hypothalamus then releases signals that either increase or decrease food intake. How appetite is controlled is not completely understood, but the more that is learned about it the more it becomes understandable why weight loss and maintenance are difficult. A variety of signals from the nervous and endocrine systems and signals from the stomach and intestines are all involved. For example, recent research reported that after weight loss, the stomach releases more of a hormone called ghrelin. This causes a message to be sent to the hypothalamus to increase hunger.

A number of research studies have shown that after weight loss, a number of factors make maintaining that weight loss difficult. One study showed that after weight loss, the body compensated by needing fewer calories to maintain weight. So if two individuals weigh the same but one person has recently lost weight, that person will require fewer calories to maintain that weight than somebody who has always weighed that amount. The majority of calories that a person needs are for what is called basal energy needs. That is the number of calories needed to survive when you are at complete rest. It appears that after weight loss, the body can reduce the number of calories needed for basal energy. Other studies have shown an increased desire for fatty foods after weight loss.

Most people like to believe they can have some control over lifestyle habits, but we all live in an environment that makes weight-loss maintenance difficult. Every day we are bombarded with TV food ads and super-sizing of portion sizes. So it takes a "super-size" program to help people keep the weight off. For example, in one recent three-year study, people who had prediabetes (at high risk for developing diabetes) were put on a weight-loss program. At the beginning of the study, one group of participants was just told to lose weight and received some general information on losing weight. A second group took part in an intensive education program that lasted 24 weeks, followed by monthly contact with "lifestyle coaches." This was the successful group, winding up with only half the number of people with Type 2 diabetes as the group that was given just general information.

283.
Are meal replacers helpful for weight loss?

First of all, what is a meal replacer? It is a prepackaged meal, snack bar, or formula product, which usually contains 200–300 calories, primarily from carbohydrate and protein, although vitamins, minerals, and fiber may also be added. When eaten once or twice daily to replace a meal, it can result in weight loss. Research has shown that weight loss can be as much as 11% of starting weight over two years, but meal-replacement therapy must be continued if weight loss is to be maintained. About one-third of the individuals who start on a meal-replacement program are reported to discontinue using these products and gain back the weight they have lost.

Liquid meal replacements are an artificial way of eating, so it is not the best way to lose weight. It is only a short-term solution and difficult to sustain. A registered dietitian can give you the support you need for weight loss, either in a group or individual setting.

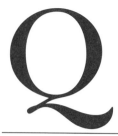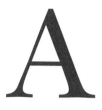

284.
How do weight-loss drugs work, and are they safe for people with diabetes?

Researchers reasoned that since appetite is regulated by the hypothalamus (a center in the brain), it might be possible to develop drugs that would influence this control center. One of the first medicines used this way was a combination of fenfluramine and dexfenfluramine. Although use of these drugs did result in successful weight loss in persons with Type 2 diabetes, the manufacturer pulled the drugs from the market because of their effects on the heart. Sibutramine (Meridia) is now available and also suppresses the appetite by acting on signals in the brain. In one research trial, people taking sibutramine lost, on average, 9 pounds more than those treated with a placebo. The drug works better if people are careful about what they eat and do regular physical activity. However, like many other drugs, it must be continued to maintain beneficial effect.

Orlistat (Xenical) is another weight-loss drug currently on the market. It inhibits pancreatic lipase (an enzyme necessary for fat digestion and absorption), and as a result a portion of food fat that is eaten is not absorbed. If too much fat is eaten, diarrhea can be a problem. Research trials report that persons can lose, on average, about 7% of their starting weight. Although the weight loss is modest, even this small amount of weight loss can lead to improvement in glucose control.

Drugs for weight loss are an active area of research, and as more is learned about appetite control, new weight-loss drugs should and will be approved for marketing.

285.
Should people with diabetes consider gastric reduction surgery?

Gastric reduction surgery can be a very effective weight-loss treatment for severely obese individuals. The most common types of surgery involve creating a small stomach pouch to receive food. Because the pouch is small, only very small meals can be eaten without pain or vomiting. In one study, people with Type 2 diabetes had lost an average of about 50

Q A

pounds in the year following surgery. More important, the majority experienced significant improvements in glucose control, and 64% of the people again had normal blood glucose levels. There are some potential adverse effects of this surgery, so anyone considering this form of treatment needs to discuss the pros and cons thoroughly with his health-care team. However, many people with severe weight problems who have tried many weight-loss techniques without success have benefited from this surgery.

286.
Can exercise help with weight loss?

Exercise by itself is unlikely to lead to much weight loss. To lose weight you have to cut back on the number of calories that you eat. However, exercise can assist with the other side of the weight-loss equation: It can increase the number of calories you use in a day. The reason it doesn't lead to weight loss is simply that most people cannot do enough exercise to burn up enough calories for weight loss. If you remember that a pound of fat has approximately 3,500 calories stored in it and that running or walking a mile burns up about 100 calories, this means an individual would have to walk or run 35 miles to burn up one pound of fat. However, exercise is important for several other reasons. Exercise improves insulin sensitivity and therefore, if done on a regular basis by persons with Type 2 diabetes, may improve blood glucose control. It also strengthens the heart and lungs and lowers blood pressure. Furthermore, for long-term maintenance of weight loss, it is essential that people do regular exercise.

287.
Can exercise help maintain weight loss?

Participating in regular exercise is the major predictor of who will maintain weight loss. Why is not completely known. Part of the reason may be that exercise burns calories and thus may prevent any decrease in the number of calories a person requires, but some researchers think exercise helps with something even more important. Namely, the discipline needed to exercise nearly every day seems to carry over to the discipline needed to monitor food intake. People

Q A

who exercise seem to do better watching what they eat. Start an exercise program slowly and gradually, and build up your endurance until you can exercise for 30 minutes nearly every day. However, to make exercise really beneficial for weight maintenance and to prevent weight gain, physical activities may need to be done for an hour a day. But it doesn't have to be done all at one time; you can accumulate 10- to 15-minute periods of physical activity throughout the day until you get to your exercise time goal.

Keeping food records of what you eat has also been shown to be helpful. There is something about having to write down exactly what and how much food people eat that makes them more careful of what they do eat. If you have diabetes, it is helpful to keep food records and blood glucose monitoring results on the same form. That way, you can see at a glance how your food intake and exercise affect your glucose control. It may seem like an effort to keep records, but all the research reports that this is essential for successful weight-loss maintenance.

Support from family, friends, and people you work with is also helpful. Family members can sabotage your best efforts by having foods around that you are trying to avoid or by encouraging you to eat more than you wish. If your family doesn't help you, it will be essential that you find some type of support or peer group that can provide support for your new lifestyle.

Stressful situations often cause people to stop exercising and to eat more, so you also need to learn ways to cope with stress. Some people learn meditation skills or progressive relaxation techniques. However, one of the best ways to cope with stress is to exercise. Over and over again, people report that exercise helps them cope by providing them with renewed vitality.

So there's no way to avoid it—maintaining weight loss starts and ends with exercise!

288.
What kind of exercise will help me lose weight?

This is an important question. About 60% of Americans face health risks associated with being either overweight or obese. The rising incidence of these conditions is largely attributed to our increasingly

Q A

sedentary lifestyle. We have become so dependent on energy-saving conveniences that we simply don't have to move very much any more. As a result, our bodies have become metabolically sluggish, and we easily put on excess pounds.

The good news it that we can reverse this trend by building more physical activity back into our daily lives. People who successfully lose weight and keep off unwanted pounds have learned how important it is to incorporate regular, moderate physical activity into each day. The most important message about physical activity and weight loss is just to get moving! If you burn more calories through activity than you consume through your diet, you will lose weight.

Perhaps the easiest way to begin increasing your activity level is to walk more whenever you can. Walking is an activity that almost everyone can do comfortably, and progress can be easily measured if you wear a small pedometer to count steps throughout each day. As you gradually increase your pace and build up the amount of time that you walk, you will steadily increase the number of calories you burn. As a result, you will lose weight and body fat. Other forms of aerobic activity, such as cycling, swimming, or low-impact aerobic dance, are equally beneficial. Weight training or other resistance exercises can help increase muscle strength, stamina, and endurance. These activities may also help prevent loss of lean muscle that often occurs with both aging and weight loss.

It is not so much what kind of activity you do but rather how much you do that makes a difference. Initially, try to do 150 minutes of activity per week, or 20–25 minutes per day. Increase your activity level until you are able to do 200–300 minutes of activity per week, or about 30–45 minutes per day. Your long-term goal should be to burn around 2,000 calories per week through activity.

289.
What's the difference between the "fat-burning" and "cardiovascular training" ranges that I see listed on my treadmill?

The best advice is to simply ignore the ranges listed on your treadmill and just exercise for as long as you can at an exercise intensity that feels "somewhat

Q A

hard" to "hard." The manufacturers of exercise equipment like to perpetuate the myth that in order to lose body fat, you have to "burn" more body fat during your exercise. However, what really matters to weight loss is the total number of calories that you expend doing an activity, not the type of fuel that your body is using more of during it.

Your body uses a mixture of carbohydrate and fat at rest and during exercise. At rest, depending on your diet and recent exercise status, most people use about 60% fat and 40% carbohydrate. As you begin to exercise, your body begins to use a greater percentage of carbohydrate, regardless of your exercise intensity. By the time you reach the so-called "fat-burning" range, your body is already using much more carbohydrate than fat. At even higher intensities (the so-called "cardiovascular-training" range), carbohydrate use increases until it reaches 100%. So, essentially, you never use much fat during exercise. However, you do use more fat for the remainder of the day when you are not exercising (during the 23 hours or so of rest).

To maximize your body-fat losses, attempt to exercise for as long as you can at a level that you can sustain. If you only have 30 minutes to exercise, work out at a harder level. If you don't like to push yourself too hard, try to exercise for 45–60 minutes to expend the same number of calories.

290.
I have Type 2 diabetes, am obese, and am thoroughly frustrated. I have tried every exercise and diet plan you can think of, not to mention health clubs, hypnosis, and various pills, but nothing has changed. What I need is the energy and stamina to exercise. Where do I get that?

Your problem, unfortunately, is all too common. Many people struggle with weight loss and exercise. Of course, exercise does give you energy and stamina, but how do you go about getting that energy when you're too tired to start?

Here are a couple of points to keep in mind. The first is that even without any exercise at all, you can

Q A

lose weight. People lose weight all the time without any exercise by modifying their diet. To get started, ask your doctor for a referral to a registered dietitian who is also a certified diabetes educator. Usually, with just minor modifications in diet, individuals can achieve some weight loss. Research proves that losing just 10% of your body weight can make you much healthier. But you can start to feel better with even less weight loss than that.

As for your exercise, try small, manageable steps. If you start with goals that are too ambitious, you set yourself up to fail. By small, manageable steps, I mean goals such as 5–10 minutes of walking a day. Think about how you spend your day and identify a few moments where you can increase your activity. For instance, if you ride a bus, try walking a few extra blocks before boarding or getting off a few blocks before your destination; park your car at the far end of the parking lot and walk to your destination; or take a walk at lunch instead of sitting at your desk. The point here is to increase your physical activity before starting more formal exercise. Research shows that gradually integrating activity into your daily routine is a very good beginning toward a more active lifestyle. The bottom line is that making decisions about physical activity that you can accomplish leads to more and more activity.

Keep in mind, too, that the guidelines for physical activity in the United States are to accumulate 30 minutes of moderate physical activity on most, if not all, days of the week. That means you can do it all at once, or in blocks of 10 minutes three times a day. Moderate intensity is when you feel warm and slightly out of breath. Walking is an excellent choice because it is convenient (you can do it anywhere), it requires no equipment except a pair of sturdy shoes, and the risk of injury is very low.

As you become more active, you might decide to formalize your walks. One good approach is called "five minutes out, five minutes back." What you do is plan a time to walk, walk for five minutes from your starting point, then turn around and walk back. Each week, increase your activity level by walking for an extra 2–3 minutes in each direction. So it would

Q   A

become 7 minutes out, 7 minutes back, then 9 minutes out, 9 minutes back, and so on. Before you know it, you'll be up to 30 minutes.

The best way to get started, whether you choose to increase your physical activity or do more formal walks, is to set weekly goals and write them down. Be as specific as possible. Write down the day(s) of the week, the time of day, and the minutes of activity. Writing down your goals will help you know what to expect, plus you'll have records of what you do. And once the plan is written down, you can always move things around if you get busy.

Remember that you can achieve weight loss without Herculean amounts of physical activity, and any activity is better than none. A modest weight-loss program that includes a healthy diet and increasing your physical activity, even if it's only a few minutes a day, is a great place to start. Don't overwhelm yourself with having to do too much. You will succeed if you are organized and methodical and your goals are practical. Don't try to make up for years of inactivity all at once. Be realistic, pace yourself, and within just a few weeks, you will begin to get some of your energy back and feel better. And more important, your success will help you feel good about yourself.

291.
My doctor told me to lose weight to control my blood glucose, so I started an exercise program three months ago. I have not lost as much weight as I expected from all my exercise (only five pounds), and I'm feeling very frustrated. What's going on?

You should be congratulated on losing any weight at all. As for your frustration with the small amount of weight you have lost, concentrate on losing body fat rather than on dramatically lowering your actual scale weight. Think of your body weight as being partly from fat and partly from lean body mass, which includes things such as your muscles, bones, organs, and water. Fat weighs less than muscle, so if you are watching your diet and exercising regularly, it is likely that you are both losing some fat weight and gaining some muscle. In actuality, then, some of your fat

Q   A

losses are being masked by your muscle gain. It is not that unusual for people's weight to stay the same or even go up for a while after starting to exercise.

The best advice is to stick with what you are doing. Eventually you will see your body weight come down as the muscle increases level off. Keep a closer watch on how well your clothes are fitting—you might only lose five pounds but drop down by two sizes! Remember, almost all individuals who have been successful with losing weight and keeping it off engage in regular exercise of some sort.

292.
I am about 150 pounds overweight, and I was recently diagnosed with Type 2 diabetes. My doctor told me to exercise to lose weight to help lower my blood glucose, but it's really hard for me to do most exercise. What can you suggest for someone in my situation?

You really need to find some exercise that you can do. Dieting alone can help with weight loss, but a recent study of people who lost significant amounts of weight and kept it off revealed that almost all of them also did some type of regular aerobic exercise.

The exercise that you do does not need to be vigorous (like jogging) in order for you to lose weight. Mild and moderate exercise done for a more extended time (45–60 minutes or more) can be effective. If your extra body weight is keeping you from walking, then try an activity that is minimally weight-bearing or non-weight-bearing such as swimming, water aerobics, running or walking in water, stationary cycling, using an elliptical strider, or circuit weight training.

The key to weight loss is consistent exercise. Try to work out five or six days per week for as long as you can. If you start to get bored with an activity, try alternating it with other activities to keep it fun and interesting. Also, try to be more active in your daily life by adding in small amounts of activity throughout your day. Get up from your desk once an hour and walk around for five minutes, for instance. Every little bit of activity counts when you are attempting to lose weight.

Q A

293.
My friend walks every day. After her latest visit to her doctor, she now tells me that she is fit. But it's obvious that she is overweight. Is it possible to be "fit and fat"?

More and more evidence shows that moderate levels of physical activity have positive effects on cardiovascular disease, weight control, and diabetes. Virtually every study of cardiorespiratory fitness shows that the fittest people—those who can walk the longest on a treadmill, for instance—are healthier than unfit people, even if the fit person is overweight. In this case, "healthier" means having lower cholesterol, triglycerides, blood pressure, and blood glucose levels—and living longer.

Often the emphasis is on weight loss to get healthier, but there is evidence to show that even if you are overweight, you can be healthy, as long as you are fit. In many studies, fitness was achieved by people who walked at a moderate pace of 3–3½ miles per hour. In some cases, they accumulated the desired 30 minutes throughout the day, while in other cases they did it all at once.

7
Exercise and Fitness

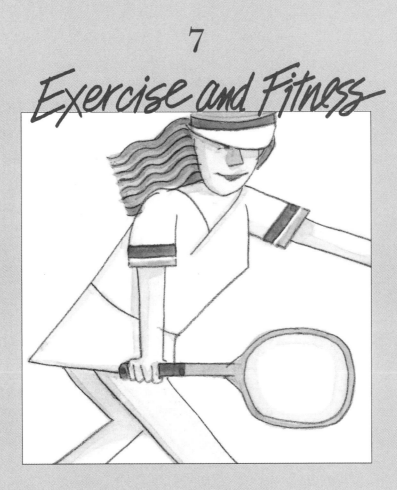

Getting Started

294. After 20 years of being mostly sedentary, I am now overweight and have Type 2 diabetes. I have decided finally that I need to start exercising. How should I go about starting?

295. Is it necessary for me to see my physician before I start a moderate exercise program?

296. How can I find out if there are any exercise programs specifically geared toward individuals with diabetes in my area?

297. My doctor told me that I need to exercise, but I just do not have enough time in my day to do it. What would you suggest I do to become more physically active?

298. How much physical activity is enough to benefit my health?

299. How do I know if I am doing too much activity?

300. I hate exercising alone. What other options do I have?

301. I am thinking about joining a fitness center. What should I look for in a facility?

302. What should my exercise goals be?

303. I have never exercised in my life, and I am now a senior citizen. Is it too late for me to start? Can exercise still help me improve my health?

304. I am 52 and have used insulin for the past 25 years. So far, I have no diabetes-related complications, but I know I don't eat right or exercise enough. How can I start taking better care of myself when it's so hard to change?

305. My work, family, and household responsibilities keep me so busy that I have very little time to exercise. What can I do that won't take up much time but will still benefit my health?

306. I've heard there are new recommendations for exercise. Is this true?

307. I've heard that many health factors are the result of genetics. If this is true, why should I bother exercising?

308. I am a smoker, but I exercise daily, keep my blood glucose under control, and eat well. Isn't this good enough?

309. I have gestational diabetes. Do I need to exercise?

Prevention and Control

310. I have been a regular walker all my life, but I still developed Type 2 diabetes. Isn't exercise supposed to prevent it?

311. My biggest fear with diabetes is that I will have to start taking insulin shots. Can exercise help prevent that from happening?

312. My grandmother, my father, and my sister all have Type 2 diabetes, and I have been told that puts me at risk. Can regular exercise really prevent me from developing it?

313. I have heard that increasing muscle and losing fat can improve diabetes control. Is this true?

314. I already have Type 2 diabetes, and I am supposed to be controlling it with diet and exercise. If I start exercising regularly, can I make it go away?

315. I have heard that exercise increases your blood flow and blood glucose use. If I exercise regularly, will my blood glucose be in better control?

316. My blood glucose is under good control when I eat correctly and take my oral medicine. Do I really need to exercise, too?

317. I take insulin. What is the best time of day for me to exercise?

The Right Stuff

318. I see all kinds of special exercise equipment advertised on TV. What special equipment do I really need to buy?

319. Do I need to buy special exercise clothing?

320. What about shoes and socks? What should I look for?

321. I have seen advertisements for special shoes made just for people with diabetes. Do I need these for exercise?

322. I frequently exercise outdoors. I have the appropriate socks, shoes, and clothing, but is there anything else I need to think about?

323. People keep telling me that I am supposed to wear "proper footwear" when I exercise to prevent problems with my feet. What exactly is the definition of "proper footwear"?

324. I enjoy jogging, but sometimes my legs hurt afterward. Is it still okay for me to run?

Activities and Techniques

325. I have friends who jog or run, but I find that running is too intense for me. Is walking okay?

326. I have seen people wearing weights while they jog or walk. Is this something I need to do?

327. I used to be an avid runner, but now I have a "trick" knee. What other activities can I do?

328. My local community center offers water aerobics classes. Would this be a good choice for me?

329. My community center offers yoga classes. Could this be a good exercise option for me?

330. I am interested in building muscle. What types of exercise can help me do this?

331. I am interested in lifting weights. How should I start?

332. What type of weight training is advised for someone like me, an overweight individual with Type 2 diabetes and chronic hypertension (high blood pressure)?

333. My doctor advised me that swimming would be the best exercise for me because of the neuropathy in my feet, but I hate to swim. Are there any other activities I can do instead?

334. I don't like running or swimming, but I love to play golf. Is this considered exercise?

335. I spend a lot of my free time gardening, but my husband says this doesn't count as exercise. Is there any physical benefit to gardening?

336. I don't do any regular exercise, but I like to shop. Is walking in the mall enough exercise, or do I need to do more than that?

337. Is engaging in maximal or near-maximal exercise like sprinting or heavy weight lifting good for people with diabetes?

338. When exercising outdoors is not a good option, what are some alternatives?

339. My back often bothers me. Are there any exercises I can do to help with this?

340. I have both diabetes and arthritis. Can exercise help me?

341. I usually walk during the week, but on weekends I like to cycle. How can I figure out if I am getting the same benefit and burning the same number of calories when I do different activities?

Stretch!

342. I've read that I should stretch before I exercise. What does this mean?

343. Sometimes I wake in the morning feeling stiff and even a little sore. Is there anything I can do about this?

344. What are the benefits of stretching?

345. My joints feel stiff when I start to exercise and for a while after I finish. Is there anything I can do to make them more flexible?

Safety Issues

346. My neighbor told me about something called the "talk test" to exercise safely. What is it exactly, and should I use it during exercise?

347. The last time I exercised when it was hot, I nearly passed out. When I checked my blood glucose, it was 200 mg/dl, so I know it wasn't due to hypoglycemia. What might have caused it?

348. I often get a little dizzy just when I stop exercising. What causes this, and can I do anything to prevent it from happening?

349. I want to exercise, but I am afraid of injuring myself. What can I do?

350. I am a 62-year-old woman with diabetes, and I am worried about developing osteoporosis. Is exercise safe for me?

351. Now that my Type 1 diabetes is under control, my doctor has given me the go-ahead to start bodybuilding again. Which bodybuilding supplements can I use, and which should I avoid?

352. I have had hip replacement surgery, and I am worried that exercising might not be safe for me. What can I do?

Staying Motivated

353. I know I need to exercise, but I just can't seem to find the motivation to exercise consistently for more than a month or two. Do you have any helpful suggestions?

354. A friend of mine keeps a journal of exercise. Is this something I need to do?

355. What are the advantages of keeping a diabetes and physical activity log? What should I include in the logs I keep?

356. Whenever I do one activity consistently for a while, I get an injury (like tendinitis or sore joints) and have to stop. Is there anything I can do to prevent this from happening?

357. I have been exercising regularly, but now I have a cold. Is it all right for me to take a few days off?

358. I exercise regularly when I am at home, but I also travel often. How can I keep up my exercise routine while traveling?

Blood Sugar Highs and Lows

359. How often should I test my blood glucose when I exercise?

360. I have heard that the oral medicines I take for my diabetes will not have any adverse effect on my blood glucose during exercise. Is this true?

361. I take insulin injections, and sometimes even mild exercise like walking makes my blood glucose go too low. Is there any way that I can prevent this from happening?

362. Is there anything I can do besides eating snacks to keep myself from becoming weak, shaky, and hungry after sustained physical work?

363. My doctor recently put me on an insulin pump using pretty high doses of insulin all the time. Now my blood glucose often gets low when I am just out walking the dog. Is there anything I can do to prevent this from happening?

364. I have heard that people with diabetes can easily become hypoglycemic when they exercise. Is "having a low" something that everyone with diabetes has to worry about, or just people who take insulin?

365. How can I avoid hypoglycemia from exercise?

366. I have had diabetes for a long time, and I no longer sense or feel "lows." What can I do to help make sure my blood glucose level is in a safe range when I exercise?

367. If I become hypoglycemic, what should I do?

368. What about special sports drinks and snack bars? Should I use them to keep my blood glucose level from going too low? Can they help boost my energy level when I exercise?

369. Even though my blood glucose level was 256 mg/dl yesterday when it was time for my walk, I went anyway. My glucose went down to 192 mg/dl by the end of my walk, but I felt tired the whole time. Did I do the right thing?

370. I often find that my blood glucose level is higher in the morning, before I have eaten anything, and even when I exercise. Why is this happening?

371. Sometimes after I do some weight training, my blood glucose goes up. Why does this happen?

372. I was always under the impression that exercise reduces blood glucose levels. However, by the time I finish my exercises, my blood glucose level has risen 20 points. Why does this happen?

Exercise and Your Heart

373. I found out that I had Type 2 diabetes when I was in the hospital with a heart attack. Is it safe for me to exercise?

374. When I exercise, I sometimes feel short of breath, and my heart feels like it is pounding in my chest. Is this normal?

375. My diabetic father had a heart attack while exercising when he was 55 years old. Now I am 55 and planning to start exercising. Do I need to worry that the same thing will happen to me?

376. I have heard that there are good and bad types of cholesterol. What are they, and how can exercise affect how much of them I have?

377. My doctor recently put me on a new drug. Now whenever I exercise, my heart rate is no higher than 110 beats per minute, although I used to be able to get it up to 135. Is this a side effect of the medication?

378. I developed diabetes 10 years ago. I also have a lot of other health problems, including high blood pressure, high cholesterol, pain in my legs when I walk, and cataracts. Is there any kind of exercise that is safe for someone like me to do?

Exercising With Complications

379. What if I have diabetes complications? Is it still safe to exercise?

380. I have just been told that I have retinopathy. What are good exercise options for me? Are there types of exercise that I should avoid?

381. I have just been told that I have protein in my urine and that my kidneys are affected by diabetes. Is it safe for me to exercise?

382. I know that people with diabetes can have a lot of problems with their feet. Can exercise help prevent any of these problems?

383. When I walk, the bottoms of my feet start to feel numb. What should I do about this?

384. I have neuropathy, but it does not cause much pain. Instead, it prevents me from walking well, and I have problems with balance. Is there anything I can do to improve my ability to walk and to keep my balance?

385. My feet are somewhat numb due to peripheral neuropathy, and I just lost my left big toe due to a chronic infection. Can I still safely do walking or jogging as my main form of exercise?

386. My heart-rate response to exercise may be blunted by the diabetic autonomic (central nervous system) neuropathy that I have. Can I still use my heart rate to monitor exercise intensity, or is there another way that would be better?

387. I have been told that I have diabetic gastroparesis (delayed emptying of the stomach into the intestines). Will this condition affect my blood-glucose response to exercise?

Q A
Getting Started

294.

After 20 years of being mostly sedentary, I am now overweight and have Type 2 diabetes. I have decided finally that I need to start exercising. How should I go about starting?

Before you start, it is best to have a physical exam and possibly an exercise stress test to rule out heart disease and determine what would be a safe exercise intensity for you to begin with. You already have two risk factors for the development of heart problems (a sedentary lifestyle and Type 2 diabetes), and you may have more as well.

If you are not able to have a checkup, then start out very slowly and at a low intensity. Do very mild aerobic exercise, such as walking, stationary cycling, or swimming. Your exercise intensity should feel "fairly light" to "somewhat hard" and should be done at no more than 50% of your estimated maximal heart rate. (Your maximal heart rate can be roughly estimated as 220 minus your age.) Your initial exercise frequency should be three days per week (with at least one day of rest between each exercise day). Exercise for 20 continuous minutes or two 10-minute sessions with a rest period between.

Eventually, you can slowly increase your exercise (over 10–12 weeks) up to a maximum intensity of "hard," or 75% of your estimated maximal heart rate, five to six days per week for 45–60 minutes per exercise session. At all times, be aware of any possible symptoms of heart disease (chest pain, pain radiating down your arm, neck, or jaw, unusual shortness of breath, heart palpitations, dizziness), and stop exercising immediately if any of these should occur. If you do not feel well at any point, stop exercising immediately. Follow these precautions and you should be able to exercise safely and effectively.

295.

Is it necessary for me to see my physician before I start a moderate exercise program?

It depends on your risk factors for heart disease and whether you have any diabetic complications. Coronary heart disease accounts for more deaths in the United States each year than any other type of dis-

Q A

ease. The greater the number and severity of risk factors you have, the more likely you are to have heart disease. The risk factors include a family history (close male relative less than 55 years old or female relative less than 65 with heart disease), high cholesterol and other blood fat levels, hypertension (blood pressure greater than 140/90), current cigarette smoking (or quit within the past six months), diabetes, obesity, and physical inactivity. Diabetic complications such as microvascular (eye, kidney, or nerve) disease also increase your risk.

The American College of Sports Medicine recommends that you have a physical exam and exercise test prior to participating in moderate exercise only if you are in the "high risk" category (having one or more signs or symptoms of heart disease, or known heart, lung, or metabolic disease); everybody with diabetes is classified in this category due to the presence of diabetes alone. If you want to participate in vigorous exercise, though, a physical exam and exercise test are recommended for all males over 45 years old and females over 55, regardless of their other risks.

296.
How can I find out if there are any exercise programs specifically geared toward individuals with diabetes in my area?

Most exercise programs geared specifically toward people with chronic health problems are organized through hospital outpatient programs (for example, wellness programs), universities, YMCAs, YWCAs, Jewish Community Centers, athletic clubs, and other local groups. You might want to check with a local hospital to find out which groups offer cardiac rehabilitation programs, as these groups may also offer programs specifically for people with diabetes.

Another place to check is your local or regional chapter of the American Diabetes Association (ADA). Though the ADA itself may not offer programs, local offices may have information on where such programs are offered, or on local support groups. The national ADA can be reached at 1-800-DIABETES (342-2383), or at www.diabetes.org. Other organizations to contact for information are the Juvenile Dia-

Q A

betes Research Foundation (JDRF) at 1-800-533-CURE (2873), or www.jdrf.org, and the Diabetes Exercise & Sports Association (DESA) at 1-800-898-4322, or www.diabetes-exercise.org.

297.
My doctor told me that I need to exercise, but I just do not have enough time in my day to do it. What would you suggest I do to become more physically active?

Physical activity comes in two forms: structured and unstructured. Structured activities are those that you engage in as part of your normal exercise routine. These should conform to the recommendations of the American College of Sports Medicine and the Surgeon General: 20–60 minutes of aerobic exercise a minimum of three days per week, with almost daily exercise being more optimal, at a moderate exercise intensity or higher.

Unstructured physical activities are those done in the course of your daily activities. These may be lower in intensity that your structured activities. Remember, any activity expends calories and can help you lose or maintain your body weight. Some examples: walking up the stairs whenever possible instead of using the elevator; parking your car at the far end of the parking lot; getting up and moving around your office or job area for five minutes at least once an hour; walking places instead of driving; riding a bike to your workplace once a week. You can add a large amount of activity to every day with these types of activities. But to top off your good health, find time for a structured exercise program as well.

298.
How much physical activity is enough to benefit my health?

There is a common misconception that exercise must be vigorous and structured to be beneficial. While doing this sort of activity certainly does improve fitness and offer health benefits, the good news is that modest amounts of daily activity can also greatly benefit health.

A moderate amount of physical activity is defined as an accumulation of 30 minutes of fairly brisk activity per day—for example, walking at a lively pace. If

257

Q A

doing 30 minutes of such activity at one time is too much at first, it is fine to do shorter amounts throughout the day and gradually build up to a total of 30 minutes. It is best if you can gradually increase your exercise time until you are able to do a minimum of 10–15 minutes of nonstop activity per session.

When you have Type 2 diabetes, and especially if you are trying to lose some weight, it can be helpful to keep a "calorie burning" goal in mind. If you increase calorie burning by 150–200 calories per day, or about 1,000 calories per week, through increased physical activity, you can improve blood glucose control and lose weight.

The bottom line is that doing some activity is better than doing none, and choosing to do a little bit more activity each day is better than choosing to do less.

299.
How do I know if I am doing too much activity?

Though doing regular physical activity is associated with improvements in health, it is possible at some point to exercise too much. If the amount of activity you do or the intensity of effort required is extreme or excessive, this can certainly lead to injury and setbacks. It is important to pay attention to what your body is telling you and to increase your activity level at a gradual pace. This will help assure that you don't overexercise. Even a competitive athlete must train sensibly and allow for adequate periods of rest and recovery to achieve optimal performance.

Here are some warning signs that you might be overexercising or trying to do too much too fast:
■ Feeling fatigued rather than invigorated and energized after an exercise session.
■ Taking a long time to recover and return to a comfortable, resting state after doing physical activity.
■ Being very short of breath, to the point of being unable to talk during an activity.
■ Feeling more than a mild level of discomfort. (An exercise should never feel very hard, painful, or difficult.)
■ Experiencing muscle soreness or joint aches and pains, or suffering injuries.

Q A

- Having an increased susceptibility to colds, flu, or other infections.
- Experiencing burnout and lack of interest or desire to exercise.

300.
I hate exercising alone. What other options do I have?

Lots! Any physical activity can be done with a friend; all you have to do is ask someone. If a friend isn't available (they aren't always), consider joining a gym. In addition to having plenty of other people around, most gyms offer various aerobic classes you could join. Check with local gyms to see if they offer classes at your particular fitness level.

For seniors, there are even more options for exercising with others. Many church and community organizations offer classes or put together exercise groups. You can also visit your local shopping mall before the stores open—most open their doors before store hours for people to walk. On weekends you can also visit local school tracks, where you will find any number of runners, joggers, and power walkers. There are so many opportunities.

If you still can't find anything, consider taking out an ad in the local paper or placing an announcement in your church circular. There will be plenty of people who are looking for others.

301.
I am thinking about joining a fitness center. What should I look for in a facility?

There are a number of benefits to joining a fitness center. A good-quality center should offer a wide variety of exercise options in a pleasant, safe, and unthreatening environment. It can be a great place to learn about new forms of exercise and try them out. It can also be a place to socialize and have fun, and it can be a place to get support as you attempt to make lifestyle changes. However, when you join a fitness center, you are making an investment. So do your research. You want to be certain that the decision you make is the best one for you.

Here are key considerations to keep in mind as you evaluate any fitness center you consider joining:

Q A

- Is a fitness and health assessment done when you enter the program?
- Will you be thoroughly oriented to the facility, including being shown how to use the equipment correctly?
- Is your progress monitored through record-keeping or another method, and is follow-up fitness testing done periodically?
- Are the fitness instructors or personal trainers certified by a recognized, professional association, are they knowledgeable and qualified, and are they CPR-certified?
- Are staff members supportive and friendly?
- Is the center bonded?
- Is a safety and emergency plan in place?
- Is there a variety of exercise equipment that is appropriate for your level of exercise?
- Is the exercise equipment well maintained and clean?
- Are the locker rooms clean?
- Does the center provide classes that are of interest to you and that are appropriate for you?
- Is the center convenient to your home or work?
- What is the cost of membership?
- Does the staff know how to respond to a diabetes-related emergency?
- How crowded is the center at the time of day that you plan to exercise?

302.
What should my exercise goals be?

Setting goals can help you successfully reach a desirable and healthy level of physical activity. Individual goals are stepping stones that can help you make gradual, consistent, and steady progress toward achieving this healthy level of activity.

Though the amount you are able to do initially may be much less than this, the Surgeon General suggests 30 minutes per day as a level of activity that all adults should ultimately try to achieve to improve health and prevent chronic disease. Your starting goals should guide you toward doing this amount of activity gradually. Once you are able to consistently achieve 30 minutes of daily activity, you may decide to maintain this level or you may decide to continue to

Q A

work toward more formalized exercise and achieving a higher level of fitness. Goals can keep you "on track" in either case.

Be specific when you set your goals. What level of activity do you want to reach? How you will reach this level of activity? What type of activity do you plan to do? When and where will you do the activity? And who will help you achieve your goal and how they will help? Always set yourself up for success by being realistic about what you can do. Your goals should be a bit challenging, yet they should be achievable. They should never be so hard to accomplish that they are out of reach.

Also try to think short-term. Set daily or weekly goals that help you make progress toward your desired level of activity. Be flexible and accept challenges as they come. When circumstances change, be willing to modify and reset your goals. "All or nothing" thinking can burn you out and turn exercise into a chore instead of an enjoyable activity. It's also a good idea to reward yourself for successes when you accomplish your goals.

303.
I have never exercised in my life, and I am now a senior citizen. Is it too late for me to start? Can exercise still help me improve my health?

It is never too late to take steps to improve your health and level of physical fitness. Regular participation in physical activity has been shown to benefit seniors in many ways.

Exercise can strengthen the heart and cardiovascular system. It can reduce the risk of coronary artery disease and hypertension. It helps reduce the loss of muscle and strength associated with normal aging. It improves bone strength and reduces the risk of osteoporosis and bone fractures. It improves balance and reduces risk of falling, which can prevent injury. It increases flexibility and reduces joint and muscle "tightness," which can be especially helpful to those who have arthritis. Studies even show that exercise can help maintain memory and the ability to do mental work.

An advantage of being a senior citizen is that you perhaps have more time to commit to regular physi-

Q A

cal activity now than you did in the past. Take advantage of this and make activity a routine part of each day. Seniors who live physically active lives tend to enjoy good health, the ability to do the things they want to do, and a good quality of life as they age. Start by talking with your doctor and diabetes-care provider about your desire to begin an activity routine, and have a thorough medical exam. Then identify good exercise options to begin with, set realistic starting goals, and gradually make progress toward increasing your activity level.

304.
I am 52 and have used insulin for the past 25 years. So far, I have no diabetes-related complications, but I know I don't eat right or exercise enough. How can I start taking better care of myself when it's so hard to change?

The problem you have is complex, and trying to fix it all at once can be discouraging. The best way to solve such a problem is to break it down into smaller, more manageable parts. Start by looking at it as a combination of issues: poor eating habits and lack of exercise. Tackling one part at a time can help you to take better care of yourself.

Changing your eating habits can start with examining what you currently eat. This way, you can see where changes might be beneficial and make them gradually. For example, if you find you tend to eat foods that are high in saturated fat and cholesterol, which can contribute to insulin resistance and increase the risk of heart disease, you might decide to eat smaller portions of those foods or find lower-fat alternatives for them. If you discover your vegetable intake is low, you might start by adding a vegetable to your dinner menu every other day, or every third day if that's what you can manage. If you'd like help or guidance in modifying your diet, consider making an appointment with a registered dietitian who is also a certified diabetes educator.

The second issue is exercise. You probably already know a lot about the physical benefits of exercise, but you may not realize that exercising regularly, however moderately, can also give you an emotional boost. Peo-

Q A

ple who exercise regularly tend to feel more upbeat. When you are ready, make a commitment to do some exercise regularly. Since you haven't been physically active, start small. Have your doctor assist you in selecting the type and amount of exercise to do at first. If your budget can stand it and you think you might like some encouragement, you might consider working out with a certified personal trainer. With regular exercise, you will be surprised at how quickly you can increase your strength, endurance, and sense of well-being.

305.
My work, family, and household responsibilities keep me so busy that I have very little time to exercise. What can I do that won't take up much time but will still benefit my health?

You are not alone in facing the challenge of finding enough time to exercise. For many people, lack of time is a barrier to a successful exercise program. The good news is that you can greatly improve your health by adjusting your usual daily routine and learning to fit small amounts of physical activity in.

First, let's clarify the difference between physical activity and exercise. Exercise is a formalized, structured, and planned form of activity. Regular exercise certainly does improve physical fitness and health, but it requires that you take time to change into exercise clothes, work out, and sweat, then shower afterward—all of which can be barriers to "sticking with it." Physical activity, on the other hand is *any* movement that uses muscles and increases calorie burning. The great thing about physical activity is that it is unstructured and can fit into your daily routine in many ways. Here are some good examples of how to increase your daily physical activity:

■ Walk for 10 minutes during your lunch break at work and take the stairs instead of the elevator. (As a matter of fact, walk wherever you can.)

■ Load groceries and packages into your car yourself instead of accepting help.

■ Do your own yard work instead of hiring someone to do it.

■ Do household chores, like vacuuming the floor vigorously.

Q   A

- Make family time active time—play, walk, swim, or hike with your children or grandchildren instead of sitting on the sidelines.
- Limit TV and computer time.
- Avoid sitting for more than 30 minutes at a time. Get up and move often.

Simply look for small opportunities to do things in a physically active way throughout each day. Gradually work up to a total of 30 minutes of daily activity; this will greatly benefit your health.

306.
I've heard there are new recommendations for exercise. Is this true?

The Institute of Medicine, an arm of the National Academies, recently issued new guidelines for the United States and Canadian governments. They recommend at least one hour of daily moderate exercising for most people. Moderate exercise includes walking, slow swimming, and leisurely bicycling, and the daily hour can be broken up into several sessions during the day. This recommendation replaces the U.S. Surgeon General's 1996 recommendation of 30 minutes of exercise at least 3 times per week.

What does this mean for people with diabetes? No one is certain yet. The new guidelines are designed for average people to get the best health benefits. For the moment, most health-care providers continue to recommend that people with diabetes get 30 minutes to an hour of moderate exercise on most days.

307.
I've heard that many health factors are the result of genetics. If this is true, why should I bother exercising?

While it's true that genetic markers can have a significant impact on your health, the idea of "you are either born with it or you aren't" is false. Though some people may make significant health gains in a shorter period of time, nearly everyone can benefit from some type of increased physical activity. Studies have shown that moderate exercise can decrease the risk of, or possibly lessen the effects of, complications. Exercise can also help control blood glucose,

Q   A

cholesterol, triglycerides, and other factors that contribute to overall health. Don't depend on excuses like bad genes or other reasons, such as being "big-boned," to keep you away from regular exercise.

308.
I am a smoker, but I exercise daily, keep my blood glucose under control, and eat well. Isn't this good enough?

Absolutely not. It's good that you have such an otherwise healthy lifestyle, but why not go the extra mile? Consider this: A smoker who exercises reduces his risk of cancer by 13%, but a smoker who quits and doesn't exercise reduces his risk by 90%. Smoking itself is the overwhelming factor here.

Smoking also causes other health problems. It increases the risk of cardiovascular disease. Combined with other risk factors, such as diabetes, that risk is greatly increased. Smoking also increases blood pressure, decreases exercise tolerance, and causes emphysema and chronic bronchitis.

Stopping smoking can be very difficult for many people, but that's not a good reason for not quitting. Talk with your health-care team about how you can quit, and, please, do it soon.

309.
I have gestational diabetes. Do I need to exercise?

Exercise is important for women with gestational diabetes. Not only can frequent exercise help control blood glucose levels, it can help curb appetite that might result in later weight gain.

It is important, however, that you not exercise too vigorously. The American College of Obstetricians and Gynecologists recommends that women with gestational diabetes have an exercise heart rate that is 25% to 30% lower than that for women who do not have diabetes. Moderate activity is the key here. You should especially avoid any activities where you might fall or any kind of sports activities where physical contact might result. Walking and stationary bicycling are both excellent activities for women with gestational diabetes.

310.
I have been a regular walker all my life, but I still developed Type 2 diabetes. Isn't exercise supposed to prevent it?

Regular exercise has been associated with a lower risk for developing Type 2 diabetes (a 58% decrease in a recent study), but other factors may have precipitated your diabetes that exercise alone could not overcome. You may have a strong family history of diabetes, deposited fat around the abdomen, or poor eating habits; any of these factors could have contributed to the development of your diabetes.

Type 2 diabetes is predominantly an insulin resistance syndrome. Your body may make plenty of insulin but may not use it well, thus necessitating a greater insulin production to try to overcome this resistance. Elevated blood glucose results when your level of insulin resistance exceeds your insulin production. In addition, all individuals with Type 2 diabetes also experience some beta-cell (the cells in pancreas that make insulin) failure.

It is possible that your walking helped reduce your insulin resistance and kept you from developing diabetes sooner. But diabetes is not always preventable. However, continuing to engage in regular exercise now that you have diabetes will help with your blood glucose control, and you will continue to gain other health benefits as well.

311.
My biggest fear with diabetes is that I will have to start taking insulin shots. Can exercise help prevent that from happening?

Whether you have to take insulin shots depends on several factors. The reason that you would ultimately have to go on insulin injections if you have Type 2 diabetes is that your pancreas can no longer produce enough insulin to overcome the insulin resistance that you have. Type 2 diabetes is essentially an "insulin-resistant state," and individuals with Type 1 diabetes may have some insulin resistance as well. Being resistant means that the insulin that you produce does not work as effectively as it should, and it takes more insulin to have the same effect on blood glucose.

Q A

If you want to avoid taking insulin injections, then you will need to try to lower your level of insulin resistance. Obesity is one factor that contributes to insulin resistance; if you can lose some body fat, your level of insulin resistance should decrease. Another contributing factor is diet. It is well established that a diet high in refined sugar and/or fat (especially animal fats) can contribute to insulin resistance. A third factor is being sedentary. An active person is constantly replacing depleted muscle glycogen (stored carbohydrates in muscle), and insulin sensitivity is usually heightened during this period of recovery from exercise (from several hours up to two days, depending on exercise intensity and duration). Physical activity can also help build muscle mass, which is a more metabolically active tissue that requires lesser amounts of insulin to work.

If you have to go on insulin injections, don't despair. It may be that you were genetically inclined to experience insulin resistance and more beta-cell (pancreatic cells that make insulin) failure. In that case, no amount of exercise is likely to prevent the need for insulin injections.

312.
My grandmother, my father, and my sister all have Type 2 diabetes, and I have been told that puts me at risk. Can regular exercise really prevent me from developing it?

Yes, regular exercise does appear to lower your risk for developing Type 2 diabetes. The results of a recent study of people with impaired glucose tolerance (a prediabetic state) engaging in 30 minutes of moderate aerobic exercise five days per week showed that they lowered their risk of developing diabetes by 58%. These people moderated their diets as well, and most of them lost some body fat.

Type 2 diabetes has strong genetic components, meaning that it tends to run in families. Having any near relative (parent, sibling, grandparent) with this type of diabetes increases your risk significantly. Maintaining a normal or near-normal body weight and being physically active can reduce your chance of developing diabetes substantially. Although not everybody with Type 2 diabetes is overweight, over 80% of

Q A

them are when they are diagnosed. Having fat located primarily in the abdomen, in particular, is associated with a greater diabetes risk.

However, in the early stages of diabetes, blood glucose control can often be achieved with proper diet and regular exercise. Several prospective studies have shown that even moderate walking helps decrease diabetes risk. In other words, being physically active, even if you are not engaging in vigorous exercise, can help prevent the development of Type 2 diabetes.

313.
I have heard that increasing muscle and losing fat can improve diabetes control. Is this true?

Excess body fat and physical inactivity are health risk factors that many Americans face. These risk factors contribute to the high incidence of heart disease, hypertension, and Type 2 diabetes in our population. The good news is that a moderate weight loss of just 10–20 pounds can improve insulin sensitivity and blood glucose control for many people with diabetes.

Though weight loss is important, the kind of pounds one loses is also important. This is where physical activity fits in. Exercise burns fat, builds muscle, and gives your body a "metabolic boost"—something that restricting calorie intake alone can't do. Muscle is metabolically active tissue that not only uses glucose as an energy source but also burns fat—and fat is primarily stored, excess calories. By using glucose, muscle helps lower the production of insulin by the liver and aids in the overall control of diabetes.

Keep in mind that moderate lifestyle changes add up. When it comes to better health, simple changes can make a big difference. Be sensible and moderate about your calorie and food intake. And try to do 30 minutes per day of physical activity, or enough to increase calorie burning by 150–200 calories per day.

314.
I already have Type 2 diabetes, and I am supposed to be controlling it with diet and exercise. If I start exercising regularly, can I make it go away?

You can control your blood glucose and keep it in the normal range, but you still will always have Type 2

Q A

diabetes. Your diabetic symptoms and elevated blood glucose levels will recur as soon as you stop working hard to control them. To develop Type 2 diabetes in the first place, you probably developed a resistance to insulin first, but your blood glucose levels did not become elevated until your pancreas started being unable to make enough insulin to compensate for the insulin resistance.

Exercise can potentially reduce the severity and symptoms of diabetes by decreasing insulin resistance. If your body becomes more sensitive to insulin, the amount of insulin you produce may be enough to cover your needs. However, the effects of each bout of exercise last only one to two days, with only one day being more likely. Therefore, you will need to exercise at least every other day to benefit fully.

In many cases, exercise is not enough to overcome insulin resistance when it is combined with lowered insulin production. Body-fat losses and healthy dietary changes may also be needed to control blood glucose levels. Even then, in many cases of long-standing diabetes, diabetes drugs (including, possibly, insulin injections) will also be needed to control diabetes. In any case, you should still include exercise as part of your diabetes regimen, as being physically active can reduce your risk for diabetes-related complications.

315.
I have heard that exercise increases your blood flow and blood glucose use. If I exercise regularly, will my blood glucose be in better control?

Most studies have shown that regular exercise can help lower your overall blood glucose levels (measured by glycosylated hemoglobin, or HbA_{1c}). It is true that exercise itself increases blood glucose use during the activity. Your body has two mechanisms to take up glucose from your bloodstream and get it into your cells: One is the mechanism that occurs when insulin binds to cells and facilitates glucose being taken up; the other is glucose uptake directly due to muscle contractions during physical activity. The increases in blood flow to your muscles and skin ensure that more blood glucose has the opportunity to be taken up during exercise. Theoretically, exercise should always help

Q A

lower your blood glucose levels, at least during and possibly for a short time after the activity.

However, exercise intensity can also affect the blood glucose response; you may elevate your blood glucose with intense exercise such as heavy weight training, although the effect is only temporary (lasting 1–2 hours). In addition, if you want your overall blood glucose level to end up being lower, you must be careful with your diet since the type and quantity of food that you eat can have the same or an even bigger effect on blood glucose levels than exercise.

316.
My blood glucose is under good control when I eat correctly and take my oral medicine. Do I really need to exercise too?

Congratulations on being able to achieve good control using only two out of the three cornerstones of diabetes management (diet, medication, and exercise). Over time, however, you may find that you are no longer able to accomplish this and, other than changing the kind of medicine you take, exercise will be your last remaining diabetes management tool.

Exercise gives you other important health benefits that help control diabetes, such as improved insulin action in the body (sensitivity to insulin), easier body-weight maintenance, and body-fat loss. If you are overweight and sedentary, you are experiencing some insulin resistance (that is, the insulin that your body makes is not working as effectively as it should); if your pancreas at some point becomes unable to produce enough insulin to compensate for this resistance, your blood glucose control will worsen without exercise.

Most disease states attributed to aging are really diseases of a sedentary state. In addition to the possible blood-glucose-lowering benefits of exercise, regular physical activity can lower your risk for, prevent, or possibly reverse other chronic conditions such as heart disease, hypertension (high blood pressure), obesity, colon cancer, depression, premature death, and diabetes complications.

317.
I take insulin. What is the best time of day for me to exercise?

The best time of day for anyone to exercise is at a convenient time, because ease and convenience con-

Q A

tribute to sticking to an exercise routine. However, when you take insulin it is extremely important that you understand the action time of your insulin (see below) in relation to your scheduled exercise time. When you understand this, you can make good decisions about how to manage your blood glucose in any exercise situation.

The way your blood glucose level changes when you exercise is a reflection of the level of insulin circulating in your blood. If you have a lot of insulin circulating and actively working to lower your blood glucose, you are likely to see a big fall in your blood glucose values when you exercise. This happens if you exercise during "peak" insulin action. Conversely, if you exercise when your circulating insulin level is low (for example, in the morning, before you take your insulin), you may experience an unexpected rise in blood glucose. If your blood glucose remains at a fairly stable level when you exercise, your circulating insulin level is well adjusted for the activity you plan to do.

There are several management strategies that can help you maintain optimal blood glucose levels when you exercise. Schedule your activity sessions for times when your insulin is not peaking. This will reduce your risk of experiencing hypoglycemia. If you cannot schedule your activity like this, adjust your insulin; decrease your dosage if its peak action time coincides with your planned exercise time. (Always discuss insulin adjustments with your doctor first.) Eat additional carbohydrate before and during exercise.

Action Profiles of Available Insulins

INSULIN	ONSET OF ACTION	PEAK OF ACTION	DURATION OF ACTION
Lispro	10–20 minutes	1–3 hours	2–4 hours
Aspart	10–20 minutes	1–3 hours	3–5 hours
Regular	30–60 minutes	2–4 hours	5–8 hours
NPH	1–2 hours	5–7 hours	13–18 hours
Lente	1–3 hours	4–8 hours	13–20 hours
Ultralente	2–4 hours	8–10 hours	8–30 hours
Glargine	——	No Peak	Up to 24 hours

Q A
The Right Stuff

318.
I see all kinds of special exercise equipment advertised on TV. What special equipment do I really need to buy?

Making a decision about investing in exercise equipment can be quite confusing. Though you can find good and reliable information on TV, in magazines, or on the Internet, there is a lot of false and misleading information about exercise equipment there, too. The truth is that all you really need, beyond a safe and comfortable place to exercise, is good-quality footwear and comfortable clothing that fits well, is appropriate for the activity you plan to do, and is suitable for the climate in which you exercise. When you stick with exercise such as walking, calisthenics, and stretching, the investment required is minimal.

However, you may decide you want to expand your exercise program and purchase some equipment for home use. Exercise equipment such as dumbbells, ankle weights, exercise balls, resistance bands, or fitness videos can be inexpensive and fairly simple to use. It also can be very pricey and complex—for instance, a home gym or equipment such as a treadmill or stair-climbing machine. Thoroughly research any piece of equipment you consider purchasing, and try it out before you buy it. Make certain you know how to use it correctly, that it is comfortable to use, and, above all, that you enjoy using it. Store salespeople should tell you how to use any piece of fitness equipment.

No matter what your budget, be leery of any product that seems too good to be true. Avoid products that make any of these claims:
- An effortless, sweat-free workout
- Amazing results immediately
- Sculpt or slim a specific area of the body
- Loss of weight and inches while you exercise using the equipment or wearing a special type of clothing

319.
Do I need to buy special exercise clothing?

The most important qualities to look for in exercise clothing are comfort and appropriateness for the cli-

Q A

mate and for the activity you plan to do. Exercise clothing such as sweats, shorts, T-shirts, and exercise tights are all good options, but casual, loose-fitting shirts, blouses, slacks, and shorts can work too.

When you exercise in a warm climate, wear lightweight, light-colored, loose-fitting clothing. Cotton and linen are ideal fabrics because they absorb moisture and breathe. They allow sweat to evaporate, which helps keep you cool. Never dress in heavy sweats or clothing made of rubber or plastic with the idea that you will "sweat off" excess pounds. You can quickly become overheated and suffer heat illness, which can become a medical emergency.

When you exercise in cold weather, dress in layers. Layered clothing provides better insulation from the cold than a single bulky coat or jacket does. You can remove layers as you warm up and add them back if you feel too cool during exercise. Polypropylene and other high-tech fabrics that both insulate and wick moisture away from your skin are ideal to wear as an underlayer. Remember, too, that you can conserve a lot of body heat by wearing a hat on cold days.

320.
What about shoes and socks?
What should I look for?

Selecting suitable footwear for exercise is very important. You should choose good-quality shoes and socks that are appropriate for the activity you plan to do. Today's athletic shoes are specifically designed and structured for almost every sport. It is important to look for shoes that are specifically designed for your activity. Shoes that have silica-gel or air midsoles and built-up heels are good choices for weight-bearing activities like walking. Shoes with these features are designed to absorb impact and reduce stress on your feet and joints. Shoes should also have good arch support to help hold your feet in a good position during exercise.

Cotton tube socks or other thick athletic socks are not the best choice for exercise because they can wrinkle in your shoe, rub, and cause blisters. Socks that have a constructed heel and toe design and are made of polyester or a cotton-polyester blend material are a better choice. Socks with these features tend

Q A

to reduce friction and rubbing in your shoe and reduce the risk of developing blisters. Some socks are made of specialized materials that pull moisture away from your skin. Though more expensive, these are a good choice, too.

321.
I have seen advertisements for special shoes made just for people with diabetes. Do I need these for exercise?

Many magazines advertise specially made shoes for people with diabetes. These shoes claim to offer better support and reduce the risk of injury when exercising. They are sometimes custom-made and can be very expensive.

The good news is that you probably do not have to make a special investment in these kinds of shoes. Studies have shown that they do not offer any advantage or substantially reduce the risk of injury more than a pair of ready-made shoes. It is important, however, that you invest in a good pair of ready-made shoes for exercise. While the price of running shoes or cross-training shoes has increased in the last few years, it is worth investing in a pair that fit snugly, support your arches and your ankles, and will feel comfortable for extended periods of time. Many exercise shoes may seem expensive, but the cost is nominal when you consider that you will avoid injuries later.

322.
I frequently exercise outdoors. I have the appropriate socks, shoes, and clothing, but is there anything else I need to think about?

Have you thought about sunscreen? Many people who exercise outdoors don't give it a second thought, but even a mild sunburn can contribute to an increased risk of skin cancer.

Look for a sunscreen with an SPF (sun protection factor) of 30 or greater. Also look for one that blocks ultraviolet light of both types, UVA and UVB. And use sunscreen whenever you exercise outdoors—a sunburn can happen on even the cloudiest and coldest days, not just in the middle of summer.

Q A

323.
People keep telling me that I am supposed to wear "proper footwear" when I exercise to prevent problems with my feet. What exactly is the definition of "proper footwear"?

"Proper footwear" is well-cushioned, good-fitting athletic or walking shoes that would be less likely to rub and cause blisters or calluses on your feet when you exercise. The use of silica-gel or air midsoles in shoes as well as polyester or cotton-polyester socks to prevent blisters and to keep your feet dry to minimize any potential trauma is recommended as well. Whether you have peripheral neuropathy (numbness or loss of sensation in your feet) or not, monitor your feet closely both before and after exercise for blisters and other potential trauma that you may or may not feel.

Diabetes (and specifically peripheral neuropathy) is the leading cause of toe, foot, and lower-limb amputations in the United States, and neuropathy is the most common diabetes-related complication. An undetected, untreated blister has the potential to become infected, and if you have loss of sensation, you also have a lesser capacity to heal such infections because the small blood vessels (capillaries) in your feet do not receive normal blood flow. In this case, an ounce of prevention is truly worth a pound of cure.

324.
I enjoy jogging, but sometimes my legs hurt afterward. Is it still okay for me to run?

The rule with any exercise is to stop if something hurts. In this case, however, the pain in your legs might be caused by a number of different factors.

First, make sure you have the right kind of shoes for jogging. A good pair of running shoes will provide both arch support for your feet and adequate cushioning to absorb the impact from running.

Another possible reason for injury may be the surface you are running on. Hard surfaces such as cement or asphalt can be particularly hard on joints and shins. If you find you have pain in either your knees or your shins, consider running on softer sur-

Q A

faces, such as grass. You can also switch to a treadmill; most treadmills have a cushioned surface to help absorb the repeated impact of your feet against the running surface.

If your legs still hurt after changing your shoes and running surface, check with your doctor to see if other problems might be to blame.

Activities and Techniques

325.
I have friends who jog or run, but I find that running is too intense for me. Is walking okay?

Many people find running difficult for different reasons. Sometimes people worry about injuries like twisted ankles or shinsplints. Sometimes it's simply that running and jogging can easily wind some people. Whatever the reason, running isn't for everyone.

Walking can provide many of the same benefits as running or jogging. It will be necessary, of course, for you to spend more time walking than you would need to if running in order to get the same benefits—45 minutes of brisk walking compared to 30 minutes of light jogging, for example, or walking every day instead of jogging every other day. But be assured that walking can provide every bit as good a workout as running, and it can be just as challenging.

326.
I have seen people wearing weights while they jog or walk. Is this something I need to do?

The idea behind wearing wrist or ankle weights, which strap on using Velcro, is to make the activity more difficult and thus to expend more calories or make better health gains. In reality, this is rarely the case. In fact, ankle or wrist weights may actually be counterproductive. Not only are ankle and wrist weights generally too light to provide any kind of strength benefits (stick with lifting weights to do that), they can actually slow you down so much that you may not reap the benefits of aerobic training. Skip the ankle or wrist weights and just get out there and walk or jog.

Q A

327.
I used to be an avid runner, but now I have a "trick" knee. What other activities can I do?

Basically, you want to pick activities that place less stress on your knee. Running on asphalt or pavement places extremely high repeated force on your lower-extremity joints. Over time, or when an injury has occurred, the joints being stressed are less able to handle the wear and tear caused by repeated foot strikes on such hard surfaces. An alternative is to find a "softer" place to run, such as grassy surfaces, a cushioned track, or a treadmill. Most treadmills are made to absorb some of the foot-strike forces by being considerably more flexible and elastic than a road or sidewalk would be.

An alternative solution is walking briskly instead of running, as the stress on the knee and other lower-extremity joints is considerably less with walking. Elliptical strider and cross-country skiing machines also minimize joint stress because your feet never lose contact with the striders. In addition, you might elect to do more non-weight-bearing exercises such as cycling, stationary cycling, rowing, swimming, walking or running in water, water aerobics, or chair or floor exercises. These activities place substantially less stress on all of the lower-extremity joints and may help you avoid further problems with your knee.

If you decide to run some anyway (whether outside or on a treadmill), it is advisable to cross-train, that is, do different activities on successive days: Monday, run; Tuesday, row; Wednesday, water aerobics; Thursday, stationary cycle; Friday, run, Saturday, swim; and Sunday, no exercise—day of rest.

328.
My local community center offers water aerobics classes. Would this be a good choice for me?

Water aerobics can be suitable for many people, but it can be especially good for people with certain medical conditions. Since water aerobics is a non-weight-bearing exercise (meaning that your feet and legs do not support most of your weight), people who normally are not able to stand or walk easily can find water aerobics easier. Also, water aerobics is not a high-impact exercise, so people with nerve damage,

Q A

arthritis, or other joint problems may find it more comfortable.

Even while water supports your weight, it provides a great deal of resistance for your muscles to work against. Think about how much more energy it takes to walk through water than it does to walk along the beach. Water resistance is what makes it so hard. When you work on land, you only work against gravity. But water provides resistance in all other directions. This can result in improved joint mobility and muscle strength.

Not only do many community and senior centers offer water aerobics classes, so do most YMCAs and YWCAs.

329.

My community center offers yoga classes. Could this be a good exercise option for me?

Originally from India, yoga is a form of stretching and breathing that increases muscle tone, flexibility, and strength. It can be an excellent exercise option. In addition to other benefits, yoga can help reduce stress and increase muscular coordination.

There are many different types of yoga. Some concentrate on simple breathing and flexibility while others can be very strenuous and physically demanding. It is important to speak with a yoga instructor before beginning a new class. The good news is that there are many yoga classes offered specifically for seniors. Make sure you pick a class that is right for your fitness level.

330.

I am interested in building muscle. What types of exercise can help me do this?

Resistance exercise most effectively increases muscle mass and strength. When you do resistance exercise, you use your muscle strength to work against an opposing force. Forms of resistance exercise include using either weight machines or lifting free weights, calisthenics, and exercises that use resistance bands, elastic tubing, or exercise balls to create resistance.

During the adult years, there are a number of good reasons to include resistance exercise in a well-planned fitness routine. Resistance exercise, sometimes called "strength training," can increase muscle

278

Q A

strength and endurance, improve muscle tone, help maintain bone strength and prevent fractures, improve balance and agility, build lean muscle, help with weight control, improve glucose tolerance, and increase the body's sensitivity to insulin.

331.
I am interested in lifting weights.
How should I start?

Weight lifting can be very beneficial to your health, but as with any form of exercise it is important to exercise safely. Talk with your physician about your desire to begin a weight-training program and have a thorough medical exam before you begin. The purpose of an exam is to make sure your heart and cardiovascular system are in good shape, your blood pressure is well controlled, and that you don't have retinopathy or other diabetes complications that could be aggravated by weight-lifting activities. It is also important to identify and address possible orthopedic limitations.

The next step is to learn. Weight training requires a certain amount of skill and technique. It is best to have a trained person show you how to use weights safely and correctly. If you exercise in a fitness center, a trained staff member should be able to work with you. If you decide to do home exercise, investing in a few sessions with a reputable personal trainer may be beneficial. Fitness videos and "how to" exercise books can also be useful resources.

Here are some weight-training guidelines to keep in mind. Always do a 5–10 minute warm-up before you begin and after you end each training session; a short period of light exercise helps get the blood flowing before heavy exercise and allows the muscles to rest after straining them. Start slowly and gradually increase the effort required to do an exercise; use no more than 2–5 pounds of weight for upper-body exercises and 5–10 pounds of weight for leg exercises. While lifting, focus on proper technique, use slow movements, and remember to breathe freely. Never hold your breath while lifting, as this may cause you to lose consciousness.

A well-designed program should include 8–10 different exercises that focus on all the major muscle groups. Initially aim for 6–10 repetitions (lifts) of each exercise, then gradually increase to 10–15 repe-

Q

A

titions, and then to 15–20. Start with one set (series of repetitions) of each exercise, then increase to two to three sets of each exercise per session. Allow a short rest interval between each set. Train two to three days per week, with rest days in between.

332.
What type of weight training is advised for someone like me, an overweight individual with Type 2 diabetes and chronic hypertension (high blood pressure)?

Since you already have high blood pressure at rest, you will need to be especially careful when you engage in any weight training or resistance training, as the rise in your blood pressure due to exercise may be exaggerated, or relatively greater, compared with someone without hypertension. Furthermore, if your blood pressure goes too high during an activity such as a heavy lift when you may hold your breath, your risk for having a stroke or other cardiovascular event is increased.

Accordingly, it would be best for you to engage in only mild to moderate weight or resistance training, emphasizing more repetitions (10–15) with a lighter weight or lower resistance. Doing so should allow you to keep your blood pressure at less dangerous values. The recommended frequency for such training is two to three days per week, and 8–12 exercises utilizing all of your major muscle groups (upper and lower body) should be included in your program. Also, you would want to progress slowly with your training, increasing the amount of weight you lift only after you can lift your current weight more than fifteen times in your final set (most people do two to three sets of 10–15 repetitions on each exercise).

333.
My doctor advised me that swimming would be the best exercise for me because of the neuropathy in my feet, but I hate to swim. Are there any other activities I can do instead?

Yes. Your doctor obviously wants you to avoid activities that put a lot of pressure on your feet (weight-bearing activities) since you would not be able to feel any injuries to your feet, such as blisters, calluses, or infec-

Q A

tions. However, swimming is not the only non-weight-bearing activity that you could do. If you do not mind water in general, you can purchase a belt to hold you up (a specific floatation device) so that you can walk or run in the water without getting your face and head wet. Many health clubs and YMCAs also offer water aerobics classes, which involve arm and leg movements in shallow water. Although your feet would touch the bottom of the pool during water aerobics classes, your weight in water is much less, and the stress on your feet would be considerably reduced.

Many other activities are non-weight-bearing as well, such as cycling or stationary cycling, using a rowing machine, chair exercises, floor exercises, some weight training, and resistance training with bands. You may also be able to purchase exercise videos that show you how to do many of these activities with minimal stress on your feet.

A final note: If you do undertake any weight-bearing activities, make sure to inspect your feet daily for signs of trauma, and treat any such symptoms as soon as they develop to prevent worse problems with your feet.

334.
I don't like running or swimming, but I love to play golf. Is this considered exercise?

Any form of physical activity is good for you, but some are definitely better than others. Running or swimming may not be for you, but golf is certainly exercise—as long as you're doing it right. If you are walking the course, golfing can burn as many as 345 calories per hour. Carry your own clubs and that number rises dramatically—to 470 calories per hour! But avoid taking a golf cart or hitching a ride, since this can burn as little as 270 calories per hour—about as much as cleaning the house.

335.
I spend a lot of my free time gardening, but my husband says this doesn't count as exercise. Is there any physical benefit to gardening?

Gardening can be a powerful calorie-burner. Studies show that shoveling, hoeing, spading, tilling, and

Q A

mowing can improve your aerobic capacity and help build muscle tone, strength, and a better sense of balance. Indeed, you can burn as many calories in an hour of gardening as you can cycling at 10 mph or using a rowing machine. For example, a 180-pound man can burn approximately 350–450 calories doing an hour of yard work, depending on which activity he does and how much effort he puts into it. If he were to do 20 minutes of work three times during the day, he would burn between 120 and 150 calories per workout. A 150-pound woman doing the same activities would burn slightly less, about 300–400 calories per hour.

Have you ever wondered how much energy certain around-the-house activities require?

■ Chopping wood, stacking firewood, plastering, or mowing the lawn is equivalent to playing golf or walking at 3.5 mph.

■ Mopping, painting, weeding, raking, or trimming hedges is equivalent to weight training, playing volleyball, or playing doubles tennis.

■ Scrubbing floors, digging, hoeing, or tree trimming is equivalent to rowing on a machine, swimming a slow crawl, or playing singles tennis.

336.
I don't do any regular exercise, but I like to shop. Is walking in the mall enough exercise, or do I need to do more than that?

Any physical activity that you can add to your day is far better than none. The activity that you do in a day can be either structured (like a one-hour walking workout) or unstructured (like walking from your car into the mall). However, either type of activity adds to your total daily energy expenditure.

The main differences between mall walking and a more structured walking session may be the exercise intensity and the resulting training effect you get from the activity. If you are stopping to window shop or just ambling through the mall, you will not experience as much of a cardiovascular training effect as you would from walking briskly.

A brisk walk will probably help lower your blood glucose levels better than shopping alone could.

Q A

Keep in mind, though, that the more energy you expend each day, the easier you can control your body weight, and a lower body weight may help lessen the potential harmful effects of diabetes by improving your overall blood glucose control. So if you are not going to exercise regularly, at least do your shopping! If you want even better blood glucose control, do both.

337.
Is engaging in maximal or near-maximal exercise like sprinting or heavy weight lifting good for people with diabetes?

Probably not. "Maximal" or "near-maximal" exercise involves coming close to reaching your maximal heart rate (which can be calculated by subtracting your age from 220). In addition to activities such as sprinting or heavy weight lifting, shoveling snow, other forms of hard physical labor, and climbing stairs rapidly can cause you to reach this high heart rate level.

Having your heart rate go so high may not be good for several reasons. By itself, diabetes increases your risk for heart disease, which could result in a heart attack during heavy exercise. Your risk may actually be even higher if you smoke cigarettes or have other risk factors such as high cholesterol, high blood pressure, or advanced age. If you are going to engage in heavy exercise, it may be wise to have a physical exam and exercise stress test before participating.

To know if you are exercising at this intense level, you can measure your heart rate and compare it with your estimated maximal rate. If your heart rate reaches 80% or more of your estimated maximal rate, you are doing heavy exercise. To gain the optimal effects of cardiovascular training, your exercise need not be more than moderate (about 50% to 75% of your maximal heart rate).

338.
When exercising outdoors is not a good option, what are some alternatives?

When the outdoor weather is inclement, it is a very good idea to have an indoor exercise plan as a backup. This prevents poor weather from becoming an excuse for physical inactivity. In the summertime,

Q A

extreme heat, high humidity, and poor air quality are all good reasons to choose an indoor exercise option. In the wintertime, extreme cold can make indoor exercise a much safer and more agreeable choice than outdoor activity.

Good indoor exercise options include the following:

■ Joining a fitness center. If you live in a southern area where the summers are very hot or a northern area where the winters are very cold, investigate the possibility of joining during the months when the weather is the most extreme.

■ Becoming a mall walker. Though you can do brisk walking at a mall at any time, many malls sponsor mall walking groups. Participants walk before the stores open in the morning.

■ Investigating options in your community. Many churches, hospitals, community centers, and schools offer fitness and exercise classes to their communities.

Also consider exercise options that you can do in your own home: calisthenics and stretching, light weight lifting with free weights (or using an exercise band or ball to do some strengthening work), or exercise videos that are appropriate for your fitness level. You might also purchase a piece of exercise equipment like a stationary bicycle or a treadmill to have in your home.

339.
My back often bothers me. Are there any exercises I can do to help with this?

Back pain, and especially lower back pain, is very common. It can have any number of causes, which is why we recommend that you speak with your health-care provider about whatever symptoms you may be experiencing. Make sure that it's all right to exercise before you do anything else.

If your doctor gives you the OK, one thing you can try to do is strengthen your lower back. Nearly every kind of exercise activity employs some muscles in the lower back—the stronger these muscles, the longer and more comfortably you can exercise. In addition, a stronger lower back can help ease the aches and pains caused by some forms of arthritis.

Q   A

A simple exercise to strengthen the lower back is to lie face down on the floor with your arms over your head. (Imagine flying through the air like Superman and you will have a good idea of the position.) Raise your arms and legs off the floor while arching your back and hold this position for 3–4 seconds. Return to the original position and repeat this exercise 10 times. Once the 3- to 4-second interval becomes easy, gradually increase the time you can hold your back arched. While you are not moving your body very much with this exercise, you are putting added tension on the muscles in your lower back.

340.
I have both diabetes and arthritis. Can exercise help me?

Besides giving general health benefits and improved blood glucose control, regular exercise can help relieve some of the symptoms associated with arthritis. Low-impact exercises that do not stress the joints can strengthen muscles and tendons, which in turn can result in improved flexibility and mobility and decreased aches and pains.

Yoga, bicycling, swimming, stretching exercises, and light resistance training (lifting weights) can all be beneficial. For specific exercises, consult your health-care professional. There are also numerous books on exercises for people with arthritis.

It is important to avoid exercises that can place heavy stress on joints, as these may aggravate symptoms of arthritis. Running, for example, especially on asphalt or a similarly hard surface, can cause more problems than benefit. Walking, on the other hand, should be fine.

341.
I usually walk during the week, but on weekends I like to cycle. How can I figure out if I am getting the same benefit and burning the same number of calories when I do different activities?

First, remember that any amount of physical activity you do is beneficial, and varying your physical activity routine is a very good idea! It keeps exercise from becoming routine and uninteresting, it allows you to work and strengthen many different muscle groups,

Q A

and it helps prevent overuse injuries associated with doing the same exercise routine over and over again.

One way to estimate that you are getting the same cardiovascular benefit and are burning the same number of calories with different activities is to monitor your heart rate. Heart rate is an indicator of how strenuous an activity is, and as heart rate increases so does oxygen uptake and calorie burning. To get equal benefit and burn the same number of calories, you can either choose to do slower, less intense activities for a longer period of time or do faster (or more intense) activities for a shorter amount of time.

This is a helpful guideline: Light activities increase heart rate by less than 10–20 beats per minute and burn under 200 calories per hour; moderate activities generally increase heart rate by 20–40 beats per minute and burn 200–400 calories per hour; and vigorous activities increase your heart rate to over 60% of your maximal heart rate and burn over 400 calories per hour.

Calorie burning for different activities varies, and the amount of effort required determines how much time it will take to achieve the same benefit. Here is an example: If a 170-pound man usually walks three miles in an hour, he will burn about 350 calories. If he decided to swim instead, it would take him 35 minutes of swimming with moderate effort to achieve the same level of calorie burning. If he decided to cycle at a pace of 9 miles per hour, it would take him 45 minutes to burn about 350 calories.

Stretch!

342.
I've read that I should stretch before I exercise. What does this mean?

Whether you are engaging in aerobic activities, like jogging or bicycling, or strength exercises, such as weight lifting, stretching is an important part of your exercise routine. Not only can stretching help prevent injuries, it can actually improve your performance.

By taking a few minutes before exercising to stretch the muscles in your body, you can improve both flexi-

Q&A

bility and blood flow. Especially as we grow older, our bodies' muscles and connective tissues become more rigid. If you begin exercising right away, these tight muscles and other tissues could easily become overextended, leading to tears and sprains. In addition, tight muscles could prevent a full range of motion, thereby reducing the benefits of certain exercises (especially strength exercises).

Gently stretch the muscles of the body before beginning any activity. Neck and shoulder muscles can be stretched by rolling the head in both clockwise and counterclockwise directions, and by gently pulling the head toward either shoulder and holding the position. The arms and chest can be stretched by pulling one arm across the chest and holding it with the opposite hand behind the elbow; you can also put one arm over your head and reach down with that hand toward the small of your back. To stretch leg muscles, brace yourself against a wall and push against the floor with one leg fully extended behind you—be sure to keep your foot flat on the floor to feel the full benefit of this stretch.

You can find more stretching ideas in various exercise books and magazines. Just keep in mind that the key to any stretch is to be gentle and hold the stretch for 15–20 seconds at a time.

**343.
Sometimes I wake in the morning feeling stiff and even a little sore. Is there anything I can do about this?**

A difficult workout the day before might be to blame for morning muscle soreness. It may also be a symptom of arthritis. If the pain becomes acute or if the achy feelings continue, see a doctor.

The good news, however, is that stretching may be able to help with your morning soreness. Before you get out of bed, try the following stretches to help loosen the muscles in your body:

■ Knees to your chest: While lying on your back, pull your knees as close to your chest as you can. Hold this position for about 20 seconds. Do this three times.

■ Arching your back: Lie on your stomach. Raise your chest and head (you can use your arms) but

Q A

keep your stomach and legs on the mattress. Hold this position as long as you can. Do this twice.
■ Full stretch: Many of us do this without even thinking. Lie on your back with your arms raised over your head. Reach as far as you can with your arms and legs to stretch out the chest, back, and stomach. Hold this position for a few seconds, then repeat.
■ Holding the mattress: While lying on your back, stretch your arms to each side and grasp the sides of the mattress in each hand. Once you have a firm handhold, try to raise your back off the mattress. This one can be difficult, so do not hold this position very long.

Whenever you stretch, be sure to breathe deeply and regularly. And always quit if you begin to feel any kind of pain.

344.
What are the benefits of stretching?

Maintaining flexibility is an important part of overall fitness, yet stretching is an all-too-often neglected form of exercise. As we age, our muscles and joints lose elasticity and become more prone to tightness, stiffness, and injury. This is why taking time to stretch is so important.

Stretching can have important benefits. It increases flexibility, the ability to move joints freely and comfortably through a wide range of motion; it reduces the risk of muscle pulls and joint injury; it relieves muscle tension, pain, and stiffness; it reduces risk of back pain; and it is relaxing.

Stretching exercises should always feel gentle and relaxing. Move into a stretch just until you feel mild muscle tension. Keep stretching comfortable; if you feel discomfort or pain, ease off a bit. Hold each stretch steadily for 10–20 seconds, relax, then repeat the stretch two or three times.

Avoid "bobbing," "bouncing," or straining. Focus on doing relaxed breathing while stretching (avoid holding your breath). Think pleasant, relaxing thoughts, or listen to quiet music as you stretch.

Q A

345.
My joints feel stiff when I start to exercise and for a while after I finish. Is there anything I can do to make them more flexible?

Stiffness and loss of flexibility are natural consequences of aging. However, diabetes accelerates the rate at which this occurs through the increased presence of *glycosylation* endproducts. When your blood glucose is elevated, some of the excess glucose attaches itself to proteins in the body, such as in joints, on cartilage, in collagen, and other places, which then become "glycosylated." This results in irreversible changes to these proteins, making them stiff and inflexible.

You can compensate for some of your loss of flexibility by doing stretching exercises two or three days per week (this is recommended for everyone). Proper stretching involves holding stretches for 10–30 seconds, without bouncing, and stretching the major muscle groups of the upper and lower body. You can stretch before and/or after exercising; stretching afterward is often easier as joints and muscles are already warmed up and slightly more flexible then. You may also want to include range-of-motion exercises along with your stretching routine. These exercises involve actively moving your joints to the fullest extent in every direction possible, sometimes using light weights or resistance bands to increase strength as well.

Safety Issues

346.
My neighbor told me about something called the "talk test" to exercise safely. What is it exactly, and should I use it during exercise?

The "talk test" is an easy, effective way to monitor your exercise intensity. While it cannot determine if your exercise intensity is too low, it can alert you to the fact that you are exercising at a harder level than you need to. If you are exercising, you should be able to converse freely with an exercise partner or other person. If you cannot talk normally because you feel

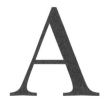

too winded, you have exceeded your *ventilatory threshold* (exercise intensity at which your breathing rate increases greatly), and you are exercising at a level that is too hard.

It is not necessary to work out higher than your ventilatory threshold to gain cardiovascular fitness and the benefits of regular exercise. In fact, in terms of diabetes control, you are better off exercising at a level that is lower than this threshold, because engaging in intense physical activities may cause your blood glucose levels to increase for up to two hours following exercise. Thus, your blood glucose levels are more likely to decrease during moderate exercise, but increase during intense, near-maximal work. Using the "talk test" will help you monitor your exercise and keep it from being harder than it needs to be.

347.
The last time I exercised when it was hot, I nearly passed out. When I checked my blood glucose, it was 200 mg/dl, so I know it wasn't due to hypoglycemia. What might have caused it?

Exercising in a hot environment, especially when the humidity is high, can cause you to become faint for several reasons. First, when it is hot and you are physically active, you have increased blood flow to your skin and muscles as your body tries to cool itself. Exercise itself increases your body's heat production, and the hot environment may cause you to heat up even more. This heat has to be released for you to avoid some type of heat exhaustion or heat stroke. A greater blood flow to these peripheral areas means that you may have more blood in your legs and arms, but less returning to your brain. A lack of adequate blood flow to your head can cause you to pass out, especially if you are exercising and stop without cooling down properly (continuing an activity at a low intensity for at least five minutes before stopping).

Another reason for your faintness could be dehydration. You normally lose some body water when you sweat. When exercising in the heat, you tend to sweat more and your body loses even more water. When you lose enough, your body has a limited amount of blood that can be circulated because some of the

Q   A

water you lose is from your bloodstream. As a result, you may not have enough blood to send to both your peripheral areas and your head at the same time. Your body may try to shut down some of the blood flow to your active muscles to preserve it for your heart and head, but doing so will only increase your heat retention and worsen the problem.

Prevention is key. Drink adequate amounts of water (or other noncaffeinated beverages) before, during, and after exercise in the heat. A good rule of thumb is to drink 6–8 ounces of fluid before starting and every 15–30 minutes during an activity. You should also try to keep your blood glucose under control, as elevated blood glucose levels can increase your water losses (due to more frequent urination) and contribute to dehydration. Remember, you will already be 1% to 2% dehydrated before you become thirsty, so start drinking before your thirst increases.

348.
I often get a little dizzy just when I stop exercising. What causes this, and can I do anything to prevent it from happening?

When you exercise, blood flow to your active muscles and skin increases, partly because various capillaries (the smallest blood vessels) open, which may be closed at rest. Overall blood flow can increase by a factor of five or more, which means that a lot of blood is flowing into your active limbs. If you stop exercising suddenly without properly slowing down your pace first (that is, cooling down), it is very likely that some of your blood will pool in your extremities (feet, lower legs, and hands) because of the combined effects of greater blood flow and gravity. Dizziness results when an insufficient amount of blood is making it uphill to your brain against gravity. If blood flow to the brain is severely compromised, your body will get itself horizontal to restore flow (that is, you will faint).

To prevent dizziness following exercise, cool down properly before stopping completely. Spend at least five minutes continuing your activity, but at a much easier pace (for example, walking after you have been jogging). Doing so allows the blood flow to begin to readjust and compensate to maintain blood delivery

Q A

to the brain. Another preventive measure is to stay adequately hydrated by drinking water or other fluids before, during, and after physical activity, especially if it is prolonged or done in the heat. Dehydration can result in a lesser amount of blood being available to circulate back to the brain, and poorly controlled diabetes contributes to dehydration.

Another possible reason for the dizziness is diabetic autonomic neuropathy (central nervous system damage). If you have this condition, you are more prone to dehydration, and an adequate cool-down period is essential.

349.
I want to exercise, but I am afraid of injuring myself. What can I do?

If you wear proper footwear and clothing, perform your chosen exercises safely, and keep away from forms of exercise where you might fall and seriously injure yourself, you can avoid almost all injuries that can interfere with regular exercise and daily activities. Even the most diligent of us may sometimes suffer minor injuries, however, so it is important to keep in mind the RICE rule: rest, ice, compression, and elevation.

Rest. Pay attention to your body. If something hurts, your body is telling you to stop. Don't use the injured body part until it feels better. Not giving an injury enough rest can delay healing and even make the injury worse.

Ice. Swelling causes more pain and slows healing. The faster you get ice on the injured area, the less pain and swelling you will have. Fill a plastic bag with crushed ice or use an ice pack. Cover the ice pack with a wet cloth to avoid freezing the skin. Apply the ice for 10–15 minutes three to four times per day after the injury occurs.

Compression. Wrapping the injury in an elastic-type wrap can also help reduce the swelling. Make sure it's not so tight that it cuts off your circulation: Your fingers and toes should not tingle or lose their color.

Elevation. Raise the injury above your heart whenever possible. For example, if you've hurt your ankle, lie down and elevate it on a pillow. Elevating an injury may stop it from throbbing.

Q A

If the pain is acute, or if it continues for longer than a few days, see your doctor immediately to rule out a more serious injury.

350.
I am a 62-year-old woman with diabetes, and I am worried about developing osteoporosis. Is exercise safe for me?

Not only is exercise safe, but it can be beneficial. Weight-bearing activities, such as walking, running, climbing stairs, and lifting weights, can help maintain bone mass and lower your risk for developing osteoporosis. In addition, by strengthening muscles and improving balance and flexibility, regular physical activity can reduce your risk of falling and bone fractures.

Before you start an exercise program, though, consult your physician to determine the level of exercise that is safe and appropriate for you.

351.
Now that my Type 1 diabetes is under control, my doctor has given me the go-ahead to start bodybuilding again. Which body-building supplements can I use, and which should I avoid?

People with diabetes should be very wary of nutritional supplements. Many advertised bodybuilding supplements employ deceptive marketing tactics to make their products seem more effective than they actually are. Some may take published research out of context, claim "universal testing" when no research has been done, make false statements about research currently being performed, reference research inappropriately, and make dubious claims about the efficacy of their ingredients. In recent years, manufacturers have touted the benefits of chromium picolinate, magnesium, and creatinine, but there is little scientific evidence that these products provide anything beyond a placebo effect for users. Some recent supplements containing a combination of ephedra and caffeine (or ma huang and guarana) have even proven to cause severe problems and, in some cases, death. It is advisable for people with diabetes to avoid most, if not all, bodybuilding supplements.

Q A

If you are interested in bodybuilding or other intense physical training, you should consult your diabetes health-care team about the best way to approach this kind of exercise. Most athletes increase the amount of protein they eat, but this can present a problem for people with diabetes as it can add to stress on the kidneys. Most dietitians will recommend an increase in your intake of complex carbohydrates, but this will require careful monitoring of your blood glucose levels to keep your diabetes under control.

352.
I have had hip replacement surgery, and I am worried that exercising might not be safe for me. What can I do?

The first thing to do is talk with your physician. He or she can tell you how much activity is enough. Be sure to ask about specific exercises that will be easier on the hip joint, and also about exercises that can help strengthen the muscles and tendons around the joint.

There are a few guidelines for exercising after a hip replacement surgery. Always allow yourself plenty of time to recover from the surgery, and do not begin any exercise program without first consulting your doctor. Also check with your doctor before doing any exercises that involve the lower body. Avoid crossing your legs or locking your knees, as both can place undue stress on the hip joint. Also avoid any exercise that involves bending at the hip at more than a 90° angle, as this, too, can result in stress on the joint.

Staying Motivated

353.
I know I need to exercise, but I just can't seem to find the motivation to exercise consistently for more than a month or two. Do you have any helpful suggestions?

Motivation to stick with an exercise program can be found in many different places. Here are some of the keys to sticking with it: choosing physical activities that are enjoyable, realistic, feasible, and easily accessible; setting attainable goals and exercise schedules; choosing appropriate exercise and equipment to

Q   A

avoid injury; exercising with a partner; and employing alternative activities to reduce boredom with a single activity.

Face it, exercise has to be fun or you will not end up doing it for any length of time. It also needs to be convenient and accessible. In addition, choosing activities with your limitations in mind is important; for example, if you have loss of sensation in your feet, a non-weight-bearing activity would be more appropriate to avoid injuring your feet unknowingly. If you are the type of person who has trouble with motivation, find a partner who can help motivate you; if you know that your "partner" is waiting for you to show up for a walk, you are more likely to follow through to avoid disappointing him or her. Also, consider setting up a series of different activities to break up the monotony of repeating the same routine day after day.

Finally, you need to understand the difference between failure and backsliding. If you deviate from your exercise schedule, or skip a session, it should not be viewed as a failure. It is normal to take days off, especially since you should be considering your exercise as a long-term, permanent lifestyle change. When unexpected days off occur, consider them as a temporary backslide and return to your normal schedule as soon as possible.

354.
A friend of mine keeps a journal of exercise. Is this something I need to do?

It's not a bad idea. Keeping an exercise log can be useful for a variety of reasons. It is an easy way to keep track of what exercise you have been doing, and it can come in handy if a physician asks for a sample of recent physical activity. If you lift weights, keeping a log means you don't have to remember what amount of weight you lift for each exercise. And if you're trying to lose weight, an exercise log and a nutrition diary (writing down everything you have eaten for each day) provide simple ways to calculate how many calories you have eaten and expended for a particular day.

More than that, though, an exercise log can provide a good psychological incentive to adhere to a program of regular exercise. When you write down every time you exercise, you are able to see a record

Q A

of what you have accomplished. Once you build a significant record after exercising every day or every other day, you can see by your log that you have really started to accomplish something. And if you begin to slip, maybe by missing a few days of exercise, your log will let you catch yourself before it gets worse.

355.
What are the advantages of keeping a diabetes and physical activity log? What should I include in the logs I keep?

Record-keeping is an important part of diabetes management in general. When you are diligent about record-keeping, you gather important information about your diabetes management and blood glucose control. You and your diabetes care provider can use this information to make informed decisions about how to fine-tune your management. When exercise is part of your lifestyle, record-keeping plays an especially important role in helping you to maintain optimal blood glucose levels in various exercise situations.

Here are key pieces of information that should be included in a diabetes and physical activity log:
- Results of your blood glucose tests throughout the day, including those that you take before, during, and after exercise.
- Information about when you take your diabetes medicines and the dosages, including any adjustments you make for exercise.
- What you eat for meals and snacks (including extra carbohydrate for exercise), and the timing of your meals and snacks in relation to the time of day that you exercise.
- The time of day you exercise, the intensity or effort required, the duration of your exercise session, and the type of activity you performed.

356.
Whenever I do one activity consistently for a while, I get an injury (like tendinitis or sore joints) and have to stop. Is there anything I can do to prevent this from happening?

It sounds like you are experiencing *overuse injuries*, which are more common in people with diabetes.

Q A

Overuse injuries are the result of repeated or excessive stress being placed on a particular joint or joints. These injuries often involve inflammation and swelling around the overused areas. With diabetes, you have an increased likelihood of glycosylation (excess blood glucose "sticking" in these areas) that may contribute to the stress in these areas.

One way to prevent such injuries is to vary your activities, or "cross train." If you like to do both running and cycling, for example, you could run or walk three days per week and cycle on alternating days. Doing so will give you a greater overall fitness level, as each type of training specifically increases your fitness for doing that activity alone. It is also important to give your joints and muscles an adequate amount of recuperation time; overuse injuries are more likely to occur if you do not rest one day or more per week or at least participate in a different activity on each day.

Finally, your physician may recommend that you use NSAIDs (nonsteroidal anti-inflammatory drugs) such as aspirin and ibuprofen, but not acetaminophen, to help reduce the inflammation and swelling. Using these over-the-counter drugs prudently can help prevent such problems. In an extreme case of pain and inflammation, your physician may recommend a cortisone shot in the affected area, but keep in mind that such treatment may temporarily worsen your blood glucose control.

357.
I have been exercising regularly, but now I have a cold. Is it all right for me to take a few days off?

If you are fighting off a cold, you likely will not be at your physical peak. As long as you resume your exercise routine when you are feeling better, there is no reason you cannot take a few days off to recover. On the other hand, many people find that exercising (though at a lower level than normal) can help alleviate some of the immediate symptoms of a cold, such as a stuffy head.

To decide if it's all right to exercise, think about your symptoms and determine whether they are located in the head or in the rest of the body. If you have a stuffy nose, sinus trouble, or a sore throat, for example, then exercise is probably all right. Try exercising at about half your normal intensity. As long as you continue to feel all right, you can continue to exercise.

If, however, your symptoms are located in other areas of your body, you may want to avoid exercising until your symptoms are gone. Fever, a cough, diarrhea, or a general achy feeling are all indications of a more widespread infection, for which the body needs rest. If you exercise, you could prolong the infection or worse. This is especially true if you are running a fever, as it is easy to dehydrate yourself through exercise at times like these. Once these symptoms pass, you can resume your workout again.

358.
I exercise regularly when I am at home, but I also travel often. How can I keep up my exercise routine while traveling?

Exercising on the road need not be difficult. Many hotels have either a swimming pool or a fitness center with weight machines, treadmills, and stationary bicycles. When making hotel reservations, ask what kind of facilities are available and whether they require an extra charge for use.

If you aren't staying at a hotel, or if you don't want to spend your vacation time in your hotel gym, look for ways to build physical activities into your travel days. Think about walking while sightseeing instead of taking a tour bus or rental car. Avoid elevators and take stairs whenever possible. Remember, any kind of physical activity is better than nothing.

Blood Sugar Highs and Lows

359.
How often should I test my blood glucose when I exercise?

The frequency of blood glucose monitoring for times when you exercise depends on a number of variables. One of the most significant variables is the type of diabetes medicines you take. If you take insulin or one of the oral drugs (sulfonylureas or repaglinide) that increases your risk of hypoglycemia, you should always monitor before and after exercise.

Q A

The purpose of monitoring at these times is twofold. First, it tells you whether your blood glucose is in a safe range for the activity you plan to do and allows you to make decisions about how to correct out-of-range values. Second, it provides important feedback about how your blood glucose changed during your activity and whether adjustments in medication dosages or carbohydrate intake were effective. Based on this feedback, you can fine-tune adjustment strategies to further optimize your management with exercise.

If you engage in vigorous or prolonged activity (over 45 minutes) or more than a typical amount for you, additional testing is warranted. Testing once or twice during your activity is advisable so that you can get an idea about how your blood glucose is responding. It is also a good idea to do additional testing for several hours after prolonged or strenuous exercise because blood glucose levels can continue to fall for up to 24 hours and even 36 hours after unusually rigorous activity.

If you manage your diabetes with diet and exercise or you take one of the oral medicines that does not raise the risk of hypoglycemia, periodic blood glucose monitoring can still be beneficial in helping you understand how your blood glucose changes with activity. Anytime you suspect either hyper- or hypoglycemia, stop to test and treat appropriately.

360.
I have heard that the oral medicines I take for my diabetes will not have any adverse effect on my blood glucose during exercise. Is this true?

That depends on the type of medicine you take. Physicians prescribe many different types of drugs to people with diabetes—some that target the pancreas to increase insulin production, some that increase insulin sensitivity in the body, some that keep the liver from overproducing glucose at night when you are fasting, and others. Some of the sulfonylureas (which increase insulin production and may decrease insulin resistance) last a long time (24–72 hours) and have a greater potential for causing lower blood glucose levels both during and after exercise, especially

Q A

an activity that is strenuous or prolonged. Diabinese, DiaBeta, and Micronase, in particular, are more likely to cause hypoglycemia because of their longer action time. Another commonly prescribed drug, Glucophage, acts primarily on the liver and, as such, is unlikely to cause low blood glucose levels. Most of the other insulin sensitizers are also not likely to increase your risk for hypoglycemia.

It is still recommended that you monitor your blood glucose more frequently around exercise to determine your response and to prevent or correct a potential low blood glucose level. If you begin a regular exercise program, check with your physician to see if you need to lower the dose of your diabetes drugs, especially if you want to avoid having to eat extra carbohydrate (if you are trying to lose weight through exercise and diet).

361.
I take insulin injections, and sometimes even mild exercise like walking makes my blood glucose go too low. Is there any way that I can prevent this from happening?

Think of insulin this way: You always need some in your body, but too much insulin in your body during exercise can cause your blood glucose to plummet. You *can* prevent low blood glucose from occurring during exercise, but it takes some planning or some preventive measures before and/or during your activity.

For spontaneous exercise, your only option is to increase your carbohydrate intake if you find your blood glucose going low during or after the activity. For moderate aerobic exercise, you may need to eat an additional 10–15 grams of carbohydrate for every 30–60 minutes of exercise. The only way you can know the exact amount you will need is by testing your blood glucose levels frequently (before, perhaps during, and after exercise) to determine your individual response.

For planned exercise, you may have to eat some extra carbohydrate, or you may be able to reduce the dosage of the insulin that will be in your body during the activity. For example, if you take only NPH in the morning and the exercise is after lunch, then reduc-

Q A

ing your morning dose by one unit would be appropriate (to start). Keep in mind, however, that if you do not end up doing the exercise, your blood glucose level may be higher since you reduced your insulin dose. If you take Humalog, NovoLog, or Regular insulin injections for meals, you may be able to reduce the dose given 1–2 hours before exercise by 1–2 units for the activity.

362.
Is there anything I can do besides eating snacks to keep myself from becoming weak, shaky, and hungry after sustained physical work?

Feeling weak, hungry, and shaky can be a warning sign that your blood glucose is falling too low with activity. However, it is important to verify that this is truly what is happening. Always have your blood glucose meter with you and test when you get this feeling. If you are experiencing hypoglycemia, or a low blood glucose level, be prepared to treat it with a rapidly absorbable carbohydrate source such as fruit juice or glucose tablets. Your goal, however, is to prevent this from happening repeatedly when you are active.

The best way to correct a pattern of hypoglycemia with activity is to be a "diabetes detective." Collect and record as much information as you can about your diabetes management and look for clues about why you might be experiencing hypoglycemia. Keep track of your blood glucose level before, during, and after physical activity. Write down the time of day that you are physically active, how long you exercise, and how hard you work. Also write down what time you take your diabetes medicines, what dosages you take, and what you eat for your meals and snacks and when.

You may need to change the time of day that you exercise. Exercising one to two hours after a meal is usually safe because blood glucose levels are higher after you eat. Exercising when diabetes medicines are "peaking," or most active, is more risky because you are more likely to experience a large fall in blood glucose with activity during these times.

Talk to your diabetes-care provider to make certain that the dosages of your diabetes medicines are prop-

Q A

erly adjusted and that you are taking them at the best time in relation to your scheduled activity. Also check to see that your meal plan is incorporating enough carbohydrate to balance your level and time of exercise.

363.
My doctor recently put me on an insulin pump using pretty high doses of insulin all the time. Now my blood glucose often gets low when I am just out walking the dog. Is there anything I can do to prevent this from happening?

There are a number of methods to prevent low blood glucose when using an insulin pump. First and foremost, you will need to check your blood glucose readings more frequently—before, during, and after exercise—to establish a pattern. For example, suppose you start with your blood glucose at 150 mg/dl, and it consistently drops by 40–50 mg/dl after 30 minutes of walking the dog. Then you know that you will have to make some changes, especially when you start out with your blood glucose lower than 150 mg/dl.

Next, consider the regimen changes that you can make. An insulin pump affords you the ability to decrease basal (baseline) insulin infusion during any activity. You can simply override your normal basal insulin setting by programming a temporary basal amount that is less than your normal amount; for instance, if your basal is usually 1.5 units/hour during the time you are walking, you may want to try lowering it to 1.0 units/hour during the activity. Alternatively, you can eat a small carbohydrate snack (10–15 grams) to compensate for each 30 minutes of exercise, using your blood glucose monitoring to adjust your carbohydrate intake or your basal insulin reduction.

Finally, you may also want to consider giving a smaller bolus amount for meals or snacks eaten within an hour before walking the dog. If your circulating insulin levels are too high when you are walking, your blood glucose levels are more likely to fall. Also, to be on the safe side, make sure you carry glucose tablets, candy, or raisins with you on your walk to treat any symptoms of hypoglycemia.

Q A

364.

I have heard that people with diabetes can easily become hypoglycemic when they exercise. Is "having a low" something that everyone with diabetes has to worry about, or just people who take insulin?

Though exercise-related hypoglycemia is a concern for many people who have diabetes, not everyone is at risk of experiencing a "low" (blood glucose below 70 mg/dl) with activity. Your diabetes management, and especially the kind of diabetes medicines that you take, influence your risk of experiencing hypoglycemia with exercise.

If you control your diabetes with meal planning and exercise but do not take glucose-lowering drugs, your risk of hypoglycemia is low and is really not any greater than it would be if you did not have diabetes.

If you take oral glucose-lowering drugs, your risk of hypoglycemia may be higher depending on which drug you take. Some do moderately increase risk while others do not. Drugs that increase the risk of hypoglycemia include sulfonylureas and repaglinide (brand name Prandin). Drugs that do not raise your risk level include alpha-glucosidase inhibitors (Glyset, Precose), biguanides (metformin [Glucophage]), and thiazolidinediones (Actos, Avandia).

If you take insulin injections, your risk of hypoglycemia with activity is increased.

If you do take insulin or one of the oral drugs that raises hypoglycemia risk, be aware that prolonged periods of activity, vigorous activity, and low starting blood glucose increase the possibility that you will experience hypoglycemia. Also, if you are new to a fitness program, if you exercise during the time your insulin or oral medication is "peaking," or if it has been a long time since your last meal, you are at a higher risk for hypoglycemia during exercise.

To be on the safe side, check with your doctor or diabetes-care provider before you design an exercise plan.

Q A

365.
How can I avoid hypoglycemia from exercise?

The best way to prevent hypoglycemia when you exercise is to do extra blood glucose monitoring. Then you'll know if your blood glucose is in a good range for the activity you plan to do. If you know your blood glucose is lower than it should be, you can take corrective action. The most immediate option is to eat extra carbohydrates. You can also learn to adjust your insulin or oral medication, but always discuss appropriate adjustments with your diabetes-care provider first. Both of these options can help prevent hypoglycemia during and after exercise.

Doing additional monitoring during and after exercise can help you understand how your blood glucose responds to various forms of activity and to different exercise situations. When you understand how your blood glucose responds, you can make better decisions about how to adjust your diabetes management to maintain optimal blood glucose levels during and after exercise sessions. Again, the options are to eat extra carbohydrate before and periodically during exercise, reduce your insulin or oral medication before you begin activity, or a combination of the two. You can also exercise one to two hours after meals or snacks, a time when blood glucose levels tend to be rising, or you can alter the time of day that you exercise in relation to when you take your medication to avoid "peak" times.

The information you gather when you do additional testing gives you valuable feedback about how well the adjustment strategies you tried worked and whether they helped maintain your blood glucose level in an optimal range throughout an exercise session. You can use this information to further fine-tune your adjustment strategies.

366.
I have had diabetes for a long time, and I no longer sense or feel "lows." What can I do to help make sure my blood glucose level is in a safe range when I exercise?

It sounds like you have hypoglycemia unawareness, a loss of the typical warning signs of hypoglycemia,

Q A

which can create a risky situation when you exercise. You must learn to do what your body used to do for you and find new ways to alert yourself to the possibility of low blood glucose. The best way to do this is to be very diligent about monitoring your blood glucose before, during, and after exercise. Frequent testing will alert you to a falling blood glucose level and give you a chance to consume carbohydrate before you become hypoglycemic.

Another level of safety is added if you exercise with a "buddy" who knows about your diabetes. This person should be able to recognize unique warning signs of hypoglycemia such as paleness, confusion, slurred speech, irritability, or lack of coordination. A buddy should be informed about what to do to assist you if your blood glucose is low enough that you are unable to help yourself. Finally, you should always wear medical identification and carry a rapidly absorbable carbohydrate to treat hypoglycemia should it occur when you exercise.

367.
If I become hypoglycemic, what should I do?

Though your first round of defense is to take steps to prevent hypoglycemia from occurring when you exercise, it is important to know how to treat low blood glucose (below 70 mg/dl) appropriately, should it occur. This is what you should do:

Stop your activity immediately and check to determine what your blood glucose level is. If your blood glucose level is under 70 mg/dl, consume 15 grams of a rapidly absorbable carbohydrate source such as glucose tablets, fruit juice, or raisins, wait 15–20 minutes, and recheck. If your blood glucose is 80–120 mg/dl when you retest, it is safe for you to resume your activity. If it is still under 80 mg/dl, consume an additional 15 grams of carbohydrate, wait another 15–20 minutes, and recheck. Resume your activity when your blood glucose reading is at least 80 mg/dl. Continue to consume extra carbohydrate as needed to keep your blood glucose in your goal range for the rest of your exercise session.

If your blood glucose is 70–100 mg/dl when you first test your blood glucose, consume 15 grams of a rapidly absorbable carbohydrate source and continue

Q A

your activity. Continue to consume additional carbohydrate as needed to keep your blood glucose in your goal range. If your blood glucose is over 100 mg/dl when you first test, and you have no symptoms of hypoglycemia, continue your activity and consume additional carbohydrate as needed to maintain your blood glucose level in your goal range.

368.

What about special sports drinks and snack bars? Should I use them to keep my blood glucose level from going too low? Can they help boost my energy level when I exercise?

Special sports drinks and snack bars can be useful, but they are certainly not necessary to keep your blood glucose level from going too low when you exercise. Carbohydrate is the nutrient that fuels working muscles and helps maintain your blood glucose in a good range during exercise. Though most snack bars and sports drinks are good sources of carbohydrate, so are fruits, diluted juices, low-fat yogurt, and breads and starches. Any of these foods can fulfill the same role as carbohydrate sources—and at less cost.

However, snack bars and sports drinks do offer some advantages. They are portable and easy to carry along with you, and they are a convenient way to take in controlled amounts of carbohydrate during prolonged periods of activity. Sports beverages are also formulated to supply fluid and appropriate amounts of electrolytes as well as carbohydrate. (Look for a sports drink that supplies no more than 14 grams of carbohydrate and 125 milligrams of sodium per eight-ounce serving.)

Snack bars and beverages that are formulated specially for diabetes are also becoming popular in the marketplace. Some of these (Extend Bar and NiteBite) are specifically designed to prevent hypoglycemia by causing a slow, sustained glucose release after you consume them. They may be helpful as snacks before or after exercise, but they are not appropriate treatments for hypoglycemia, which requires a carbohydrate source that raises your blood glucose level quickly.

Q A

369.
Even though my blood glucose level was 256 mg/dl yesterday when it was time for my walk, I went anyway. My glucose went down to 192 mg/dl by the end of my walk, but I felt tired the whole time. Did I do the right thing?

Though exercise usually has a blood-glucose-lowering effect, if you attempt physical activity when your glucose is very elevated, it can remain at a high level or rise even higher when you exercise. If your blood glucose is high before exercise, do some problem-solving to figure out the reason before you start your planned activity. Here are some questions to ask yourself:

■ Did I take the correct dosages of my medicines and did I take them on time?

■ Have I been sticking with my meal plan, or could extra food be contributing to my elevated glucose level?

■ Am I feeling stressed?

■ Could I be getting a cold or the flu, or do I have an infection of another kind?

When your blood glucose level is over 250 mg/dl, you should always test your urine for ketones before you start to exercise. If the test is negative and you think your blood glucose is high because of stress or eating extra food, exercise will usually help lower your blood glucose. However, if ketones are present in your urine, you should delay exercising. The combination of hyperglycemia and ketones tells you that you do not have enough circulating insulin available to meet your body's needs. This means that glucose, an essential energy source for exercise, can't enter your muscle cells.

If you exercise in this situation, you may experience an increase in your blood glucose and ketone levels and raise your risk of diabetic ketoacidosis. You may also become dehydrated. Hyperglycemia causes excessive urination, and exercise causes sweating. Both contribute to significant fluid loss. If you exercise when you are dehydrated, you increase your risk of becoming overheated and of overstressing your cardiovascular system. You might feel tired and

Q A

fatigued when you exercise. This not only leads to a difficult and unpleasant exercise experience but also makes you more prone to injury.

If your blood glucose is over 300 mg/dl, it is too high to exercise safely. Be certain that your medications and meal plan are well adjusted and that there is not some other cause for your hyperglycemia that needs to be corrected. It is best to establish reasonable control before you resume your activity routine.

370.
I often find that my blood glucose level is higher in the morning, before I have eaten anything, and even when I exercise. Why is this happening?

Exercise usually has a blood-glucose-lowering effect, but sometimes blood glucose unexpectedly rises in the early morning. There are a couple of possible explanations for this.

One is that circulating levels of hormones that counter insulin's blood-glucose-lowering action tend to be higher in the morning. High levels of these hormones, called *counterregulatory hormones*, can contribute to insulin resistance and morning hyperglycemia in some people, an event called the *dawn phenomenon*. These hormones can also prevent the usual lowering of blood glucose you expect to see with exercise.

Another possible explanation is that if you exercise before taking your morning dose of insulin or oral medication, your circulating insulin level will already be low. When your insulin level is low, the liver produces more glucose than the body's tissues are able to take up and use for energy. Even when you exercise, you must have enough insulin available to allow your muscles to take up and use the glucose they need to do their work. If this amount of insulin is not available, your blood glucose level can rise when you exercise.

371.
Sometimes after I do some weight training, my blood glucose goes up. Why does this happen?

You are actually experiencing a normal response. Studies on people with both Type 1 and Type 2 dia-

Q A

betes have shown that very intense exercise such as weight training or near-maximal aerobic exercise (sprinting) can actually cause an immediate rise in blood glucose due to the body's hormonal response to such physical efforts. Such exercise causes the release of several hormones in your body that increase your liver's production of glucose and reduce your muscles' uptake of glucose. The effects of these hormones can easily exceed your body's immediate need for glucose, and thus blood glucose rises.

While this rise in glucose can last for an hour or two after exercise, once the hormonal effects wane, increased replacement rates of muscle glycogen (carbohydrates stored in muscle that are used during exercise along with glucose) can cause your blood glucose to be lower later, potentially resulting in hypoglycemia (low blood glucose). Monitor your blood glucose frequently at regular intervals after exercise to make sure that hypoglycemia does not occur.

372.
I was always under the impression that exercise reduces blood glucose levels. However, by the time I finish my exercises, my blood glucose level has risen 20 points. Why does this happen?

During exercise, muscle cells draw on stored glucose (called glycogen), blood glucose, and free fatty acids for energy. To maintain the body's blood glucose level, the liver releases glucose it frees from its glycogen stores and makes from other sources. But in a person with Type 2 diabetes, the body has difficulty regulating its blood glucose level because either it's not able to make enough insulin or its cells are less sensitive to insulin. When someone with poorly controlled Type 2 diabetes (running constantly high blood glucose levels) starts exercising, his blood glucose level can go even higher, because when the liver releases glucose into the bloodstream during exercise, the cells still have a problem getting enough insulin or responding properly to insulin, so the blood glucose is not absorbed. In this case, exercise of long duration or high intensity at night can even lead to high blood glucose the next morning.

Q   A

In contrast, for someone in good health with a well-controlled blood glucose level (indicating the body has sufficient insulin available), exercise can be effective in helping the cells become more sensitive to insulin and in using blood glucose during exercise. In such a person, it's reasonable to expect the blood glucose level to drop after exercise as the cells replenish their glycogen stores by taking up blood glucose.

To prevent exercise-induced high blood glucose, people with diabetes should check their blood glucose level before engaging in exercise. If it is over 240 mg/dl, it's best to recheck the level 15 minutes into exercise. If the level starts to drop, it's a sign the body has enough insulin available to help muscle cells absorb glucose from the blood. If the level doesn't drop, it's best to stop exercising, drink plenty of water, and follow your treatment plan for treating high blood glucose as set up by your diabetes educator.

Exercise and Your Heart

373.
I found out that I had Type 2 diabetes when I was in the hospital with a heart attack. Is it safe for me to exercise?

Many people have their diabetes diagnosed in the emergency room or the hospital while being treated for a heart attack. It is estimated that a third of all people with diabetes are currently undiagnosed; since diabetes hastens the development of heart disease, it is not surprising that a stressor such as a heart attack will finally make the diabetes easily detectable.

It is safe for you to exercise once your physician gives you the green light to begin. However, you still need to approach exercise with extreme caution. At first, it would be best if you exercised in conjunction with an outpatient cardiac rehabilitation program. These programs offer medical supervision and immediate access to heart monitoring. At least initially, your primary concern with exercising is prevention of another heart attack, not your diabetes control.

After you have been exercising safely for a while, you may then choose to continue on your own or

Q A

with another community-based exercise program with less intensive medical supervision. Remain alert for any signs or symptoms of recurrence of heart problems, and see a doctor immediately if any symptoms should occur.

374.
When I exercise, I sometimes feel short of breath, and my heart feels like it is pounding in my chest. Is this normal?

Whenever you exercise, your heart rate increases, and if it increases enough you may be more aware of the rapid beating of your heart in your chest. However, your heart rate can be abnormally elevated (tachycardia) due to medication effects or abnormal contractions of your heart (cardiac arrhythmias). The shortness of breath you are experiencing could be perfectly normal, especially if you are out of shape, as you may be working out above your *ventilatory threshold,* the exercise intensity at which your breathing rate increases greatly. However, it may also be symptomatic of other health conditions such as lung obstructions (emphysema, chronic bronchitis, or asthma), heart failure (due to a weakened heart muscle), or reduced blood flow to your heart (coronary ischemia).

Diabetes alone is a risk factor for heart disease. Consequently, if you continue to have shortness of breath or rapid heart palpitations, you would be well advised to have a check-up with your physician to determine whether the cause of your symptoms is anything abnormal. In the meantime, you may want to reduce your exercise intensity, as doing so should lower your heart rate and lessen your symptoms of breathlessness.

375.
My diabetic father had a heart attack while exercising when he was 55 years old. Now I am 55 and planning to start exercising. Do I need to worry that the same thing will happen to me?

Actually, yes. The fact that your father had a heart attack at the age of 55 gives you a strong risk factor for heart disease. The fact that he had diabetes also puts you at risk for developing it, if you do not have it

Q A

already. Before you start exercising, you will want to consider several things to determine how to proceed safely.

First, consider your current training status. If you have already been exercising, but stopped for three months or less, then you have already experienced some health benefits by lowering the amount of work your heart has needed to do. If you have been sedentary, then you now have two risk factors for heart disease.

Second, consider your other risk factors for heart disease. You already have one from your father's heart attack at an early age. You will want to determine if you have any others. Advancing age (even 55) increases your risk, as does being male, smoking cigarettes, hypertension (high blood pressure), elevated cholesterol levels, being sedentary, obesity (especially extra abdominal fat), and emotional stress. If you have two or more risk factors, for your own safety, you may want to see your physician for a physical and an exercise stress test before beginning a moderate to vigorous exercise training program.

Finally, consider the exercise that you intend to do. If it is just a mild to moderate walking program, you may be all right even without a prior physical exam (even though it is still recommended) if you only have one or two risk factors, but you will want to start out slowly and be aware of any symptoms of heart disease (chest pain on exertion, excessive shortness of breath). For brisk walking or weight training, though, you will want to get checked by your doctor to get a clean bill of health first.

376.
I have heard that there are good and bad types of cholesterol. What are they, and how can exercise affect how much of them I have?

In addition to various blood fats, you have two main types of cholesterol in your bloodstream: low-density lipoproteins (LDL) and high-density lipoproteins (HDL). The LDL cholesterol is the bad type to have too much of because LDL is the most likely to contribute to plaque formation, vessel blockage, and heart disease. The stress of hyperglycemia resulting from poorly controlled diabetes makes the LDL even more damaging to artery walls by oxidizing it, which triggers inflammation and, ultimately, plaque formation. Conversely, the good type of cholesterol is HDL, which acts as a cholesterol removal system in the blood. In addition to having hyperglycemia, people with Type 2 diabetes often have lipid abnormalities such as elevated levels of triglycerides (blood fats) and LDL cholesterol. It is important to increase HDL levels as much as possible while lowering LDL levels to prevent heart disease and other vascular disease.

Exercise can affect the levels of these types of cholesterol, especially the HDL. Being physically active increases HDL levels, and being inactive causes them to decrease. LDL appears to be affected more by dietary intake of saturated fat and cholesterol (both of these increase LDL levels) than by exercise; a healthier diet can cause LDL levels to decrease. For an overall healthier heart and optimal blood lipids, engage in regular exercise and eat a healthier diet. Some individuals have genetically driven high cholesterol or blood fat levels that are not treatable with diet and exercise alone. If you are one of these people, you may need to see your physician to discuss the possibility of taking drugs to help lower your cholesterol.

377.
My doctor recently put me on a new drug. Now whenever I exercise, my heart rate is no higher than 110 beats per minute, although I used to be able to get it up to 135. Is this a side effect of the medication?

Very likely. One class of drugs in particular, beta-blockers, is designed to keep your heart rate lower at rest and during exercise. Beta-blockers target the heart and inhibit receptors that, when activated, normally increase your heart rate and the strength of your heart's contraction. With less frequent and weaker heart contractions, the total amount of blood pumped out by your heart is lessened; by lessening the work done by your heart in this manner, it is less likely that you will develop *ischemia*, a severely reduced blood flow to your heart, during exercise.

Q   A

Some examples of beta-blockers are propranolol, atenolol, and metoprolol.

The restrictions that this class of drugs poses on your heart's response may reduce your exercise tolerance somewhat—especially if the drug is propranolol, as this drug targets other receptors around your body and not just those in the heart. The other two mentioned are second-generation beta-blockers that target the heart more directly and may not interfere with exercise quite as much.

People taking beta-blockers are still able to exercise and monitor their exercise intensity effectively. The Rating of Perceived Exertion scale, where you rate how hard you believe you are exercising with a number between 6 for "no exertion," and 20 for "maximal" exertion, is still valid to use, even though heart rates will be lower than expected while using beta-blockers. Ask your doctor about the level at which you should be exercising.

**378.
I developed diabetes 10 years ago. I also have a lot of other health problems, including high blood pressure, high cholesterol, pain in my legs when I walk, and cataracts. Is there any kind of exercise that is safe for someone like me to do?**

Yes, believe it or not! These are some of the things you need to consider first, though, before choosing the type of exercise to do: With diabetes, high blood pressure, and high cholesterol, you have three definite risk factors for heart disease. If the pain in your legs is caused by peripheral vascular disease (artery blockage in your legs), then you have another risk factor. With these known risks and your current age, you would be well advised to have a physical exam and possibly an exercise test before you start an exercise training program.

For you, mild to moderate aerobic exercise (walking or cycling, for example) would be most beneficial. You can also safely engage in weight training or resistance training as long as your focus is on lower-weight, higher-repetition training. You need to avoid high-intensity work, including heavy yard work, shov-

Q A

eling snow, or heavy weight lifting, however, because of the excessive stress these activities place on your heart and your vascular system as a whole. Furthermore, pain in your legs when you walk indicates that you probably have some blockage of the arteries in your lower legs limiting your blood flow there, giving you another reason to avoid strenuous exercise. Use your pain as a guide to let you know when you are exercising too strenuously; slow down a little if your leg pain becomes more than mild. Finally, if your cataracts are limiting your vision, then exercising indoors on a treadmill or stationary cycle or in a swimming pool would likely be safer for you than walking or riding outdoors.

You can still attain many of the health benefits of exercise, though, and engaging in regular activity may help alleviate some of the health problems that you already have.

Exercising With Complications

379.
What if I have diabetes complications? Is it still safe to exercise?

It is always a good idea to check with your doctor before beginning an exercise program. He or she should be able to direct you toward exercises that are best for people with diabetes. Certain exercises may be safer for you than others.

If you have proliferative retinopathy (eye disease), you should avoid high-impact aerobics, heavy weight lifting, and anything that involves straining or jarring movements. You should also avoid any exercise that places your head lower than the rest of your body.

If you have neuropathy (nerve damage) with loss of sensation in your feet or legs, you should avoid all weight-bearing exercises and stick to activities such as swimming, bicycling, rowing, and chair exercises. Repetitive exercises that place pressure on the feet, such as using a treadmill, walking long distances, and jogging, may lead to foot ulcers and fractures. If you have nephropathy (kidney disease), it's a good idea to avoid high-intensity or strenuous exercises.

Q A

380.
I have just been told that I have retinopathy. What are good exercise options for me? Are there types of exercise that I should avoid?

When you have retinopathy, or any other diabetes complication, it is important that you take extra care to make sure the activities you plan to do will benefit your health without worsening your complication. When it comes to retinopathy, the most important precaution is to have regular eye exams. Your level of retinopathy should be carefully assessed so that exercise recommendations, as well as limitations, can be specifically and individually outlined based on the findings of the exam. That said, the following are general, sensible guidelines to keep in mind when you have retinopathy:

Moderation is the key to safety. Most moderate forms of activity are safe and beneficial for people with retinopathy. Aerobic activities like walking, stationary cycling, swimming, low-intensity machine rowing, or stair climbing are good options. Weight lifting or other resistance exercises are usually safe if you use a low amount of weight or light resistance and a high number of repetitions. Stretching is also good.

Activities that involve vigorous bouncing or jarring, heavy lifting (especially with the upper body and arms), straining or holding your breath during exertion, isometric exercises, or lowering the head below the waist are best avoided. Examples of high-risk exercise include those that are strenuous and anaerobic, such as sprinting and heavy weight lifting with a high amount of weight or resistance and a low number of repetitions. High-impact activities such as jogging, running, or high-impact aerobic dance and vigorous contact sports such as football or basketball are also risky. These forms of exercise can increase both blood pressure and the pressure in the eye, which can cause trauma and injury to already "fragile" eyes.

381.
I have just been told that I have protein in my urine and that my kidneys are affected by diabetes. Is it safe for me to exercise?

When you have diabetes, physical activity is an important part of your management because it helps

Q A

improve both blood glucose and blood pressure control, which in turn reduces your risk of developing complications of diabetes such as nephropathy.

However, when you have protein in your urine (proteinurea) and your kidneys are affected by diabetes, there is a dilemma. Exercise causes a temporary rise in blood pressure which is associated with short-term changes in kidney function and a temporary increase in the amount of protein that is lost in the urine. Just what the exercise-related changes in kidney function mean in terms of progression of nephropathy is still being debated. By keeping your blood glucose and blood pressure at optimal levels, the changes in kidney function that occur with exercise are less severe than they would be if your control were less than optimal.

Mild or moderate forms of activity are the safest exercise options when you have proteinurea because they result in a limited increase in blood pressure. Good choices include walking, water exercise, stretching, light calisthenics, or light weight lifting. Very vigorous or prolonged activities such as intense endurance events, heavy weight lifting, isometric exercise, or heavy work that causes excessive straining can greatly increase both blood pressure and urine protein loses. They are therefore not the best and safest options. Remember to discuss your plans to begin a new exercise program with your diabetes-care provider before you begin.

**382.
I know that people with diabetes can have a lot of problems with their feet. Can exercise help prevent any of these problems?**

Regular exercise can help prevent or improve foot problems in people with diabetes. To understand how and why, you need to look at the cause of changes in diabetic feet.

Diabetic foot problems include numbness in the toes and foot, chronic and shooting pain, abnormal calluses, and, sometimes, ulcerations that are resistant to healing. There is no question that diabetes-related foot problems are the leading cause of lower-extremity amputations today. Most of these changes are due to insulin resistance and sustained elevations in blood glucose levels; the resulting reduction in blood flow

317

Q   A

to the feet causes damage to the tissues and the nerves in those areas.

The good news is that a recent study demonstrated that people with diabetes who exercise regularly have improved blood flow to their feet, although their responses were still less than in people without diabetes. Engaging in regular exercise may not be able to completely reverse foot problems once you have them, but it may still improve them. And regular exercise may help to prevent such problems from occurring in the first place.

383.
When I walk, the bottoms of my feet start to feel numb. What should I do about this?

Experiencing numb feet when you have diabetes should always be taken seriously, and this is especially true when you exercise. Numbness can be a symptom of peripheral neuropathy, a serious complication of diabetes. It can also be related to poor blood supply to your feet, the result of atherosclerosis. To reduce the risk of serious foot injury, it is important for all people with diabetes to have annual foot exams that include an assessment of circulation, reflexes, foot structure and mechanics, and sensation.

Because peripheral neuropathy affects how you sense, feel, and position your feet, it is important that you take special care to protect them when you exercise. Have a thorough foot exam before you start a new activity routine and discuss best exercise options with your doctor. Protect your feet by investing in good-quality shoes that are properly fitted and appropriate for the activity you plan to do. Break in new shoes gradually and wear clean socks that fit smoothly into your shoe. (Make sure you wear protective footwear when you do water sports.) And examine your feet by looking at them and touching and feeling them before and after every exercise session. Report any redness, swelling, blisters, calluses, or signs of injury to your physician.

The safest exercise options when you have peripheral neuropathy are non-weight-bearing activities such as swimming, bicycling, rowing, armchair exercises, stretching, or moderate strength and resistance activities such as weight lifting or calisthenics.

Q   A

The least safe exercise options are prolonged, high-impact, or strenuous activities that are weight-bearing. Examples include walking long distances, jogging or running, high-impact aerobics, climbing stairs, treadmill exercise, jumping, or playing sports such as tennis or basketball.

384.

I have neuropathy, but it does not cause much pain. Instead, it prevents me from walking well, and I have problems with balance. Is there anything I can do to improve my ability to walk and to keep my balance?

Tai chi, yoga, and stretching exercises can help you walk better and improve your balance with minimum impact on your feet. Here is another good way to improve balance: Stand on one leg like a stork, resting your raised foot on the inside of the opposite knee. Most people can stand this way for only 15–30 seconds at first, but try to work up to standing on one foot for 2–3 minutes at a time. Do this three times a day, and your balance and walking will improve.

If you have access to the necessary machinery, try doing leg exercises such as knee extensions, leg presses, and leg curls to strengthen your walking muscles. If you don't have access to this equipment, ask your doctor for exercises you can do at home using ankle weights, or ask for a referral to a physical therapist. Your insurance should cover this service.

If you don't have much pain because your feet are numb, be careful not to do pounding, weight-bearing exercises such as jumping jacks or running. Swimming, biking, and rowing are alternatives that will keep you fit and minimize the impact on your feet.

385.

My feet are somewhat numb due to peripheral neuropathy (nerve damage), and I just lost my left big toe due to a chronic infection. Can I still safely do walking or jogging as my main form of exercise?

Continuing with frequent walking or jogging may be asking for trouble. For one thing, these forms of exer-

Q   A

cise are weight-bearing and, consequently, put a lot of stress on your lower extremities. In addition, with loss of sensation in your feet, you may be unaware of any blisters or calluses that develop on your feet because of this kind of exercise. These areas can then become infected (which you also may not feel), and you then run the risk of further amputations of your toes or other areas of your feet. The fact that you have already had an infection in your toe that was not able to heal properly increases your risk for a similar situation to occur with your remaining toes.

The type of exercise that would be safer for you is anything non-weight-bearing, including swimming, running in water, water aerobics, stationary biking, rowing machines, and the like. These exercises have a much lower chance of causing blisters, calluses, or other foot traumas that could develop into an infection. If you do engage in weight-bearing activities, then make sure that you inspect your feet daily for even minor trauma and are vigilant about your foot care. If you cannot inspect your own feet easily, ask someone else to do it for you.

386.
My heart-rate response to exercise may be blunted by the diabetic autonomic neuropathy that I have. Can I still use my heart rate to monitor exercise intensity, or is there another way that would be better?

Diabetic autonomic neuropathy (DAN), damage to non-consciously controlled bodily processes, does have effects on your resting heart rate (usually elevated) and your heart-rate response to exercise (usually blunted). Undoubtedly, if you usually aim for a target heart rate during exercise, that target would need to be lowered to prevent you from working out too vigorously.

A recent study demonstrated that people with DAN can effectively use the "heart-rate reserve" method to monitor exercise intensity. This method involves, first, measuring both your resting heart rate (upon waking) and your maximal heart rate; with DAN, you would need to actually measure rather than estimate

Q A

your maximal heart rate since DAN may have blunted your maximal value. Your heart-rate reserve (with DAN) is the difference between maximal and resting heart rates. Once you have calculated this difference, add a percent of heart-rate reserve to your resting heart rate to arrive at the new target value. It is still appropriate to exercise at a certain percentage (50% to 85%) of this value.

Example: If your resting heart rate is 95 beats per minute, and your measured maximal heart rate is 155 beats per minutes, your heart-rate reserve is 155 – 95, or 60 beats per minute. If your goal is 50% of heart-rate reserve, add (0.50×60) plus 95 beats per minute to arrive at a target heart rate of 125.

An alternative method of monitoring exercise intensity with DAN is to use the Rating of Perceived Exertion (RPE) scale. One version of the scale goes from 6 ("no exertion") to 20 ("maximal exertion"). Even with DAN, an acceptable cardiovascular training range would be from 12 to 16 ("somewhat hard" to "hard") for your overall subjective feeling of how hard you are working.

387.
I have been told that I have diabetic gastroparesis (delayed emptying of the stomach into the intestines). Will this condition affect my blood-glucose response to exercise?

Gastroparesis is caused by damage to the nervous system related to diabetes and is another outcome of diabetic autonomic neuropathy (DAN). In this particular condition, the movement of food and fluids through the stomach and the intestinal tract is abnormal and can result in alternating bouts of diarrhea and constipation.

Gastroparesis may slow the digestion and absorption of carbohydrates that you eat to prevent or treat low blood glucose that can result from exercise. Since exercise increases blood glucose use, the potential for much more severe hypoglycemia exists if ingested carbohydrates are not processed in time. Conversely, after exercise, your blood glucose can rise too high once all the food is finally absorbed.

Q A

Ask your diabetes doctor about medicines that may ease the symptoms of gastroparesis. Check your blood glucose frequently when you exercise. Make sure to take in only small amounts of food or carbohydrate prior to exercise, and allow a little extra time after eating before you start to exercise. Also try to begin your exercise session with your blood glucose level slightly higher than it would normally be at the start of a session. If low blood glucose should occur, treat it with glucose tablets or another form of readily absorbed carbohydrate (regular soda or sugared candy).

8
Medications

Oral Drugs and Supplements

388. How do glyburide (Micronase, DiaBeta, Glynase PresTabs), glipizide (Glucotrol, Glucotrol XL), glimepiride (Amaryl), nateglinide (Starlix), and repaglinide (Prandin) work, and what are the side effects?

389. How does metformin (Glucophage and Glucophage XR) work, and what are the side effects?

390. How do acarbose (Precose) and miglitol (Glyset) work, and what are the side effects?

391. How do rosiglitazone (Avandia) and pioglitazone (Actos) work, and what are the side effects?

392. With all of the oral diabetes medicines on the market today, how do doctors decide which one (or ones) to prescribe?

393. Do people with diabetes need to take vitamin supplements?

394. Are there any supplements people with diabetes shouldn't take?

395. Are there any drugs that can raise blood glucose levels?

396. Can I take birth control pills?

Insulin Injections

Frequently Asked Questions

Q A

388.

How do glyburide (Micronase, DiaBeta, Glynase PresTabs), glipizide (Glucotrol, Glucotrol XL), glimepiride (Amaryl), nateglinide (Starlix), and repaglinide (Prandin) work, and what are the side effects?

All of these diabetes drugs share a common thread in that they stimulate your pancreas to produce more insulin. In Type 2 diabetes, the body doesn't use insulin properly, which causes the pancreas to over-work. Eventually the pancreas cannot make enough insulin to meet the body's needs, and over time it wears out and makes less and less insulin. Insulin is necessary because it allows glucose to leave the blood-stream and enter the cells, where it provides fuel for your body. These diabetes pills stimulate your pancreas to produce more insulin, which helps lower your blood glucose level.

The main difference between these drugs is the length of time they work in your body. Glyburide, glipizide, and glimepiride all stimulate the pancreas for 24 hours, whereas nateglinide and repaglinide stimulate the pancreas just after a meal for 2 to 3 hours. Some people just need a boost in insulin after they eat while others need more insulin around the clock.

Side effects of glyburide, glipizide, and glimepiride include hypoglycemia, weight gain, and photosensitivity (meaning that you may be more likely to get sunburned, so you need to use sunscreen when exposed to sunlight). Hypoglycemia (low blood glucose) is very common and can occur if you eat less than usual, skip a meal, exercise vigorously, take certain antibiotics, or drink alcohol. If you feel symptoms of hypoglycemia (such as shaking, sweating, or lightheadedness), check your blood sugar, eat a snack, and call your doctor. If you experience hypoglycemia often, your doctor may need to change your medicine dose or switch your prescription to a different drug. Simply eating more to prevent hypoglycemia is not a good idea, because it will cause you to gain weight. Hypoglycemia is rare with nateglinide and repaglinide.

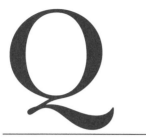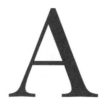

389.
How does metformin (Glucophage and Glucophage XR) work, and what are the side effects?

Type 2 diabetes has three features: failure of the pancreas to make enough insulin, resistance to insulin, and release of too much glucose by the liver. One of the liver's jobs is to store glucose in your body as glycogen and release it from storage when you need it, such as between meals and overnight. The signal for the liver to stop releasing glucose is increased levels of insulin in the blood. Under normal conditions, insulin in the blood means that blood glucose levels must be high already, so the liver doesn't need to release more. In Type 2 diabetes, this system is broken, and large amounts of glucose continue to be released into the bloodstream by the liver. Metformin causes the liver to be more sensitive to the presence of insulin, thereby slowing down the release of stored glucose from the liver and helping to keep your blood glucose within range.

The difference between Glucophage and Glucophage XR is that Glucophage works for 12 hours and is usually taken twice per day, whereas Glucophage XR works for 24 hours and should be taken with the largest meal of the day.

The possible side effects of metformin include a metallic taste in the mouth, upset stomach, nausea, and diarrhea. Most people have no side effects with metformin or report only having loose stools when they first start taking metformin. Other people have to stop taking metformin because they cannot tolerate the diarrhea.

Certain people cannot take metformin because they have heart, kidney, or liver disease. Metformin should be stopped before you have a diagnostic test with iodinated dye such as an angiogram or IVP (intravenous pyelogram) in order to prevent a potentially fatal side effect called lactic acidosis. Forty-eight hours after the test, you would have a blood test to check your kidney function and would restart metformin based on the results.

Q   A

390.
How do acarbose (Precose) and miglitol (Glyset) work, and what are the side effects?

When we eat a meal, our food moves from our stomach into our intestines where it is broken down. The nutrients in our food, such as carbohydrate, are absorbed into the bloodstream from here. Normally, it takes about 20 minutes from the time you take a bite for this to start happening. Acarbose and miglitol slow down the time it takes carbohydrate to be absorbed into the bloodstream by blocking the enzymes that break down starches and certain sugars into glucose. As a result, your blood glucose doesn't rise as sharply after each meal. For these pills to work, it is important to take them with the first bite of your meal.

Studies so far have shown that these drugs lower after-meal blood glucose levels by about 50 mg/dl. However, between meals, they only lower glucose levels by about 25 mg/dl to 30 mg/dl, which is less than other drugs. People who take acarbose or miglitol, therefore, either do not have very high blood glucose or take the drug in combination with something else.

Possible side effects of acarbose and miglitol include gas, bloating, and diarrhea. It is possible to minimize these side effects by starting with a very small dose and slowly increasing to the desired level. Some studies indicate that acarbose might impair absorption of other drugs, either by causing the drugs to pass through the intestines too quickly or by binding to the drugs so they can't be absorbed into the body. In most cases, this effect is of little consequence, but for drugs that must remain within a narrow dosage range, such as digoxin, the interaction may be more significant. It's best to talk to your doctor or pharmacist about any possible interactions and watch for signs that your other medications are becoming less effective.

391.
How do rosiglitazone (Avandia) and pioglitazone (Actos) work, and what are the side effects?

Type 2 diabetes has three features: failure of the pancreas to make enough insulin, release of too much glucose by the liver, and resistance to insulin. Rosiglitazone and pioglitazone work by making the muscle

Q   A

and fat cells more sensitive to the action of insulin. They are most effective in people who still produce fairly high amounts of insulin. Because these medications change the cells, it may take at least four weeks before you will notice lower blood glucose readings.

The side effects of rosiglitazone and pioglitazone can include mild to moderate edema, or water retention, and weight gain. Some people may experience cold symptoms, headache, or muscle pain. These drugs may also reduce the effectiveness of birth control pills. They carry a warning to have liver enzymes measured by a laboratory blood test every two months for the first year and periodically thereafter. This warning was issued because a similar medication, troglitazone, caused many cases of severe liver injury. Troglitazone was taken off the market in 2000. But because rosiglitazone and pioglitazone are in the same class as troglitazone, the FDA acted to protect the consumer. To date, rosiglitazone and pioglitazone have not caused liver injury.

392.
With all of the oral diabetes medicines on the market today, how do doctors decide which one (or ones) to prescribe?

Many doctors follow an algorithm, or flowchart, in selecting diabetes drugs. If diet and exercise alone cannot control a person's diabetes, a physician can choose from among five different classes of oral diabetes medicines, which allow the choice of drug to be tailored to the individual needs of the person with diabetes. Sulfonylureas and meglitinides act on the pancreas to facilitate insulin secretion. Thiazolidinediones act on muscle to enhance insulin sensitivity and glucose uptake. Metformin, a biguanide, acts on the liver to decrease glucose output. Alpha-glucosidase inhibitors slow absorption of carbohydrate from the intestines. Physicians also prescribe insulin, either alone or in combination with oral agents.

Often, a slender person is started with a sulfonylurea, while an overweight person may be started with metformin. Sulfonylureas can cause weight gain, which might be undesirable in a heavier person. Metformin does not cause weight gain when used alone and may cause some weight loss.

Q A

Age and kidney functioning also influence choices. Metformin is eliminated through the kidneys, so people with kidney disease or declining kidney function (as can happen with age) may not be good candidates for metformin. Sulfonylureas can cause hypoglycemia, which can be more serious in older people.

If the first drug is not fully effective, a second one may be prescribed. Many people now are on "triple therapy" with three different drugs. When diet, exercise, and oral medicines do not provide optimal blood glucose levels, insulin injections are added.

393.
Do people with diabetes need to take vitamin supplements?

You do not need to take any special vitamins or minerals just because you have diabetes. If you are eating a balanced diet with a variety of foods, your nutrient needs are likely to be met. There is no research to date that indicates that certain vitamins or minerals will improve your diabetes control, except in rare cases of chromium deficiency. (Chromium deficiency, however, is very rare in this country, and adding extra chromium to the diet where there is no deficiency is of no benefit.)

Certain groups of people may benefit from a taking a multivitamin because their diets may not provide adequate amounts of certain nutrients. These individuals include the elderly, pregnant or breast-feeding women, strict vegetarians, and people on very low calorie diets (less than 1,200 calories per day). Older people with diabetes, and most women, can benefit from taking 1,000 to 1,500 milligrams of calcium each day to reduce osteoporosis. Women of child-bearing age should consider taking a folic acid supplement to prevent birth defects.

If you are concerned about your vitamin or mineral intake, check with your dietitian. If your diet is lacking some important nutrients, he or she may recommend a supplement.

394.
Are there any supplements people with diabetes shouldn't take?

Yes, there are some vitamin supplements and herbs that can have negative effects on diabetes control. Certain supplements can have effects on blood glu-

Q A

cose control. Glucosamine, which is sold to improve joint health, may make insulin resistance worse or raise blood glucose levels. Ginseng, which is sold as a memory aid and energy booster, may cause a low blood sugar reaction if you take diabetes pills. Also, it is possible that echinacea, which is supposed to boost the immune system, may make Type 1 diabetes and other autoimmune diseases worse. St. John's wort, which is sold to treat depression, may make your sensitivity to sunlight worse if you take sulfonylurea diabetes pills.

And there are some herbs no one should take: chaparral, coltsfoot, comfrey, ephedrine (ma huang), germander, jin bu huan, lobelia, phenylalanine, sassafras, L-tryptophan, and yohimbe. These herbs have had serious side effects, such as liver damage and even death.

It is important to remember that even though many of these products are touted as being "natural" and safe, they have an effect on the body and can even be dangerous. In fact, because these products do not undergo rigorous testing that the Food and Drug Administration requires for pharmaceuticals, we don't know all the risks associated with supplements.

Finally, you should always consult with your doctor before starting a supplement. It is also important to let your doctor know what supplements you do take, and discuss whether any of them could have an effect on your diabetes care. Doing so is especially important if you are taking any medications, are pregnant, or have a chronic disease.

395.
Are there any drugs that can raise blood glucose levels?

Prescription and over-the-counter drugs can indeed affect your blood glucose level. Some drugs can raise your blood glucose levels, and some will cause them to drop. Others may also interfere with how your diabetes pills work. If you have concerns about a specific medication you are taking, check with your doctor or pharmacist about the effect it could have on your diabetes.

The following classes of drugs are known to raise blood glucose:

Q A

■ Diuretics, especially if taken in high doses, such as Diuril, Hydrodiuril, Lasix (used to treat fluid buildup);
■ Epinephrine (used to treat allergic reactions) and epinephrine-like drugs (cold, flu, and allergy medicines);
■ Lithium (used to treat manic depression);
■ Phenobarbital or phenytoin (Dilantin) (used to treat epilepsy and other nervous system disorders);
■ Steroids, such as prednisone and cortisone (used to reduce inflammation); and
■ Thyroid preparations (used to treat reduced or absent thyroid function).

Other medications that can potentially raise blood glucose include estrogen and birth control pills, and preparations used as appetite suppressants.

Be sure your diabetes health-care team knows about all the prescription and over-the-counter medications you are using. And when you start a new medication, test your blood glucose regularly to see if it affects your blood glucose control. If you feel that it does, check with your doctor or pharmacist about whether you need to change it or adjust the dose.

396.
Can I take birth control pills?

That depends. Some women shouldn't take birth control pills because they have a family history of breast and ovarian cancer. Birth control pills can also cause circulation and blood-clotting problems, especially in women who smoke. Some doctors also recommend against taking birth control pills if you have uncontrolled high blood pressure or high cholesterol levels.

Women with diabetes sometimes find they have difficulty controlling their blood glucose levels when they take birth control pills. Even without birth control pills, the changes in hormone level that occur during the menstrual cycle can raise blood glucose levels, and this effect may worsen with birth control pills. In fact, one study found that 67% of women who took oral contraceptives had changes in premenstrual blood glucose levels. If you do take birth control pills, you may have to work with your doctor to adjust your diabetes treatment plan to keep your blood glucose levels under control.

Q   A

Using some form of birth control, whether you choose oral contraceptives or something else, is important for women with diabetes. Planned pregnancies give babies the best chance of good health.

Insulin Injections

397.
I'm afraid of injections.
What can I do?

It's perfectly natural not to want to inject yourself. People are reluctant to inject insulin for many reasons. You may be fearful that injecting will hurt. You might just be squeamish about sticking yourself. Or the idea of having to go on insulin therapy may be troubling to you.

Whatever the reason, there is assistance available to help you overcome your reservations. If it's the puncture that bothers you, you may want to try a device that is designed to make it easier to self-inject. Some devices hide the needle so you can't see it, while others use a spring-loaded action that inserts the needle for you. As for pain, those who inject insulin will attest that the punctures for blood glucose monitoring cause more discomfort than the very fine insulin needles.

For some people, facing what insulin therapy means to them is enough to stop them from taking injections, even though they know it may be the best treatment option for them. For some, insulin therapy is an emotional threshold they are unwilling to cross. Others believe that if they need insulin therapy, their diabetes has become more serious and they equate it with a grave prognosis. Unfortunately, diabetes is already serious, whether you treat it with diet and exercise alone, oral drugs, or insulin.

Many people don't want to begin insulin therapy because they believe taking injections will be too inconvenient. While it's true that swallowing a pill is much easier, new pen-type insulin delivery systems have minimized the inconvenience of insulin therapy.

If you are advised to make the transition to insulin therapy, make your concerns known to your healthcare team. They will be able to ease your fears and help you find solutions to your concerns.

Q A

398.
How does insulin work?

Insulin is a hormone that is released by the beta cells in the pancreas in response to various stimuli, including elevated blood glucose. One key purpose is to control the blood glucose rise that occurs right after a meal. There are several body systems important in blood glucose regulation in addition to the pancreas, including the liver and the muscles. After a meal, when your blood glucose level rises, insulin acts on the liver by signaling it to stop converting glycogen (the stored form of glucose) into glucose and releasing the glucose into your bloodstream. Insulin also signals the liver to take some glucose out of your blood and store it as glycogen. Insulin also prompts muscle to store glucose as glycogen. In addition to regulating blood glucose, insulin has major effects on the way cholesterol levels are controlled, the way blood vessels behave, and the way certain tissues respond to several other signals.

In Type 1 diabetes, the pancreas is not able to make insulin at all, so people have to inject it throughout the day.

In Type 2 diabetes, the body becomes resistant to the effects of insulin. The cells simply don't recognize that it is there and, as a result, the insulin can't get glucose into the cells at the necessary rate. Because of this resistance, the liver doesn't recognize the signals to decrease glucose production, raising blood glucose levels even higher. Over time, your body might stop making insulin, or it may not make enough of it to keep your blood glucose levels even. Diabetes drugs, along with diet and exercise, may help the body's cells more sensitive to the action of insulin so that they can use it more effectively. However, if you have Type 2 diabetes and your body doesn't make enough insulin anymore, you may need to supplement your supply by injecting insulin.

399.
Why are there different types of insulin?

Insulin is secreted by the body in two major patterns. Throughout the day, the beta cells in the pancreas secrete insulin at a relatively constant, low level, called the basal level. After meals, the pancreas releases a dramatically higher level of insulin, called a

Q A

bolus, which stimulates the cells to make use of the glucose in your food.

Insulin manufacturers have tried to produce products that mimic the insulin patterns that your body requires. There are basal insulins such as glargine, Ultralente, NPH, and Lente and faster-acting after-meal insulins such as Regular, lispro, and aspart. Manufactured insulins are also described by how quickly they begin to take effect after you inject them, and how long they keep working in your body. The standard terms are "long-acting" (glargine and Ultralente), "intermediate-acting" (NPH and Lente), "short-acting" (Regular), and "rapid-acting" (lispro and aspart). Your body requires a mixture of basal and after-meal insulin, which is why you may need to take more than one type of insulin. If you use two kinds of insulin, you may be able to use premixed, fixed combinations of insulin; they come in three different percentage ratios (70/30, 75/25, and 50/50). A 50-unit dose of 70/30 insulin, for instance, contains 35 units of NPH insulin and 15 units of Regular insulin (that is, 70% NPH and 30% Regular). Your typical blood glucose patterns will dictate the type and dose of insulin that is best for you.

In the United States, most people use "human insulin." This type of insulin is made in a laboratory and is structurally the same as the insulin your body produces. (It doesn't come from humans.) Some people still use pork insulin, which is actually derived from pigs. However, pork insulin has limited use in this country, because it can still cause allergic reactions.

400.
How should I store my insulin?

All unopened vials, cartridges, or pens filled with insulin should be stored in the refrigerator. Most vials of insulin can be kept at room temperature for 28 to 30 days. After that, the insulin will become less potent. Most people don't use a whole vial of insulin within a month, so they refrigerate it to make it last longer. Keep in mind, injecting weak insulin that has been stored at room temperature beyond the recommended guidelines is a common cause of unexplained high blood glucose readings.

Q A

The storage guidelines for pens and pen cartridges vary according to the type of insulin and manufacturer. If you use one of these products, be sure to select the right size for your needs, so you don't waste insulin. For example, to minimize the inconvenience of injection therapy, you may choose to use a 3-cc (300 unit) pen or pen cartridge that is designed for storage at room temperature. Suppose the pen or pen cartridge can be kept at room temperature for 10 days before losing potency and you use 23 units per day; in this case, you would be wasting 70 units every ten days. If this is the case, you might be better off choosing a product with a 1.5-cc (150 unit) pen or cartridge that you will finish in less than a week without wasting insulin.

401.
What do I need to know so that I can adjust my insulin dose?

You can become adept at adjusting your insulin dose, but as with any new skill, it takes time and guidance. The key is to look for patterns. You want to avoid the knee-jerk reaction of just responding to a high blood glucose reading by raising your insulin dose. Instead, your basal insulin dose is usually adjusted based on a pattern of fasting blood glucose results. If you have one high blood glucose result and two that are within range, you would not raise your basal insulin dose because of that single high reading. It would make better sense to keep your insulin dose the same and check to see if the pattern changes.

However, you may want to adjust your mealtime insulin dose based on a number of factors. These include the grams of carbohydrate that you plan to eat, whether you plan to exercise before your next meal, and your current blood glucose level. What you want to avoid is getting into the habit of correcting elevated blood glucose readings with extra insulin so often that you are unable to see when your basal insulin dose needs to change. That's a trap many people fall into, but it's one you can avoid with guidance from your health-care team. Your doctor or other provider can help you look at the whole picture and not lose sight of your basal insulin needs. With guidance, you can gain confidence in your insulin adjustment skills.

Q A

402.
Does it matter where I inject my insulin shot?

Where you inject insulin is as important as when you inject it for two reasons: First, you can damage the tissue under your skin if you inject insulin in the same place every time. This damage can cause inconsistent absorption of insulin at these sites. Second, different body regions absorb insulin at different speeds.

Some experts suggest that you inject breakfast and lunch insulin into your arms and abdomen, which absorb insulin relatively quickly, and inject supper and bedtime insulin into your buttocks and thighs, which absorb insulin more slowly. Doing so helps insulin last through the night.

Wherever you inject, make sure it's at least 1 inch from any spot you've used in the past week. You should also stay at least 2 inches away from your navel and avoid injecting in or near moles, scars, and any lumpy fat deposits caused by previous shots. The insulin won't be absorbed well at these spots. If you make a change in where you inject your insulin, be sure to test your glucose more often than usual to find out how your body responds to shots at different sites.

One reason some people don't rotate their injections sites enough may be that it is inconvenient to have to undress to expose their skin. Injecting doesn't have to be that troublesome, however. Some people do inject their insulin right through their clothes. This can be especially handy when you are at work or out where it is difficult to find a private space. Studies have shown this practice is safe and will not raise the chance of infection, as long as you are injecting through a single thin layer of clean clothing.

Frequently Asked Questions

403.
How can I remember to check my blood glucose and take my pills?

It can be hard to remember all the checks and pills that must be taken throughout the day. There are ways to keep on top of them, however. One way to help remember is to match cues with your diabetes care activities. For example, you might try linking

Q A

your blood tests or medicine doses to specific every-day events, such as getting up, eating a meal, brushing your teeth, or arriving home from work. That way, taking your pills or checking your blood glucose can become a habit that you always remember to do. Keeping your meter or pills where you will see them when doing the particular activity will help, too.

Some people find it is useful to create rituals around taking their medicines or testing. For example, you might always do your first blood glucose check between getting out of the shower and dressing. By incorporating your diabetes care into the pattern of your daily life, it will be easier to remember.

Sometimes setting up cues and patterns isn't enough. You may need a different kind of reminder. Setting a timer or an alarm may work for you. You could set the clock after each test or pill to remind you when it's time for your next test or dose. Alternatively, you may prefer to set the alarm on your clock or watch to ring at each time during the day when you need to take care of your diabetes. After each test or pill, set a timer or alarm to alert you when it's time for your next test or dose.

Finally, making a weekly schedule that shows when you should take each medicine and do each blood glucose check is a good way to stay on top of your diabetes care routine. Hang the schedule where you will see it, such as on the refrigerator or by the bathroom mirror, or slip it into your datebook. Then check off each item after you do it, so you can tell at a glance whether you've taken your dose and when the next one is due.

404.
Why do I have to take several different drugs to manage my diabetes?

Diabetes sounds like a medical condition that should be easy to treat. Just take a drug that lowers blood glucose if it is too high, or simply make changes in your lifestyle. Unfortunately, diabetes is a complex, multifaceted problem. Your body has several separate but interrelated metabolic pathways to regulate your blood glucose. The liver, pancreas, muscles, and fat cells are regulated by a complex hormonal system to control your blood glucose level. If one of these path-

Q A

ways is impaired or functions incorrectly, your blood glucose control suffers.

Having several different chemical pathways by which blood glucose can be regulated has allowed researchers to develop different classes of drugs, each working in a different way. Some drugs decrease the release of glucose by the liver, some prod the pancreas to secrete more insulin, and some work by making your body's cells more sensitive to the action of insulin. Some people require a pill to treat each feature and may take three to four different medications just to lower blood glucose. This is a good strategy when treating a disease or medical condition. If you have the opportunity to correct a problem from a couple of different directions, you have a better chance of getting the disease under control.

In addition, it is a common rule of thumb that each drug has a specific side effect profile, and often the side effects of a given drug are related to a higher dose. If a couple of drugs are used, each at a lower dose, there is less likelihood of experiencing a given side effect since each drug is at a lower level. The downside of this strategy is that the drug regimen may require the use of several pills or injections of insulin at differing times of the day.

It is a general rule that for almost any drug there is proper dose, one that will result in the desired therapeutic response. There is also a dose that will result in a greater likelihood of an adverse response or side effect. This is true for diabetes pills and insulin injections; too little drug and we are unsuccessful in the treatment of the high blood sugar, too much drug and a person may become sick from the side effects. Finding this balance is critical. For some people, this may mean taking numerous pills throughout the day or combining oral medications with injections of insulin. To avoid confusion about your dosing schedule, make sure you have an open and honest relationship with your doctor. If you are having side effects or if the drug schedule is getting too complex, talk with your doctor about these problems. He or she would rather take the time to address your concerns than have you miss taking your medications or taking them at the wrong times.

Q A

It's important to remember that diabetes is disease caused by several metabolic problems. No one drug is the end-all treatment for diabetes. As with many medical conditions, a proper balance of several drugs that have differing effects is the most likely way of keeping your blood glucose in good control. Your diabetes may take a little time and effort to control, but with a little enthusiasm and a good diabetes team you are very likely to do a great job of controlling this condition.

Taking multiple pills can seen inconvenient sometimes, but when you understand that each pill targets a different problem, they become much easier to swallow.

405.

I have the flu. How do I take my diabetes pills when I can't keep anything down?

Two points should be made about blood glucose during an acute illness like the flu. First, when you are under physical stress, such as an infection, your body releases stress hormones. These hormones cause glucose to be released by the liver to give you extra energy to cope with the illness. Second, if you have nausea or diarrhea, you are less likely to eat. So an acute gastrointestinal illness is like a two-edged sword: Your blood glucose can creep up as a result of the infection, but you may be unable to take your medications, resulting in a greater likelihood of high blood glucose.

The most important thing to do in such a situation is to check your blood glucose more frequently. If you know how your blood glucose is responding to your diabetes medication, your medication can be dosed better. Second, if you can't eat because you are nauseated, you may need to reduce the amount of medication you are taking to avoid low blood glucose. If you take blood glucose measurements during your illness, your doctor can advise you on how much medication to take. Third, drink plenty of water to keep yourself hydrated. It is a lot harder to maintain a proper blood glucose level and recover from an acute gastroenteritis if you are dehydrated.

During a bout of flu, you need to treat the nausea directly. There are several drugs that can help to

Q   A

check or control your nausea; a diet of simple fluids and light foods are also less likely to upset your stomach. It is best to discuss the use of these drugs with your doctor to review their doses and potential side effects. Once the nausea is controlled, it will be a lot easier for you to control your blood glucose.

If your blood glucose starts to get too high, even when you're taking your diabetes medicine, your doctor may recommend intermittent doses of short-acting insulin. The guidelines for injecting these doses may include a sliding scale (recommendations for injecting insulin based on specific blood glucose ranges), or they may include an easy formula to help you figure out how much to increase or decrease your insulin dose.

It is very important to keep in touch with your doctor during an illness that interferes with your ability to take your medicine, prevents you from eating, or results in dehydration.

406.
Should I stop taking my insulin when I'm sick and not eating?

No! The stress of being sick usually makes glucose levels go higher than usual. In fact, not only do you need to continue your usual insulin schedule, but your doctor may even advise you to take extra Regular insulin. Being sick can also raise the risk of developing ketoacidosis, a life-threatening condition that is caused by very high glucose levels. However, everybody's body is different. Illness can sometimes lower glucose levels instead, so it's a good idea to test your blood glucose often when you are sick. It is also important to test your urine or blood for the presence of molecules called ketones, which are a warning sign of oncoming ketoacidosis.

It's important to work out a sick-day plan with your doctor before you need it. Together you can determine a plan for how often you should test your blood glucose levels, how to test for ketones, what you should eat, and under what circumstances you should call your doctor. Being prepared will take the stress and confusion out of being sick.

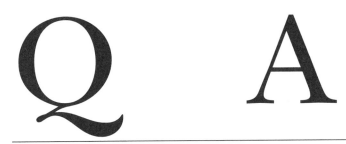

407.
How do I know if my diabetes medicine is working?

Simple. The best way to determine if your medicine is working is by measuring your blood glucose with a blood glucose meter. There is no real substitute for a blood glucose meter in helping you control your blood glucose, particularly if you are inconsistent about your diet or taking your diabetes medicine. The newer meters are smaller than ever, easier to carry, and simpler to use.

Some people claim that they have become so attuned to their blood glucose levels that they can tell when it's too high or too low. On occasion, they will rely on their perception rather than measuring their blood glucose directly. The practice of guessing your blood glucose level based on how you feel is not at all accurate and can lead to poor control. It is far better to measure your blood glucose directly and reliably with a meter than to assume that your blood glucose is well controlled simply because you are feeling all right.

To some people, lancing your finger to get a drop of blood, then using that drop to measure your blood glucose level, is a pain in the neck (and sometimes the finger), but there is no better way to get direct, immediate feedback about the current state of your blood glucose.

408.
Why do I have to take so many pills?

Type 2 diabetes has three features: failure of the pancreas to make enough insulin, release of too much glucose by the liver, and resistance to insulin. You can reduce insulin resistance through exercise, lowering your caloric intake, and losing weight. However, you may still need medicine to reach your target goals for your blood sugar. Different types of pills work on each feature of diabetes. Some drugs lower the release of glucose by the liver, some prod the pancreas into secreting more insulin, and some work by making your body's cells more sensitive to the action of insulin. Some people require a pill to treat each feature and may take three to four different medications just to lower blood glucose. The benefits of

Q A

treating diabetes effectively are the avoidance of heart disease, stroke, and the eye, kidney, and nerve damage associated with untreated diabetes.

Insulin resistance is also characterized by high blood pressure, high triglyceride and LDL cholesterol levels, and low HDL cholesterol levels. Many times, despite your efforts, your test results are not near the target goals. When this happens, you may need to take medicine. Studies have shown that these medications have had a beneficial impact on coronary artery disease. To reach a target blood pressure of 130/80 or less and protect the heart, some people require more than one blood-pressure drug. So you may be taking many pills to treat the many changes caused by the insulin resistance syndrome.

Taking multiple pills can seen inconvenient sometimes, but when you understand that each pill targets a different problem, they become much easier to swallow.

409.
My neighbor told me that chromium supplements are good for people with diabetes. Should I take it?

Several authors of medical articles have suggested that dietary chromium supplementation may be an attractive option in the management of Type 2 diabetes and could be helpful in controlling blood glucose levels in people at high risk of developing Type 2 diabetes. A systematic review of a large numbers of articles, called a meta-analysis, recently addressed that issue. This review summarized data on 618 participants from 15 different trials that reported adequate data. It showed that chromium was of no benefit in people at risk of developing Type 2 diabetes. The data for people who actually have Type 2 diabetes is inconclusive because properly controlled clinical trials have not been completed. Currently, there in no good study to show that this dietary supplement is of benefit.

This brings up the general question of using natural compounds or dietary supplements in the management of diseases. Are these products an alternative or are they complementary to the typical drugs a

Q A

doctor will use? Researchers often investigate substances that are found in nature as potential drugs to control diseases. In fact, many of the helpful drugs used today have first been found in nature, but just because they are natural compounds does not mean that they do not have toxic or adverse effects. The only way to determine if these compounds are helpful is to take them through the same rigors of a clinical trial that any drug has to go through.

At this time, clinical trials have not been done demonstrating the benefits of chromium in diabetes. Chromium is also a compound that has potential adverse or toxic effects if taken in large amounts or if it is taken by a person who is susceptible to its adverse effects. Therefore, it is best to wait for the results of these studies and use the drugs that we know are helpful and safe for the treatment of diabetes.

410.
I've heard that eating grapefruit or drinking grapefruit juice affects the action of some drugs. Does it have any effect on diabetes drugs?

Drinking fresh or frozen grapefruit juice has been shown to inhibit the metabolism of certain drugs, but not any of the drugs used to lower blood glucose. However, people with diabetes often take other drugs to manage high cholesterol, high blood pressure, blood vessel disease, impotence, and gastroparesis (slow stomach action caused by nerve damage), and some of these drugs are affected by grapefruit juice. They include felodipine (brand name Plendil), amlodipine (Norvasc), nifedipine (Adalat, Procardia), nisoldipine (Sular), verapamil (Calan, Isoptin, Verelan), simvastatin (Zocor), lovastatin (Mevacor), cilostazol (Pletal), sildenafil (Viagra), and cisapride (Propulsid).

Grapefruit juice may cause the level of these drugs in the blood to increase, which may increase the risk of side effects and other toxicities of the drug. The best strategy to prevent an interaction is to avoid drinking grapefruit juice. Another reasonable strategy is to limit the amount of grapefruit juice you drink per day and to avoid drinking it within a couple of hours of taking any drug.

Q A

411.
Will I always need to take diabetes medicine?

For most persons, the answer to this question is unfortunately yes. People with diabetes fall into two basic groups: those with Type 1 diabetes and those with Type 2 diabetes. People who produce insulin but have become resistant to its effects have Type 2 diabetes. This is typically the form of diabetes that occurs in adulthood (although the incidence of childhood Type 2 diabetes is increasing) and in people who are overweight. Type 1 diabetes occurs when too little or no insulin is produced to control blood glucose levels.

People with Type 1 will always need to take insulin to stay healthy. On occasion, people with Type 2 diabetes have been able to "beat" the disease, usually early in its course, when major efforts are made to improve their body composition. These people have dramatically reduced their body-fat content and increased their muscle mass by losing weight and improving their physical conditioning with a careful exercise program. Although this doesn't happen often, it has occurred in highly motivated individuals. Type 2 diabetes is a disease that can be modified if people make the effort to live a healthier lifestyle.

412.
How important is it to take my medicine on schedule?

The regulation of your body's blood glucose is a complex balancing act between the intake of food, the type of foods you eat, your response to your medications, and your level of physical activity. Adhering to a regular diet, a regular exercise program, and the administration of your medicines help control your blood glucose level. Diabetes is a disease that improves with control. Most of us would like to live our lives a little less formally than the care of diabetes requires. It often takes greater effort on your part, but the better you are with adhering to your medication schedule, the more successful you will be with the management of your diabetes.

344

Q A

413.
What do I do if I forget to take my diabetes medicine when I'm supposed to?

Being consistent in your diet, medications, and exercise is a key factor in controlling your diabetes. Nonetheless, many people occasionally forget to take their medicine.

It is a little difficult to give a generalized answer to this question since each person's diabetes behaves or reacts differently. In most cases, it is best to either take the oral agent or to give yourself the insulin dose as soon as possible. But if taking even a little extra insulin at the wrong time will make you hypoglycemic, or if instead you need a large dose of insulin, you will have to use a different strategy to compensate for a missed dose. If either of these descriptions fits you, it is best to call your doctor as soon as possible and be prepared to take an additional blood glucose reading with your meter to help determine the best corrective action.

414.
Why aren't my diabetes pills working anymore?

Different diabetes pills work in different ways: Some pills increase the amount of insulin your body makes, some increase the sensitivity of your cells to the effects of the insulin you already make, and others inhibit your body's ability to absorb some sugars. It is not uncommon to take three or more different pills to control blood glucose levels. Over time, people who have been on glucose-lowering pills may become less responsive to these medicines. When this happens, insulin is often added to achieve the best control.

One thing you can do to maximize the effects of glucose-lowering pills is to lose weight if you are overweight. Consulting a dietitian with expertise in diabetes can be of great benefit. Changes in your diet will often promote the weight loss you need to improve your body's reaction to diabetes pills. The bottom line is that your blood glucose needs to be controlled as well as possible. The medicines that will do the best job for you are the ones that you need. If oral drugs are just not up to the job, you will be bet-

Q A

ter off adding insulin injections—or switching over to insulin entirely—to get better control. Many new developments have made taking insulin much easier, newer preparations of insulin can be tailored to your needs much more easily, and insulin delivery devices such as pens and pumps add a new level of flexibility in administering insulin.

415.
How long do my diabetes medicines last? Is there a shelf life?

All drugs, just like foods, have a limited shelf life. But many drugs are packaged with preservatives to prevent the loss of their potency over time. Typically the pharmacy will write the expiration date on the pill bottle or the maker prints the date on the bottle. It is best to follow these dates as closely as possible. Insulin preparations are better kept refrigerated prior to opening. After the first use, refrigeration does not usually prolong its life. This varies with the maker of the insulin and the type of packaging. Storage recommendations are listed in the package insert regarding the best way to store the drug between administrations. In general, it is safe to assume that most drugs will become less effective if they are exposed to excessive heat or light, are stored improperly, or are used after the expiration date.

416.
Can I inject my insulin through my clothing?

Yes and no. Injecting through your clothing is not ideal. Your skin is a barrier to many things; it keeps good things in your body, such as fluids, and it keeps bad things out, such as bacteria. Every time insulin is injected, a small break in this barrier is made, so it is best to clean the skin to kill most of the bacteria at the injection site. This is typically done with a quick wipe of an alcohol pad over the skin prior to the injection. A clean needle is also used with each injection to ensure that no bacteria are carried into the skin.

Injecting through your clothing can obviously limit the degree of sterility at the injection site. A sterile needle will pick up bacteria as it passes through your clothing that could easily be deposited into the deeper layers of your skin. Further, the thickness of

Q A

the clothing varies the depth to which the insulin can be injected. It is best to be consistent with the depth of the injections to allow the absorption of the drug to be as consistent as possible. An injection that is not deep enough may alter the absorption of the insulin and hence its benefit.

To prevent possible infection and to promote consistency, it is better to expose the site where you will inject the insulin. However, in real life not all situations are ideal, and injecting through clothing is sometimes an expedient option. Since people with diabetes are prone to infections, though, this method is not a recommended option.

417.
I am on insulin. Can I reuse my syringes?

Again, yes and no. Ideally, it is best to use a new syringe with each injection and to clean the skin just before injecting the insulin. Using a new syringe for each injection will ensure that you have the sharpest needle possible, and therefore a pain-free injection. Reuse tends to dull the needle. However, using a new syringe for every insulin administration is not the most economical practice, and it is not always possible anyway. If you intend to reuse your syringe, briefly air-dry it, then recap. Do not clean the syringe with alcohol since this will remove the silicone that helps make each injection more comfortable. One last caveat: If you are prone to infection, reusing your syringe is not recommended; once you use it, it is no longer sterile.

418.
If I lose weight, will I be able to go off insulin and back onto diabetes pills?

This is a distinct possibility and is a function of both the severity of your diabetes and the reasons you developed diabetes. Many people with diabetes who are overweight can improve their body composition through diet and exercise. A reduction in body fat and improvements in muscle mass and function are often associated with an improvement in diabetes control. Some people have dramatically reduced their insulin requirements while others have been able to switch from insulin to pills. On occasion, people have been able to give up oral medications and control their

Q A

blood glucose with diet and exercise alone. Getting completely off medications is unlikely, but reducing the dose or changing the kind of medicine you use is very possible if a dedicated effort is made to reduce body weight and to adopt a healthier lifestyle. Changing your body composition is best accomplished by a program of exercise and diet. They work together to improve your body's ability to regulate your blood glucose level. Losing weight can be a challenge, but it is in your best interest to give it the best effort you can.

419.
I have been told that my kidneys are beginning to show a decline in how well they are working and that this may affect which medicines I take and how much. How do my kidneys affect the management of my diabetes?

People with diabetes often take a number of drugs for a variety of reasons. These drugs are metabolized and cleared from the body by the kidney and liver. In older people, there is often a decline in kidney function and a decrease in blood flow to the liver, both potentially contributing to changes in how a drug is metabolized and cleared from the body. The kidneys clear most of the insulin you use, so reduced kidney function can influence the rate at which insulin is broken down, and therefore influences insulin dosing. This is particularly true with more extreme losses of kidney function rather than with slight reductions in kidney function. It is common to have blood glucose control deteriorate as kidney function declines because very significant resistance to the action of insulin tends to co-exist in people with kidney insufficiency. When kidney function deteriorates to the point where kidney replacement therapy or hemodialysis is required, insulin clearance is markedly reduced; if the dose of insulin is not also reduced markedly, hypoglycemia may occur. People who use oral diabetes drugs will likely need to make adjustments earlier than those who rely exclusively on diabetes injections. While some oral drugs used to control blood glucose should not be used under any circumstances by people with kidney problems, others can be used if the person is monitored closely for adverse effects.

Q A

420.

Some of my friends have periods of very low blood glucose occasionally. They've been told that this is caused by some of the drugs they take. Can you explain how?

Episodes of low blood glucose can develop for a number of different reasons, but drugs are one potential contributor to the development of low blood glucose. Oral diabetes drugs that are more likely to contribute to the development of low blood glucose include the sulfonylureas (brand names Amaryl, DiaBeta, Diabinese, Glucotrol, Glucotrol XL, and the combination drugs Metaglip and Glucovance). These drugs prompt the pancreas to produce insulin. Two other drugs, brand names Prandin and Starlix, also prompt the pancreas to produce insulin but are less likely to cause low blood glucose. Drugs that make the body more sensitive to the action of insulin (such as Actos or Avandia) or drugs that slow carbohydrate digestion (such as Glyset or Precose) do not cause low blood glucose when used alone. Finally, biguanides (metformin; brand names Glucophage, Glucophage XR) control glucose production in the liver and do not cause hypoglycemia except in the extreme circumstance of prolonged fasting.

But drugs taken for purposes other than controlling blood glucose can increase the likelihood of a person developing low blood glucose through a few mechanisms. These drugs may increase the time that a diabetes medicine can exert its effect by inhibiting the rate at which the oral diabetes drug is cleared from the body. They may affect how available an oral diabetes drug is to work its action or they may change some aspect of glucose metabolism. It is also possible that some drugs may cause a defect in how the liver produces glucose that could contribute to how low the blood glucose becomes.

So drugs can contribute to low blood glucose in a variety of ways, often unexpected. This is just one of the reasons that people with diabetes should keep logs of their blood glucose levels, physical activity, and meals, among other things. Logbooks provide your health-care team with the information they need to adjust and fine-tune your individual treatment.

Q A

421.
Some of my friends take their insulin once a day, others take it three times a day, and I take it twice a day. Is my diabetes different from my friends'?

It is important to recognize that everybody's diabetes is different. But generally speaking, the difference between these individual regimens may have to do with whether you and your friends have Type 1 or Type 2 diabetes. An insulin regimen for somebody with Type 2 diabetes who still produces some insulin would not be as complex as a Type 1 regimen, which is for a person who produces no insulin at all.

What a particular individual's metabolic goals are may also influence how frequently he takes insulin, as tighter control often requires smaller insulin doses and more frequent injections. Early in the course of Type 2 diabetes, a single-dose regimen of intermediate or long-acting insulin has the theoretical advantage of not suppressing natural insulin production, which does occur with a multiple-injection regimen using short-acting insulin.

In addition, people with Type 2 diabetes either don't produce enough insulin to adequately control their blood glucose, or their bodies are resistant to the insulin that is available, or they may have both of these problems. The extent to which people with Type 2 diabetes have these problems varies considerably. This determines whether they require drugs to lower their blood glucose, and if so, the amount and type of drug required. For those who require insulin in addition to an oral drug, some require small amounts of insulin infrequently and others require large amounts with more frequent dosing. In people who use insulin exclusively to control their blood glucose levels, many factors may influence the kind of insulin regimen they follow; for instance, how quickly the insulin is absorbed and metabolized. There have been many studies of factors affecting insulin absorption and differences with type of insulin, location of injection, blood flow, and technique. All of these factors can all influence absorption.

As we stated earlier, everybody's diabetes is different. And it is those differences that determine the appropriate treatment for any particular person.

9
Successful Aging

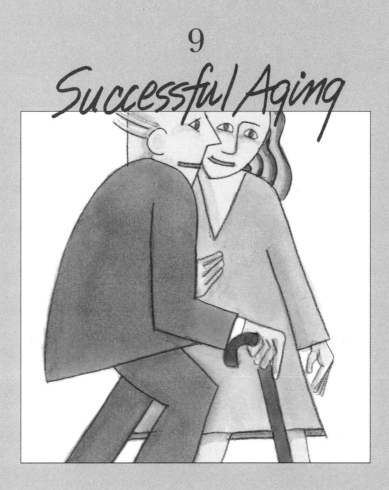

Overcoming Obstacles

422. I'm on a fixed budget. The foods I'm supposed to eat for my diabetes are much more expensive than "normal" food. Are there programs or groups that can help me?

423. My diabetes medications and supplies are expensive, and sometimes I can't afford it all. Can I skip doses or tests? Are there programs or groups that can help me make ends meet?

424. What do Medicaid and Medicare cover for diabetes?

425. Is it all right for me to continue driving? Do I need to check my blood glucose level before I drive anywhere?

426. I don't drive anymore, so it's hard to get to my doctor, pharmacist, and even to the grocery store. What can I do about that?

427. I hate the diabetes routine and the countless daily details. Since I'm getting up there in age, is taking care of my diabetes really worth all the trouble?

428. If I have a bad heart or another serious medical condition, shouldn't I be more concerned about that than my diabetes?

429. My desire to have sexual relations has declined. Is this due to my age, my diabetes, or both? Is there anything I can do to boost my desire to what it was?

430. I have had the same doctor for over 20 years. Now my family wants me to see specialists for my diabetes. Is this really necessary? I don't want to be disloyal to my doctor.

431. I am worried about my children and my grandchildren getting diabetes. How likely is that to happen?

432. With all my health problems, including diabetes, I feel like my poor health is taking over my life. Is it normal to feel this way?

433. There are just too many new things to think about with diabetes—diet, exercise, medications, and more. I don't know if I can change at my age. How do other people do it?

434. Since I retired, I am seeing a lot more of my spouse, who is driving me crazy about my diabetes care. How can I tell her to back off a little?

435. My spouse refuses to acknowledge my diabetes and how serious it is. How can I tell him that it is important and can't be ignored?

436. Since my spouse's death, I have been living alone. My children are worried about my diabetes and want me to move in with them, but I don't want to be a burden. Are there programs or groups that can help people like me?

437. Some of my friends with diabetes are using alternative therapies. One is taking chromium supplements and another is taking magnesium supplements. Should I start taking these supplements?

438. Where can I get more information about diabetes?

Diet and Meal Planning

439. Is a meal plan for an older person any different than it would be for someone younger?

440. I found a week ago that I have Type 2 diabetes. I am losing weight following my new meal plan, but I don't want to increase my food intake for fear of raising my blood glucose levels. I have never been overweight, and I'm already too thin. How much weight should I be willing to lose?

441. The meal plans I've seen don't seem to include foods that I'm used to eating. Can't I just cut down on certain foods that I already eat and figure it out for myself?

442. What do I do if I'm not feeling well and can't eat? Should I still take my diabetes medicines?

443. Should I take my diabetes medicines at mealtime or at some other time?

444. I take a number of dietary supplements and vitamins. Are there vitamins or supplements that I shouldn't take?

445. What about candy? How much is too much?

446. Can I still eat ice cream or other desserts and snacks now that I have diabetes?

447. I have given up sugary sodas, and I now drink teas and diet sodas instead. Is there anything in these drinks that I should avoid?

448. Is it all right for me to continue having my daily cocktail?

449. What should I be most concerned about avoiding: sugar, fat, or salt?

450. What about sugar-free or fat-free foods? Are they all right for me to eat?

451. There's a lot of talk about the health benefits of eating more vegetables. I like most vegetables, but not all. Which are best?

452. I know higher-fiber foods are good for my regularity. But does fiber do anything to help my diabetes?

453. I live by myself now and don't really like cooking much. It's gotten easier to pop a frozen dinner into the microwave instead. Is that all right?

454. I eat lunches at the local senior center, but they often serve all sorts of foods that I know I'm not supposed to eat, according to my meal plan. What can I do about that?

455. I get meals delivered to my home by the local Meals-on-Wheels group, but they sometimes contain foods that aren't on my meal plan. What can I do about that?

456. I'm on a fixed income and can't afford the fresh vegetables and fruits that are recommended in my meal plan. Are there less expensive alternatives that would work for me?

Fitness

457. My doctor told me to lose weight to lower my blood glucose. Do I really need to lose weight at my age? What's weight loss got to do with my blood glucose?

458. My doctor recommended that I get more exercise. I have never exercised before. Why is it important now?

459. I really don't have the money to purchase exercise equipment or special shoes and clothing. Do I need any of these things?

460. Are there specific exercise guidelines to follow?

461. I stay active all year long with gardening, golf, and walking my dog. Does this count as exercise?

462. I have recently read several articles about the importance of strength training. Is this really necessary at my age?

463. Do I need to monitor my blood glucose more frequently when I exercise?

464. Sometimes I have so much pain and discomfort in my feet that it is hard to even walk around my house. What types of exercise can I do?

465. Now that I am exercising, do I need to eat more food?

466. What time of day is best for exercising?

467. I see other people checking their pulse when they exercise. Do I need to do this?

468. I just tested my urine and found some ketones. Can I still take my walk today?

469. My doctor told me to walk for 30 minutes each day. That is too much for me. Can I walk several times each day for shorter periods instead?

470. Why do I need to stretch before and after I exercise?

Medication

471. I have Type 2 diabetes and am allergic to sulfonamides, sulfonylureas, and, indeed, any drug containing a sulfur molecule. What options does that leave me with in terms of blood-glucose-lowering drugs?

472. My blood glucose is often high in the morning, even when I haven't eaten all night. Why is that?

473. I have heard about people achieving remarkable blood glucose control with an insulin pump. Are pumps suitable for older people like me?

474. My doctor wants me to switch from pills to insulin. Is that really necessary?

475. Even though my blood pressure, blood lipids, and HbA_{1c} results are normal, my doctor wants me to start taking an antihypertensive drug, saying it will protect my eyes and kidneys in years to come. I am reluctant to take any medicine I don't really need. Is there any good reason for me to take this drug now?

476. We travel during the winter months. How do I manage my diabetes medication while I am away from my doctor?

477. Will I ever be able to stop taking medication to control my diabetes?

478. I sometimes forget to take my medication. What should I do when that happens?

479. I am on a tight budget. Can I reuse my syringes or my needles to save money?

480. I am interested in taking glucosamine and chondroitin for my joints and cartilage, but I'm not sure if they're safe for people with diabetes. Can you fill me in?

Long-Term Care

481. What are the long-term complications of diabetes that is not well controlled? How long will it take to get these complications?

482. My blood pressure is usually around 140/85 mm Hg, but my doctor has put me on blood pressure medicine to lower it, saying blood pressure control may be even more important than blood glucose control in preventing complications. Is this true?

483. I had my cholesterol checked at the mall and it was elevated. What are my next steps?

484. Does being older put me at higher risk for heart disease?

485. My doctor used the term "lipids profile." What is that?

486. Will diabetes shorten my life expectancy?

487. I have used insulin for the past 25 years. So far, I have no complications, but I know I don't eat right or exercise enough. I also know it will catch up to me some day. How can I start taking better care of myself when it's so hard to change?

488. Everything looks slightly cloudy to me. Will I lose my eyesight or go blind as I get older?

489. I have been told to check my feet daily, but I have trouble bending over. Why do I need to check my feet, and what am I looking for?

490. I sometimes have trouble walking because I cannot feel the floor. What is happening and what should I do?

491. I have had symptoms of neuropathy in my feet for eight months or so, but nothing shows up on testing. Why is this? Also, is it inevitable that the affected nerves will die? Or could they recover?

492. What can I do to prevent damage to my kidneys?

493. How does menopause affect diabetes?

494. Does having diabetes increase my risk of becoming sexually impotent?

495. What medical tests should I have to take care of myself? And how often should I get them?

496. I often leave my doctor's office confused and with an unclear memory of what he told me. What can I do about this?

497. How can I avoid problems with my medications when I seem to take so many different pills?

498. My gums are tender, and they bleed sometimes. Is there any connection between this and my diabetes?

499. Does my ethnic background affect my risk of diabetic complications?

500. Now that I am older, what do I need to do to take care of my diabetes? Will it make a difference at my age?

501. I have trouble reading the small print on my drug labels. What can I do about that?

Q A

Overcoming Obstacles

422.
I'm on a fixed budget. The foods I'm supposed to eat for my diabetes are much more expensive than "normal" food. Are there programs or groups that can help me?

All foods that are lower in fats and high in fiber are encouraged for everyone, especially for those with diabetes. However, if you are having difficulty paying for the food recommended by your doctor, nurse, or dietitian, there are governmental programs that provide assistance for eligible individuals and families. One program most people are aware of is the Food Stamp Program. The Food Stamp Program is an assistance program designed to help low-income people obtain nutritious foods. Using debit cards and other means, people can purchase breads, cereal, dairy products, fruits, vegetables, meats, fish, and poultry. This program is administered at the state and local levels, so you will need to contact your state or local government for information regarding application.

Assistance can also be obtained through the Elderly Nutrition Program. This program provides free meals to people aged 60 and over through two nutrition programs: congregate meals and home-delivered meals. Congregate or group meals are usually offered at senior centers, churches, and other community centers. People who cannot get to congregate meals are provided a home-delivered meal through "Meals on Wheels." To get more information on these two programs, contact your Area Agency on Aging. If cannot find a local Area Agency on Aging, call Eldercare Locator at 1-800-677-1116 (toll free) for assistance or go to their Web site, www.eldercare.gov.

Another assistance program is the Commodity Supplemental Food Program (CSFP). The CSFP is a program to improve the nutritional status of seniors, pregnant women, infants and children. Participants receive food boxes with items specific to their needs. The program is administered differently in participating states; contact your state and/or local government for information regarding this program.

Finally, contact your local social services, health departments or social agencies for information on local food banks and programs.

Q A

423.
My diabetes medications and supplies are expensive, and sometimes I can't afford it all. Can I skip doses or tests? Are there programs or groups that can help me make ends meet?

Diabetes care can be expensive. According to the American Diabetes Association, people with diabetes spend $13,243 per capita a year on medical expenditures. However, it is not recommended that you skip tests or medication doses to minimize costs. Monitoring your blood glucose and adhering to your medication regimen helps you achieve and maintain blood glucose levels as close to normal as possible. There are two governmental programs that assist older people pay for health-care services and supplies: Medicare and Medicaid. Medicare is a federal government health insurance program for people age 65 and older. Medicaid is a health services assistance program administered by state governments. Medicaid eligibility is based on financial need. For more information about Medicare, phone 1-800-MEDICARE (633-4227) or go to their Web site, www.medicare.gov. Contact your state government for more information about Medicaid.

If you are a veteran, you may be eligible for assistance through the Department of Veterans Affairs (VA). For more information about VA care, phone 1-800-827-1000 or go to their Web site, www.va.gov.

Finally, let your doctor or nurse know that you are having difficulty paying for your diabetes medications and/or supplies. They may know of a pharmaceutical company with a patient assistance program or local service groups that assist patients (for example, the Lions Club, Rotary Clubs, Kiwanis Clubs, or churches).

424.
What do Medicaid and Medicare cover for diabetes?

Medicare is a federal government health insurance program for people age 65 and older, and Medicaid is a health services assistance program based on financial need that is administered by state governments. In general, Medicare pays for blood glucose monitoring supplies (glucose meters, testing strips, and lancets), insulin pumps, and diabetes education.

Q A

Medicaid covers most diabetes medicines for those who are eligible. However, coverage for items and services can change. You need to discuss coverage with your doctor (or the office staff), or contact a Medicare and a Medicaid agency to determine current coverage and eligibility policies. To contact Medicare, phone 1-800-MEDICARE (633-4227) (toll free) or go to their Web site, www.medicare.gov. For information about Medicaid, contact your state government (check the government section in your local telephone directory).

425.
Is it all right for me to continue driving? Do I need to check my blood glucose level before I drive anywhere?

You need to discuss these concerns with your doctor. Usually if you have your blood glucose levels under control, then it is all right for you to drive. However, people with diabetes need to be aware that low blood glucose can have negative effects on their driving ability. Low blood glucose (also called hypoglycemia) is a blood glucose level under 60. The symptoms of low blood glucose may include shakiness, sweating, irritable mood, numbness around the mouth, nausea, blurred vision, weakness, and perhaps most important for driving, confusion and an impaired ability to react.

If you are well controlled, there are some simple precautions you need to follow to drive safely:
- Check your blood glucose level regularly.
- Always have something with you that can treat low blood glucose. Snacks that are transportable and non-perishable include regular soft drinks, juice, raisins, and glucose gel or tablets.
- Treat low blood glucose immediately.
- When on the road, do not skip meals or have late meals.

Some long-term complications of diabetes such as retinopathy may also affect your driving and are worsened by other eye diseases such as glaucoma and cataracts. Diabetes can also damage nerves and over time may impair feeling in your feet. Both could affect your ability to drive. It is important that you have an eye exam by a professional once each year and that you immediately report unusual symptoms.

Q A

Also, make sure your feet are checked for nerve damage during every office visit with your doctor.

426.
I don't drive anymore, so it's hard to get to my doctor, pharmacist, and even to the grocery store. What can I do about that?

One of the difficulties experienced by older people (and people with disabilities) who don't drive is finding reliable and convenient transportation. Friends and family are not always available, and many people don't want to burden their friends and family with all their transportation needs. Many communities are aware of this problem and offer special services or programs for older adults, such as special buses with door-to-door service or subsidies for taxi rides. Contact your local transit agency or transportation department to determine what services and programs are offered in your area.

Your community may also offer escort services that provide transportation for older adults for doctor appointments, shopping, and other errands. These services are frequently provided by service groups. Contact your local service groups (for example, the Lions Club, Rotary Clubs, Kiwanis Clubs, or churches) to see if such programs are offered in your area. In addition to these options, you might want to consider in-home services and programs such as "Meals on Wheels."

Talk with your doctor or the office staff about transportation options in your community; they may be able to direct you. For more information on the above services and programs, contact your local Area Agency on Aging and your state aging agencies. If you cannot find these resources in your area, call Eldercare Locator at 1-800-677-1116 (toll free) for assistance or go to their Web site www.eldercare.gov.

427.
I hate the diabetes routine and the countless daily details. Since I'm getting up there in age, is taking care of my diabetes really worth all the trouble?

Yes it is. Taking care of your diabetes will reduce your risk of diabetes complications and improve your

Q A

health. Managing your diabetes can be difficult, particularly when you are first diagnosed. You are asked to do many new things (changing your diet, exercising, monitoring your blood glucose level) and the routine can be tiresome. Be patient and after a while your diabetes care may not seem so daunting to you. Remember, you will have good days and bad days. Try to focus on your accomplishments in the care of your diabetes. Taking care of your diabetes might also have other advantages. For example, if you have another illness, improving your diet and getting more exercise may also help improve this condition.

If your dissatisfaction continues, you may want consider joining a diabetes support group. You can discuss your feeling about diabetes and hear how other people feel and respond to their diabetes. However, if you feel overwhelmed and are unable to cope with your diabetes care, discuss your feelings with your doctor or nurse. They can assist you directly or help locate another professional or program that can.

**428.
If I have a bad heart or another serious medical condition, shouldn't I be more concerned about that than my diabetes?**

Many people with diabetes also have other health problems or illnesses. Managing your diabetes and another disease at the same time can be challenging. However, it is important not to ignore your diabetes or your other health problems. Things you do to manage your diabetes, such as getting more exercise or improving your diet, may in fact be helpful with your other illness. If you have concerns about your different health problems or your different treatment plans, discuss these concerns with your doctor. It is important that the doctors and other medical professionals providing your care (both for your diabetes and for your other health issues) be aware of all your health problems and treatments. This allows the doctors to coordinate your care for maximum benefit. It is also crucial that they are aware of all the medicines you are taking in order to prevent harmful drug interactions.

Q   A

429.
My desire to have sexual relations has declined. Is this due to my age, my diabetes, or both? Is there anything I can do to boost my desire to what it was?

Sexual problems are not a characteristic of "normal aging," but diabetes can have a negative impact on the sexual functioning of both men and women. Impotence, the inability to achieve or maintain an erection, is a common problem for men. However, there are several effective treatment alternatives for this condition. You need to discuss this problem with your doctor and determine the available treatments appropriate for you. If you have another type of problem, discuss it with your doctor for treatment recommendations.

Women may also have sexual difficulties related to their diabetes, problems such as difficulty achieving an orgasm, vaginal dryness, and an increased number of vaginal infections. As with problems encountered by men, there are many effective treatments for these conditions: lubricants (for example, K-Y jelly) can assist with vaginal dryness, and many over-the-counter products are available to treat vaginal infections. If these problems continue, discuss your difficulties with your doctor or nurse for their treatment recommendations and guidance.

430.
I have had the same doctor for over 20 years. Now my family wants me to see specialists for my diabetes. Is this really necessary? I don't want to be disloyal to my doctor.

Your family most likely wants you to be evaluated by an endocrinologist or a diabetologist; both have special training and more experience in treating persons with diabetes. Diabetes is a complex disease; therefore, seeing a doctor who specializes in diabetes may mean better care for you.

Another option may be to see a diabetes specialist for a consultation. The specialist could review all of your issues and make recommendations. These recommendations could then be given to your doctor for implementation.

Q A

In caring for your diabetes, you may also want to consider being treated by a diabetes health-care team. A diabetes health-care team usually consists of a doctor, a nurse, and a dietitian; however, it may also include a pharmacist, a health educator, a social worker, a podiatrist, and/or an eye doctor. Providing appropriate and effective diabetes treatment is complicated and multifaceted; the health-care team is a way to provide you with the support and information you need to manage your diabetes. These different health professionals will focus on different aspects of diabetes care; for example, the doctor may focus on the effectiveness of different prescriptions, the dietitian will provide you with an appropriate diet plan, and the social worker can help you find local support services.

Your doctor wants you to have the best care possible. If seeing a diabetes specialist or a diabetes health-care team provides more effective management, he certainly would not object to refer you for additional care. If you still feel you are being disloyal, discuss your concerns with him.

431.
I am worried about my children and my grandchildren getting diabetes. How likely is that to happen?

Unfortunately, people with a parent or siblings with diabetes are at risk for diabetes. Belonging to the following ethnic groups also places you at greater risk for diabetes:

- African-Americans
- Alaska Natives
- American Indians
- Asian Americans and Pacific Islanders
- Latinos

However, being at risk does not mean your children and grandchildren will necessarily develop diabetes. A recent study funded by the National Institutes of Health, the Diabetes Prevention Project (DPP), found that proper diet and exercise can delay or prevent Type 2 diabetes in people with impaired glucose tolerance (a condition that is frequently a precursor to diabetes). Discuss your concerns with

Q A

your doctor and your family. Make sure your family is aware of their risk for diabetes and that they can lower this risk. They should discuss diabetes prevention with their doctor and have their blood glucose level checked regularly.

432.
With all my health problems, including diabetes, I feel like my poor health is taking over my life. Is it normal to feel this way?

Diabetes can be a challenging disease. If you have another illness in addition to diabetes, caring for your health problems may sometimes feel overwhelming. Given these circumstances, it is not unusual for some people to feel anxious, angry, or depressed about their health. Discuss these feelings with your doctor or nurse and ask about strategies and programs that can help you adjust and care for your health problems. Things you are doing to care for your diabetes may be helpful with your other health problems.

Some people find it helpful to discuss their problems and feelings with someone close to them (a spouse, a relative, or a friend). You could also join a diabetes support group and hear how others cope with diabetes; call the American Diabetes Association, your local health department, or local hospital for information on groups in your area. It is important to contact your doctor if depression lasts for more than two weeks or interferes with your diabetes management, as it may be due to a physical cause and require treatment.

433.
There are just too many new things to think about with diabetes—diet, exercise, medications, and more. I don't know if I can change at my age. How do other people do it?

Caring for diabetes can be complex and frustrating, even for the diabetes veteran. It can be particularly daunting for newly diagnosed people who are usually asked to alter their lifestyle dramatically. Suddenly, they are asked to exercise, change long-established eating patterns, monitor blood glucose levels, and/or take diabetes pills or insulin injections. Be patient;

Q A

you can expect difficulties (at any age) when you first start caring for your diabetes. As time goes on and you become more experienced, the tasks and routines of caring for your diabetes should become less difficult.

To hear how other people with diabetes cope, you may want to join a diabetes support group. You may find it helpful to hear others describe their concerns and how they manage the stress of diabetes management. Call the American Diabetes Association, your local health department, or your local hospital for information on groups in your area. If you continue to feel beleaguered or are unable to do the things you need to do, discuss your feelings with your doctor or nurse. They can assist you directly or help locate another professional or program that can.

434.
Since I retired, I am seeing a lot more of my spouse, who is driving me crazy about my diabetes care. How can I tell her to back off a little?

Remember, your diabetes also has an impact on your spouse, who may feel afraid and overwhelmed by your diabetes. Your spouse may feel personally responsible for taking charge of your care, which can cause further stress for both of you. An open and frank discussion with your spouse about your diabetes care and worries about your health may help. It would also be an opportunity for you to explain your concerns and discuss your spouse's role in your care management. You need to say which behaviors are supportive and which behaviors are irritating or not helpful. Remind her that you are ultimately in charge of your diabetes care, even though she may not agree with all of your decisions. Having such a discussion periodically with your spouse may also be beneficial.

Be patient with your spouse; remember that she is also under stress. It may be a good idea to bring her to your next diabetes appointment and discuss the sharing of your diabetes care with everyone concerned.

Q   A

435.
My spouse refuses to acknowledge my diabetes and how serious it is. How can I tell him that it is important and can't be ignored?

Your diabetes can be very stressful for your spouse as well as for you. Some spouses may react like yours and deny the seriousness of diabetes complications. Have an open discussion about your feelings and the seriousness of diabetes. Ask about his feelings, concerns, and understanding of diabetes. Take this opportunity to teach him about diabetes. If your spouse continues to minimize or deny the seriousness of diabetes, have him come with you to your next diabetes appointment and discuss his understanding of diabetes with your doctor.

Your spouse can be an important source of support in managing your diabetes. However, you must first determine the areas that you believe you need and want assistance and support. You then have to communicate these needs to your spouse. Your spouse should also be aware of the warning signs of high and low blood glucose and what he can do to help you with these episodes.

436.
Since my spouse's death, I have been living alone. My children are worried about my diabetes and want me to move in with them, but I don't want to be a burden. Are there programs or groups that can help people like me?

Yes, there are many agencies and resources that can provide you with information about and assistance with your diabetes care. Talk to your doctor or nurse about your diabetes management plan and goals, and identify the care areas where you feel you need additional assistance. Once that is determined, your doctor or nurse should be able to make suggestions and direct your efforts in obtaining the care or assistance you need. There are many programs and agencies that help older adults remain independent. You can also contact your local American Diabetes Association affiliate, your state Area Agency on Aging, or your local health department (city, county, or state). If you cannot find these resources in your area, call Elder-

Q A

care Locator at 1-800-677-1116 (toll free) for assistance or go to their Web site, www.eldercare.gov.

437.
Some of my friends with diabetes are using alternative therapies. One is taking chromium supplements and another is taking magnesium supplements. Should I start taking these supplements?

There is not enough data about whether chromium supplements or magnesium supplements have any effect in the management of diabetes. Because the usefulness of these supplements has not been demonstrated, they are not recommended for the treatment of diabetes.

There is no indication from recent studies that chromium supplements reduces the risk of Type 2 diabetes nor has there been a properly conducted clinical trial demonstrating benefits of chromium in the treatment of Type 2 diabetes.

Magnesium does play an important role in the body's metabolism. However, the American Diabetes Association recommends magnesium supplementation only for people with demonstrated magnesium deficiency. Eating a balanced diet should supply most people with their magnesium needs.

Discuss these and other alternative or complementary therapies you are considering with your doctor. Overuse of certain dietary supplements can lead to toxic levels and possibly adverse effects. In general, it is best to wait until clinical trials and studies prove new therapies to be beneficial before using them.

If you are interested in getting more information about these or other alternative therapies in the treatment of diabetes, contact the National Center for Complementary and Alternative Medicine Clearinghouse at 1-888-644-6226 (toll free) or to their Web site, nccam.nih.gov/health.

438.
Where can I get more information about diabetes?

There are usually many community resources available to assist you. You can contact your local American Diabetes Association affiliate, health department, or hospital for all kinds of advice—sources of diabetes

Q A

information, exercise programs, weight-loss programs, smoking cessation programs, and diabetes support groups. The Internet is another source for locating community and informational resources.

The Internet is also a source for other information about diabetes. However, the sheer volume of information available may be confusing, and it is often difficult to find reputable and unbiased sites. The following five sites are recommended for good information regarding diabetes:

- MEDLINEplus, a service of the National Library of Medicine
- www.nlm.nih.gov/medlineplus/diabetes
- Centers for Disease Control and Prevention Public Health Resource
- www.cdc.gov/diabetes
- American Diabetes Association
- www.diabetes.org
- American Association of Diabetes Educators
- www.aadenet.org
- University of Michigan Diabetes Research and Training Center
- www.med.umich.edu/mdrtc

Diet and Meal Planning

439.
Is a meal plan for an older person any different than it would be for someone younger?

Your goals of diabetes management include keeping your blood glucose at a healthy level throughout the day and maintaining a healthy weight, which will reduce your risk for heart problems and other diabetes-related complications. Because your blood glucose increases after you eat, a meal plan is one of the three major management tools (the others are exercise and medication) that help you reach and maintain a healthy weight and prevent heart problems and other problems in the future. A meal plan especially designed for you by a registered dietitian with lots of input from you will guide you on issues such as when you should eat, what kinds of food you should eat, and the amounts of food that will help you manage your diabetes best.

Q A

In general, your meal plan wouldn't necessarily differ from a younger adult's meal plan. Both would include a good selection of nutritious and tasty foods from the major food groups, foods that are good for you and your family, including many of your favorite foods. However, because your body may have less muscle mass and a lower metabolism than when you were younger, you may need fewer calories overall. So, the individualized meal plan that you and your dietitian develop will include foods that will vary in types and amounts depending on your activity level and whether you want to lose some weight to help manage your diabetes. In addition, your meal plan may vary depending on whether you cook yourself and if you are taking other medication; some drugs can interact with your diabetes medicine to compromise your diabetes management.

440.
I found a week ago that I have Type 2 diabetes. I am losing weight following my new meal plan, but I don't want to increase my food intake for fear of raising my blood glucose levels. I have never been overweight, and I'm already too thin. How much weight should I be willing to lose?

Your weight should level off soon. However, if you are always hungry or continue to lose weight when weight loss is not your goal, you need to address this issue with your doctor and dietitian. You may need to have your medication adjusted or you may need more food—or both. It is important to work with them to establish a caloric intake that is realistic and appropriate for your age, height, weight, and activity level.

441.
The meal plans I've seen don't seem to include foods that I'm used to eating. Can't I just cut down on certain foods that I already eat and figure it out for myself?

You can certainly read all of the latest information that is available on foods and their nutrient values, what the latest recommendations are for which foods

Q A

(and in which combinations and amounts) might be best for a person with diabetes, how some foods and drugs can interact with your diabetes medications and, in turn, try to figure out what might work best for you. But there's an increasing amount of information out there and lots of considerations to make in designing the best meal plan for you! Realistically, a better use of your time would be to talk with someone (preferably a registered dietitian) who's been trained to use all the latest information and techniques to develop an individualized plan—one that is most appropriate for *you* and your specific goals, activity levels, weight, general health, food choices, and other important factors. Remember, a good meal plan will include a variety of foods that are not only good for you but are also foods that you like, with recommendations on portion sizes and timing as well as ways to prepare them that make them more nutritious without sacrificing taste.

442.
What do I do if I'm not feeling well and can't eat? Should I still take my diabetes medicines?

There are many reasons you might not be feeling well, some related to your diabetes management and some not. For example, if your blood glucose levels are too high (because of certain foods or drugs, too little exercise, or stress), you may feel sick and the elevated blood glucose may put you at higher risk for other diabetes-related health problems. On the other hand, if your blood glucose too low, you may feel lightheaded, sluggish, and under the weather. To keep your blood glucose at healthy levels throughout the day, plan to take your diabetes medicine at the same times every day and eat according to your meal plan.

However, we all find ourselves feeling ill for other reasons—such as a cold or the flu—on occasion, and the thought of eating anything or taking any medicine is unpleasant. In cases like that, you should get in touch with your doctor for advice about what you can eat and how you might take your medicine without feeling even worse.

Q A

443.
Should I take my diabetes medicines at mealtime or at some other time?

Check with your doctor or pharmacist about your schedules for taking diabetes medication and other drugs. Depending on the kinds of medicines you take, mealtime may not be the best time to take them. Some of the newer diabetes drugs, on the other hand, are released over time so they can be taken at mealtime. Again, check with your doctor, and make sure he knows about all the medicines you're taking, including vitamins and herbs; sometimes it's better to take your diabetes medicine at times other than when you take your other medicines. Your doctor or pharmacist will be able to advise you on this.

444.
I take a number of dietary supplements and vitamins. Are there vitamins or supplements that I shouldn't take?

Check with your dietitian or doctor about the vitamins or other nutritional supplements you take. It is often difficult to get all the nutrients your body needs just from food alone, so a good multivitamin and selected other supplements such as calcium may be important parts of your daily routine.

The jury is still out on what vitamins or supplements may be beneficial or harmful to adults with diabetes. In general, the biggest concern about vitamins and supplements are in their composition and potential toxicity if taken in very large doses. Because vitamins and supplements are not regulated in the same way as prescription drugs, they may contain ingredients such as sugars and other binders that may be problematic for the best management of your diabetes. So again, check with your dietitian or doctor about supplements that you might want to take.

445.
What about candy? How much is too much?

Unfortunately for those of us who enjoy them, sweets may taste good but they contain very few nutrients that are useful to our bodies. To make matters worse, as we get older, some taste sensations diminish, leav-

Q A

ing others—such as our taste for sweets, in particular—intact, often increasing our desire for them!

In general, your dietitian will probably tell you to limit your intake of sweets. Remember that even sweets that are labeled sugar-free may include other ingredients (such as fats) that you'll want to limit, too. But special occasions often call for sweets of some kind, so if you do indulge, make sweets a special treat.

446.
Can I still eat ice cream or other desserts and snacks now that I have diabetes?

Yes, if you have desserts and planned snacks built into your meal plan. You might want to check the food labels to make sure the portion size and total carbohydrates match the amount suggested by your meal plan. The key is to count the carbohydrates contained in the sweets and snacks as part of your total carbohydrates for the day. Happily, ice cream is a low glycemic food! However, it is still a good idea to use reduced-fat and reduced-sugar products to cut down on unwanted calories. If your meal plan does not include a snack before bed, then consider having that small serving of ice cream as part of your dinner meal. Remember, a blood glucose level near 140 mg/dl is the target for bedtime.

447.
I have given up sugary sodas, and I now drink teas and diet sodas instead. Is there anything in these drinks that I should avoid?

Decaffeinated tea and many diet sodas are very good alternatives to regular sodas. If you like your tea sweetened, use artificial sweeteners to taste. Remember though that diet sodas often have caffeine in them. Caffeine can make you less sensitive to hunger and more anxious during low blood sugar episodes. In addition, recent studies have suggested that caffeine (in sodas, coffees, and teas) may also reduce your body's ability to process blood sugar efficiently.

448.
Is it all right for me to continue having my daily cocktail?

Your physician and dietitian will probably tell you that a little wine, beer, or a cocktail is just fine and

Q A

isn't likely to have adverse effects on your blood glucose. But it would be a good idea to limit your consumption to one drink a day (for women) or two drinks a day (for men). And drink your alcohol with food to avoid hypoglycemia or other changes in your blood glucose levels.

Remember, too, that alcohol has calories (think "weight gain"), it has little nutritional value, and excessive consumption can lead to liver damage and other cell damage. So just to be safe, check with your physician or dietitian about drinking alcohol.

449.
What should I be most concerned about avoiding: sugar, fat, or salt?

In terms of quantity, you should limit your consumption of all three. With regard to fat, it's also important to carefully select the kind you consume. Most sugary and starchy foods raise your blood glucose quickly, so it's best to reserve them for special occasions and to limit the portion size. All fats are high in calories, which can promote weight gain and damage your blood vessels. Like sugars, fats are best eaten in very small quantities. And it's important to choose beneficial fats such as olive, walnut, or canola oils, which are heart-healthy monounsaturated fats. In addition, increase your intake of omega-3 fatty acids, which are found in cold-water fish (such as salmon and tuna) and in dark-green leafy vegetables.

Finally, for many people, sodium (found in table salt as well as many processed foods) may raise your blood pressure. Non-salt condiments such as herb and spice combinations are wonderful replacements for seasoning. Be sure to check the labels to find products that are salt (sodium) free.

450.
What about sugar-free or fat-free foods? Are they all right for me to eat?

Packaging that is labeled sugar-free or fat-free is certainly appealing and suggests that the foods in them are good for you or, at least, not as bad for you! And that may be true in some cases. However, you should always check the food labels on the packages carefully before deciding to buy or eat those products. The

Q A

labels will give you important information about the calories, carbohydrate, and fats that are associated with a serving size. Often, foods that are labeled as fat-free contain other ingredients—such as sugars—that you might want to limit or even avoid. In contrast, foods that are labeled sugar-free may have more fats (and more of the wrong kind of fats) in them than you want to eat. Remember that reduced-sugar or reduced-fat foods still contain calories, so eat them in moderation.

If you are unsure about a particular product (and particularly if it's not on your meal plan), check with your dietitian. You may discover that it's a great choice for you or that there are alternative products that may be even better.

451.
There's a lot of talk about the health benefits of eating more vegetables. I like most vegetables, but not all. Which are best?

Happily, many vegetables are very nutritious and contain few calories, so your dietitian may tell you to feel free to eat as many of them as you'd like. These include lots of the leafy, green, red, and yellow vegetables which have minimal effects on your blood glucose levels. However, not all vegetables are created equal. Some vegetables—such as potatoes, corn, and many beans—are starchy and raise your blood sugar levels.

Since your meal plan was developed by you and your dietitian to include a variety of healthful foods, however, it's likely to include your favorite foods, including your favorite vegetables, and likely to exclude foods that you might have problems digesting. Your meal plan will probably suggest limiting how much and how often you eat some of the starchier vegetables.

452.
I know higher-fiber foods are good for my regularity. But does fiber do anything to help my diabetes?

Yes! Including foods with whole grains and dietary fiber in your meal plan is good for you for lots of reasons, including enhancing your regularity. Fiber food such as multigrain breads, brown rice, and whole-

Q A

grain cereals have also been shown to lower your blood glucose and your cholesterol levels (particularly total and LDL), both of which are important to your heart health. Since adults with diabetes are at greater risk for heart problems, finding easy ways to improve your cholesterol and blood pressure levels can help prevent those heart problems.

453.
I live by myself now and don't really like cooking much. It's gotten easier to pop a frozen dinner into the microwave instead. Is that all right?

There are lots of good choices available these days in the frozen dinner aisle, and in many cases frozen foods may provide as much nutrition as freshly prepared foods. Like any other foods, however, you'll want to make sure to check the food labels carefully for sugar, fat, and salt content as well as portion size. If you have any questions about the frozen dinners and whether their nutritional content is suitable to your needs, you can always ask your dietitian.

454.
I eat lunches at the local senior center, but they often serve all sorts of foods that I know I'm not supposed to eat, according to my meal plan. What can I do about that?

Meals at the local senior centers are carefully planned by nutritionists and dietitians to include a variety of foods that are targeted to the needs and tastes of the majority of older adults living in that community. They aim to combine foods from all of the major food groups, in portion sizes that are recommended for older adults, and to prepare them in ways that maximize their nutritional value. However, sometimes meals that are nutritionally sound for the majority of older adults may not be quite as sound for others. If you have questions about whether you should be eating any or all of the meals, you can ask for information about the content of the meals and alert the senior center representatives that you have diabetes so adjustments can be made to your meals.

Remember, your dietitian will rarely tell you to eliminate certain foods from your diet altogether.

Q A

Instead, you should eat foods of all sorts in moderation and look at your eating patterns over the course of a week rather than during one particular day. So, if some of the foods are not on your meal plan for that day, you can also choose to avoid them, take them home with you and freeze them for later snacks, or even share them with another person.

455.
I get meals delivered to my home by the local Meals-on-Wheels group, but they sometimes contain foods that aren't on my meal plan. What can I do about that?

As with meals at local senior centers, home-delivered meals are planned by nutritionists and dietitians to include nutritious foods from the major food groups and recommended portion sizes for older adults. If you have questions about whether you should be eating the meals, you can ask for information about the content of the meals and alert the Meals-on-Wheels representatives that you have diabetes so adjustments can be made when preparing your meals.

456.
I'm on a fixed income and can't afford the fresh vegetables and fruits that are recommended in my meal plan. Are there less expensive alternatives that would work for me?

Fortunately, many frozen or canned vegetables and fruits are as nutritious for you as fresh vegetables and fruits and are also often less expensive. As with other foods, you will want to check the food labels to make certain that these products do not contain other ingredients that you may want to avoid or limit. For instance, many frozen or canned vegetables contain additional salt and many frozen or canned fruits contain additional sugars. Try to find the frozen or canned products with low (or no) added sodium and low (or no) added sugars.

If you have questions about frozen or canned alternatives or different ways to prepare foods that are less costly, check with your dietitian.

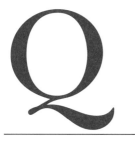 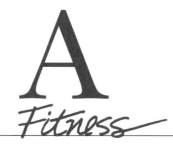

Fitness

457.

My doctor told me to lose weight to lower my blood glucose. Do I really need to lose weight at my age? What's weight loss got to do with my blood glucose?

Weight loss and increased physical activity are two of the most important components of successful diabetes management; medications are the third. That's because higher weight is one of the major risk factors for heart, kidney, nerve, and other complications that can result from diabetes. A loss of even 5% to 7% of your body weight (that's only 10–14 pounds for a 200-pound person!) can help lower your blood glucose, reduce your need for diabetes medicine, and lower your risk for other diabetes-related health problems.

Walking and other enjoyable physical activities are excellent ways to lose weight. In fact, recent studies have shown that walking improves your blood glucose level, increases your metabolic rate (which helps you to burn calories), helps you deal better with stresses in your life, and just makes you feel better.

458.

My doctor recommended that I get more exercise. I have never exercised before. Why is it important now?

There are several reasons why it is important to exercise. First, as you age, your body naturally loses muscle, or lean tissue. Lean tissue is metabolically active tissue and the more of it you have, the higher your metabolic rate. A higher metabolic rate translates into less weight gained through the years. If weight gain is a problem for you, one answer may be to increase your activity level, thus increasing your muscle mass. In addition, engaging in a regular exercise program will help your body to use insulin more effectively. This will help to lower your blood glucose, which in turn will help to reduce your risk of short-term and long-term diabetes complications. Regular exercise also acts as a natural stress reducer, antidepressant and an easy calorie burner. For many, exercise also provides a welcome social outlet when exercising with others.

Q A

459.
I really don't have the money to purchase exercise equipment or special shoes and clothing. Do I need any of these things?

Special exercise equipment is a luxury, not a necessity, and is certainly not needed to maintain an active lifestyle. One of the best (and easiest) forms of exercise is walking. Walking can be done indoors or outside, alone or with a partner, and requires no additional equipment other than a good pair of walking shoes. Well fitting shoes that provide adequate support for your feet are a necessity. Shoes that fit properly can help to ward off blisters, bunions and corns, foot and leg cramps, and back, knee, and hip pain. If you are on a tight budget with little money to allocate to exercise equipment, your first priority will be a pair of properly fitted athletic shoes. Exercise clothing is generally a matter of preference and is usually tailored toward the activity you are participating in. Comfortable, loose-fitting clothing that can be layered according to temperature needs is all that is required for exercise.

460.
Are there specific exercise guidelines to follow?

Yes and no. There are structured guidelines for exercise, and of course any exercise you do is dependent upon your medical condition, individual capabilities, and medical clearance from your physician.

Exercise specialists can design an exercise prescription for you. An exercise prescription encompasses the following:
- Type of exercise
- Intensity of exercise
- Duration of exercise
- Frequency of exercise

This plan is tailored for you based on your medical history, current fitness level, and fitness goals. It includes a warm-up and cool-down period, aerobic activities, strength training, and stretching for flexibility.

Some may not want to follow such a structured plan for exercise. A perfectly acceptable "plan" includes some form of aerobic activity such as walking for 30 minutes (either continuously or in multiple ses-

Q A

sions), 3–5 times per week; some type of strength training activity, 2–3 times per week; and stretching exercises each time you participate in an aerobic activity.

461.
I stay active all year long with gardening, golf, and walking my dog. Does this count as exercise?

Yes, and congratulations to you for maintaining an active lifestyle. There are very real fitness and health benefits from a lifestyle such as yours. Mainstream thinking in fitness used to be that exercise only "counted" when performed as part of a structured routine. We now know that every part of an active lifestyle counts toward the ultimate goal of good health. Making the daily choice to walk instead of ride, parking an extra distance from an intended location, and using the stairs instead of the elevator are all good choices that certainly add up. When looking at exercise in this light, gardening, golf, and walking your dog fit nicely into an active routine.

462.
I have recently read several articles about the importance of strength training. Is this really necessary at my age?

Strength training is important because it helps to maintain (or build) lean (muscle) tissue. Muscle tissue will help to increase your metabolic rate, which will help to prevent unwanted weight gain. In addition, the more lean tissue you maintain, the easier it will be to perform daily activities. Strength training also helps to maintain bone density and bone strength, which in turn leads to greater mobility. Greater mobility means a lesser likelihood that you will fall.

Strength training may include lifting additional weights (small dumbbells, or weight machines) or simply moving your own body weight. Examples of this include push-ups (on the floor or against a wall) and abdominal crunches. There are books and videotapes available to demonstrate proper techniques for these exercises as well as others. If a local YMCA or health club is available to you, you may want to work with an exercise specialist or athletic trainer. They can set up a strength-training program specifically designed to meet your individual needs.

Q A

463.
Do I need to monitor my blood glucose more frequently when I exercise?

Yes, you need to monitor your blood glucose before, during, and after you exercise, even if you don't feel any different. Blood glucose can drop (sometimes dramatically) during exercise, and diligent monitoring is the key to avoiding hypoglycemia. In addition, if you exercise with a partner or with a group, make sure to educate at least one person on the symptoms of a low blood glucose reaction and how to treat one if it occurs. You will need to check your blood glucose 30 minutes before exercising, just before exercising, and every 30 minutes during continuous exercise. Once you have finished your exercise session, check your blood glucose once again. Blood glucose levels can continue to drop for hours following sustained exercise; therefore, you will also want check periodically during this time, and treat a low blood glucose immediately if it occurs.

464.
Sometimes I have so much pain and discomfort in my feet that it is hard to even walk around my house. What types of exercise can I do?

There are many options for building exercise into your life that don't require you to stand or walk. Swimming is an excellent exercise, effective for both aerobic conditioning as well as muscle toning. Swimming pools are often available at a local high school, YMCA, or health club. Most facilities also offer classes specifically designed for older adults.

Another option is chair exercises. There are videotapes and books available to demonstrate aerobic exercises and muscle-toning and flexibility exercises—all performed while sitting in a chair. If exercise equipment is an option for you, stationary biking and rowing both enable you to exercise without standing.

465.
Now that I am exercising, do I need to eat more food?

You may need to eat more food once you have begun a regular exercise program. Food (caloric intake) may need to be adjusted based on several factors:

Q   A

- Are you overweight, at a normal weight, or underweight? If you are losing weight and need to maintain your weight, then additional calories may be needed.
- If you are experiencing episodes of low blood glucose, you may need to either increase your intake of food or have your medication adjusted.

Your health-care professional can help you make adjustments to your diet and meal planning.

If your blood glucose is low when you check it before you exercise, you will need to eat an extra snack before you begin. If you experience a blood glucose low while exercising, stop your exercise and treat your low blood glucose. Before resuming exercise, check your blood glucose level to make sure it has returned to a safe level.

466.
What time of day is best for exercising?

Generally, strenuous exercise is best limited to the earlier parts of the day. High-intensity activity is not recommended before going to sleep because blood glucose can continue to drop for several hours after exercise. Therefore, to avoid low blood glucose in the middle of the night or during sleep, it is best not to exercise before going to bed. This is not to say, however, that you can't participate in light activity in the evening hours. Examples of light activity include taking a stroll or a leisurely swim.

On the other hand, if your blood glucose typically runs high in the morning, exercise later in the day can at times relieve this. You will need to log your morning blood glucose readings, present this information to your doctor, and talk with him about using late-day exercise as a possible remedy for morning hyperglycemia.

467.
I see other people checking their pulse when they exercise. Do I need to do this?

Not necessarily. They are checking their heart rate; one way to determine whether you are exercising hard enough is to maintain your heart rate within a certain range. Staying within a certain range usually means that you are exercising aerobically. Aerobic means *with oxygen* and is designed to increase your respiration and

Q A

heart rate. Oxygen is needed for gaining cardiovascular benefits and for weight loss. Therefore, the goal is to exercise aerobically on a regular basis. (Anaerobic exercises, the kind typically done to increase muscle mass, are also beneficial, but for general purposes and cardiovascular fitness, we focus on aerobic exercise.)

Heart rate can be artificially lowered by some medications. Because of this, taking your pulse isn't always accurate for determining the intensity of a workout. While heart rate is still used in many circumstances, there is an easier way for you to determine whether or not you are exercising aerobically using the *talk test*. When you are exercising, you should be able to talk—to carry on a conversation while still working out at a hard or somewhat hard intensity. If this is difficult for you, you need to decrease the intensity of your workout. When you can talk comfortably during exercise, you are working in your aerobic zone, using oxygen most efficiently.

468.
I just tested my urine and found some ketones. Can I still take my walk today?

Not until ketones are no longer present in your urine. Ketones are chemicals that are released into the bloodstream when fat is used for energy instead of glucose. This can happen when there is not enough insulin circulating to help your body use glucose. If not treated (with insulin and extra fluids), this situation can progress to ketoacidosis, a serious medical condition. People with Type 2 diabetes usually do not test for ketones, as it is typically a problem in Type 1 diabetes. If you have Type 1 diabetes and have found ketones in your urine, do not exercise. After you have made the necessary adjustments (fluids and insulin), you will need to test your urine again. If no ketones are present, you can begin to exercise.

469.
My doctor told me to walk for 30 minutes each day. That is too much for me. Can I walk several times each day for shorter periods instead?

Absolutely! There are documented fitness benefits from participating in two 15-minute exercise sessions

Q A

per day or three 10-minute exercise sessions per day. If you haven't been exercising on a regular basis, it is imperative that you start out slowly to avoid injuring and overstressing your body. In addition, to make exercise a part of your daily life, you will need to find it enjoyable. It is difficult to enjoy something that is physically uncomfortable or even painful. A slow and steady start is just fine!

For some, walking 5–10 minutes at a time, three times per week, is appropriate. If this is easy for you to do, add another 10-minute session later in the day. Ultimately, you will want to work toward exercising for 30 minutes either continuously or in multiple sessions, three to five times per week. Be sure to add time for a five-minute warm-up and a five-minute cooldown to each exercise session.

470.
Why do I need to stretch before and after I exercise?

As we age, we tend to lose flexibility. The loss of flexibility makes us more prone to injury. Stretching on a regular basis helps to alleviate that loss of flexibility that comes with age. The best time to stretch is after a workout session, when your muscles are still warm from the increased bloodflow during exercise. When stretching, hold each stretch for 30 seconds and do not bounce. Stretching should not cause pain; only stretch to the point of resistance and hold that position. With continued stretching, you will see increased flexibility and greater ease while performing your daily activities.

Medication

471.
I have Type 2 diabetes and am allergic to sulfonamides, sulfonylureas, and, indeed, any drug containing a sulfur molecule. What options does that leave me with in terms of blood-glucose-lowering drugs?

For decades, sulfonylureas (pills that stimulate the pancreas to release more insulin) and insulin were the only options available to treat Type 2 diabetes.

382

Q A

They remain the most commonly prescribed treatments, but today you have other options. There are now several classes of oral drugs available, and they lower blood glucose levels in a few different ways.

Acarbose and miglitol. Acarbose (brand name Precose) and miglitol (Glyset) delay the digestion of carbohydrate, which reduces the blood glucose rise after a meal. (They do not affect the absorption of glucose or lactose, so glucose tablets or gel can be used to treat low blood glucose, if necessary.) The pills are taken just before the three main meals of the day. They are not absorbed into the bloodstream but remain in the digestive tract. Side effects such as flatulence, soft stools, diarrhea, and abdominal discomfort may occur during the first few weeks of therapy but typically abate with continued use of the drug.

Metformin. Metformin (Glucophage and Glucophage XR) works by decreasing the amount of glucose produced by the liver and by improving cells' ability to use insulin. Unlike many other diabetes drugs, metformin does not typically cause weight gain and may even bring about weight loss. It also reduces triglycerides, LDL cholesterol ("bad" cholesterol), and total cholesterol.

Gastrointestinal side effects, including nausea, diarrhea, vomiting, and flatulence, may occur at the beginning of treatment, but they usually stop with continued therapy. These side effects can be decreased by taking metformin with food 2–3 times daily or by taking the once-daily formulation, Glucophage XR.

Lactic acidosis, another possible side effect of metformin, is a rare but sometimes-fatal accumulation of lactic acid in the blood. Lactic acidosis is more likely to occur if metformin is taken in excessive amounts or by persons with poor kidney function. Symptoms of lactic acidosis include muscle pain, stomach discomfort, difficulty breathing, and increasing weakness or sleepiness. If these symptoms occur while you're taking metformin, tell your doctor right away. You should also notify your doctor before getting any x-ray tests, because special precautions may be necessary.

Repaglinide and nateglinide. Like sulfonylureas, repaglinide (Prandin) and nateglinide (Starlix) increase the amount of insulin your pancreas

Q A

releases, but they work differently from sulfonylureas. Repaglinide and nateglinide are taken 15–30 minutes before meals, three to four times daily. They are active for only a short time following meals, so you should skip a dose if you skip a meal. If you take repaglinide and eat an extra meal, add a dose; extra doses of nateglinide are not recommended.

One possible side effect of either pill is low blood sugar. The risk of developing low blood sugar increases when you drink alcohol, are very active for a prolonged period, eat less food or fewer calories than usual, or take other diabetes drugs in addition to repaglinide or nateglinide.

Rosiglitazone and pioglitazone. Rosiglitazone (Avandia) and pioglitazone (Actos) work by sensitizing the body's cells to insulin. They can be taken once or twice daily with or without meals. Possible side effects include mild weight gain, headache, and fatigue. If you take one of these drugs, your doctor will periodically do blood tests to make sure the drug is not causing any problems with your liver. You should call your doctor if you experience nausea, abdominal pain, dark urine, or yellowing of the skin while taking either rosiglitazone or pioglitazone.

One or more of these drugs may help lower your blood sugar. Taking into account any other drugs that you take and other health factors (such as allergies), your doctor will recommend the treatment that is best for you.

472.
My blood glucose is often high in the morning, even when I haven't eaten all night. Why is that?

A high blood glucose reading in the morning isn't unusual, although it does indicate that your body is not using glucose as efficiently as it should, even with your diabetes medication. Healthy before-breakfast ranges are about 80–120 mg/dl. Sometimes, however, other medications that you might be taking can reduce your blood glucose levels so much that your body will overproduce glucose as a defense mechanism. If your blood glucose readings are high in the mornings, be sure to mention it to your doctor, together with any other factors that you think might be important to know—such as recent stressful

Q A

events, certain foods outside of your usual meal plan, and other medications that you might be taking. Your diabetes medication doses—or the timing and doses of other drugs—may need to be changed to respond more appropriately to your body's needs.

473.
I have heard about people achieving remarkable blood glucose control with an insulin pump. Are pumps suitable for older people like me?

An insulin pump is a small, battery-powered device about the size of a beeper that delivers insulin into the body 24 hours a day at a rate preset by an internal program. That slow, continuous infusion of insulin helps the body to make use of the small amount of glucose that is present in the bloodstream all the time. Pump users can also override the preset infusion to deliver larger "bolus" doses of insulin to cover the glucose that comes from the foods they eat. The idea is to closely mimic the way a nondiabetic person uses insulin.

Insulin pump therapy was introduced in the late 1970's, but it wasn't used much until the technology became more sophisticated and the pumps became smaller. There has been a growing interest in the use of pump therapy since the early 1990's, when it was demonstrated that using pump therapy achieved improved glucose control compared with multiple daily injections.

Insulin pump therapy is for people who want to use intensive insulin therapy to come as close as possible to achieving normal blood glucose levels. Pumps are used most frequently used by people with Type 1 diabetes, but they can be used by people with Type 2 diabetes as well. And, to answer your question, there are no reasons for older people not to use an insulin.

Some people mistakenly believe that a pump is automatic and hassle-free. In fact, using a pump requires more care and vigilance than using traditional insulin injections. What pumps can offer, however, is lifestyle flexibility and the ability to control blood glucose very tightly. Standard insulin injection routines can be burdensome by restricting people's schedules. For example, an injection regimen that calls for one or two shots a day of longer-acting

Q A

insulin can require a person to eat his meals when his insulin is peaking. Insulin pumps, on the other hand, infuse a small amount of quicker-acting insulin continuously, so there is no real peak in insulin action with which one must synchronize meals. Pump users can schedule their meals whenever they want and simply deliver a "bolus" dose before they eat.

The fact that pumps deliver insulin continuously (much as a pancreas does) helps to avoid the blood glucose highs and lows seen with some injection regimens. And the better blood glucose levels are controlled, the lower the risk of developing diabetic complications.

Insulin pumps are not for everybody. To use a pump successfully, you must have a strong interest in achieving near-normal blood glucose levels. You'll have to work closely with a diabetes management team that is very familiar with pump therapy, and you'll have to learn and manage the equipment, including addressing the technical challenges that arise during day-to-day use. Other challenges include dealing with pump failure, infection at the site of needle insertion, and weight gain as the glucose in your bloodstream is utilized more efficiently. You would be well-advised to consider all these issues carefully before deciding whether to pursue pump therapy. If you can make the commitment and stick with it, you can enjoy excellent blood glucose control.

474.
My doctor wants me to switch from pills to insulin. Is that really necessary?

It's not uncommon to progress from pills to insulin. Different classes of diabetes drugs work in different ways: Some increase the amount of insulin your body makes, some increase the sensitivity of your cells to the effects of the insulin you already make, and others inhibit your body's ability to absorb some carbohydrates. Many people take a combination of different pills to control their blood glucose levels. This allows the action of one pill to complement the effects of others. Over time, however, many people find their response to oral medications insufficient to adequately control their blood glucose. Apparently, you have reached that point and need to start using

Q A

insulin. Usually, insulin is added to your medication regimen, and you will continue to take your pills as well. Eventually, many people transition to using only insulin to control their blood glucose.

Diabetes pills often become less effective in helping to lower blood glucose adequately when people decrease their level of activity and gain weight, which is quite common among older people. If weight gain is becoming a problem with you, it would be a good idea to consult a dietitian who has expertise in diabetes. Improvements in diet will often promote the weight loss needed to improve the effectiveness of diabetes pills, thus cancelling out the need to inject insulin. The most important thing, though, is to keep your blood glucose well controlled to avoid any complications.

When diet and exercise alone are not sufficient to control blood glucose, oral medicines have to be used. And when oral medication becomes ineffective, transition must be made to insulin, either alone or in combination with pills.

475.
Even though my blood pressure, blood lipids, and HbA$_{1c}$ results are normal, my doctor wants me to start taking an antihypertensive drug, saying it will protect my eyes and kidneys in years to come. I am reluctant to take any medicine I don't really need. Is there any good reason for me to take this drug now?

Historically, physicians only treated medical problems after they had appeared, but gradually the concept of disease prevention became more accepted. The recommendation to take an aspirin a day to reduce the risk of a heart attack or stroke is an example of such a preventive measure. Although it is not now universally recommended, your physician's recommendation is reasonable. The class of antihypertensive drug known as ACE inhibitors have shown effectiveness in reducing the vascular problems that underlie diabetic eye and kidney disease.

One way to screen for early kidney disease is to check the urine for the presence of a protein called

Q A

albumin. When it is present in small amounts (30 to 300 milligrams albumin per milligram of another substance called creatinine) the condition is known as microalbuminuria. People with diabetes should have a test for microalbuminuria done yearly by a health-care provider.

Why is this early diagnosis important? Studies have shown that ACE inhibitors can delay the appearance of microalbuminuria or delay the onset of late-stage kidney disease if microalbuminuria is already present.

In short, your physician is providing you with competent medical care.

476.
We travel during the winter months. How do I manage my diabetes medication while I am away from my doctor?

Travel is an important part of life for many older people, and having diabetes is not a reason to avoid traveling. If your diabetes is under good control at home, a little monitoring, planning, and common sense should be enough to let you maintain the same level of blood glucose control while traveling.

Monitoring your blood glucose is the foundation on which managing your medication is based. If you are taking an oral medicine, it is likely that your blood glucose control will remain similar to what it is at home unless you drastically change the amount of physical activity you engage in or the calories you consume. In this circumstance, you just need to have enough medicine on hand to handle these changes and to consider whether you need a reminder to take your medicine as your routine will likely change during a trip.

If you are taking insulin, the same principles apply. While insulin that is being used should be at room temperature, insulin that you are transporting and not currently using should be refrigerated if possible. At a minimum, insulin should not be exposed to extremes of temperature such as might happen when exposed to direct sunlight during warm temperatures in an uncooled vehicle. When you pack insulin for a trip, keep in mind that while each vial has an expiration date, after the vial is opened the insulin may lose potency in 30 days. Also keep in mind that insulin is

Q A

available in a different concentration (40 units per milliliter) outside the United States: If you need to purchase this concentration of insulin, remember that it needs to be used with the appropriate syringe, which should be available locally. Maintaining your injection schedule may be difficult when you are traveling. If you need to change the timing between when you administer your insulin and when you take in a meal, keep in mind the following guidelines: Rapid-acting insulin (Humalog and NovoLog) should be injected within 15 minutes of eating a meal, and short-acting insulin (Regular) most commonly should be administered 30 minutes before eating a meal. Consider bringing an adequate supply of syringes for your needs during a trip as the regulation of syringe purchase varies considerably from one state to another. As at home, syringes and needles should be disposed of in a puncture-resistant container. Planning for your trip should include provision for getting additional medication during your trip in the event that it is needed. This may involve getting a backup prescription from your physician, obtaining your medicine from a national pharmacy chain where your prescription can be accessed in other states, and/or establishing a relationship with a physician in the area where you travel if you go there regularly. Another thing to keep in mind when traveling is to use good common sense and to seek the advice of your health-care provider before any travel that is not routine.

477.
Will I ever be able to stop taking medication to control my diabetes?

At this time there is no cure for either Type 1 or Type 2 diabetes. When you have Type 2 diabetes and it is not controlled with diet and exercise, you will likely need to take medication to help control your blood glucose for the rest of your life. However, just as there are circumstances when an older person who usually controls his blood glucose with diet and exercise may sometimes require insulin to maintain blood glucose control, there are also circumstances when a person who takes medication to control his blood glucose may be able to control it without medication. For instance, obesity is accompanied by worsened resist-

Q A

ance to the action of insulin, but if you are overweight and lose weight you might be able to either reduce the dose of medicine required to control your blood glucose or possibly even eliminate the need for any medication. Unfortunately, many people who accomplish this kind of weight loss gain it back within one to two years, at which time the requirement for medication also returns. In people who have Type 1 diabetes, in which no insulin is produced, the requirement to inject remains for a lifetime.

478.
I sometimes forget to take my medication. What should I do when that happens?

Adherence to your medication regimen requires commitment and planning, but taking medicine on schedule is challenging for many people. This is particularly true for older people, who likely take a number of medicines in addition to those that help control their blood glucose.

When you have Type 2 diabetes, like most older adults with diabetes, it is unlikely that missing a dose of medicine will be life-threatening. Monitoring your blood glucose may be helpful, particularly when you miss more than one dose in a row. This is especially important if you use insulin. With an oral medicine, waiting until the next dose is due is a reasonable approach, but it would be best to check this approach with your doctor to be sure. People with Type 2 diabetes generally have some insulin present, and this helps buffer them from the extremes of insulin fluctuation that could occur in Type 1 diabetes when a dose of insulin is missed.

In the older person with Type 2 diabetes, a very real danger exists when you believe that you missed a dose of medicine but in reality didn't miss it. When this happens, you might take the dose you think you missed, thus exposing yourself to a serious threat of hypoglycemia as a result of overdosing. Pillboxes can help avoid such occurrences. These boxes generally have compartmentalized sections that allow the owner to store seven days of doses for three to four dosage times each day, making it easy to check that a particular dose was or was not taken.

Q A

479.

I am on a tight budget. Can I reuse my syringes or my needles to save money?

While insulin syringes and needles are designed for single-use application, you can reuse them under the right circumstances. The American Diabetes Association has taken a position of conditional support for this practice since 2001. Remember, though, that a syringe or needle is no longer sterile once it is used. So if you are prone to infection, reuse might not be a good idea. Another problem in reuse concerns the newer, thinner needles, which are designed for pain-free injections. This thinness may come at a price, however, as these needles are more likely to bend without it being visually noticeable. What you will notice when you try an injection with a bent needle is increased pain when you inject and unnecessary skin abrasion when you remove the needle after injection. It is also possible that a bent tip of a thin needle may break off at the time of injection. Both of these situations could increase the risk of skin infection. If you want to reuse your syringes and needles, make sure you talk it over with your doctor or nurse, learn how to safely recap the needles, and become familiar with potential sources of contamination.

480.

I am interested in taking glucosamine and chondroitin for my joints and cartilage, but I'm not sure if they're safe for people with diabetes. Can you fill me in?

Glucosamine and chondroitin are two dietary supplements that have received attention as complementary therapies to treat osteoarthritis. Osteoarthritis is a degenerative disease that is characterized by the breakdown of the cartilage at the joints. Cartilage is a connective tissue in the body that is composed mostly of water as well as a fibrous protein called collagen, sugar-coated proteins called glycoproteins, and cells that build up and break down cartilage called chondrocytes. Cartilage is resilient and allows for shock absorption at joints.

Glucosamine is a molecule found naturally in the body that is thought to play a key role in the production of cartilage glycoproteins by helping to stimulate chondrocyte activity. It is also theorized that glucosamine may slow down the progression of osteoarthritis.

Chondroitin is a relatively large molecule that is a component of one of the common glycoproteins essential for normal cartilage function. It may stimulate chondrocyte activity and inhibit enzymes that damage joint cartilage.

Many preparations of supplements claiming to be effective against osteoarthritis contain glucosamine alone or a combination of glucosamine plus chondroitin. Some researchers speculate that the chondroitin molecule is too large to be absorbed and used by the body when it is taken orally, which may be why some preparations include only glucosamine.

Some studies have shown that glucosamine may induce insulin resistance. The mechanism is not well understood but may range from chemical modification of cellular proteins to changes in glucose transport systems.

It is important to realize that this potential adverse effect of glucosamine has been surmised mostly from animal data. Data regarding these adverse effects in humans are not yet conclusive.

Recently, the Arthritis Foundation said that people with diabetes should check blood glucose levels more frequently when taking glucosamine since it's a type of amino sugar. People with diabetes who have osteoarthritis should inform their doctor before taking glucosamine and should closely monitor blood glucose levels and glycosylated hemoglobin (HbA_{1c}) levels after starting glucosamine to see whether doses of any diabetes medicines need to be adjusted.

Long-Term Care

481.
What are the long-term complications of diabetes that is not well controlled? How long will it take to get these complications?

The long-term complications of poorly controlled diabetes are quite serious. They include the following:

- Hypertension (high blood pressure)
- Macroangiopathy (disease of the large blood vessels)

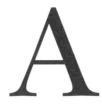

■ Microangiopathy (disease of the small blood vessels)
■ Nephropathy (kidney disease)
■ Neuropathy (nerve damage)
■ Hyperlipidemia (especially low HDL and high triglygerides)
■ Obesity
■ Insulin resistance
■ Hypercoagulability (sticky platelets, which can lead to life-threatening blood clots)
■ Glaucoma, cataracts
■ Periodontal disease

Since everybody's diabetes is unique to the person who has it, the possible onset of any one of these complications will also be unique. There are, luckily, certain steps you can take to reduce the risk of developing complications like these. First and most important is good blood glucose management. This includes knowing your numbers (blood glucose monitoring), meal planning, engaging in some type of regular exercise, and working closely with your doctor or nurse.

482.
My blood pressure is usually around 140/85 mm Hg, but my doctor has put me on blood pressure medicine to lower it, saying blood pressure control may be even more important than blood glucose control in preventing complications. Is this true?

Hypertension, or high blood pressure, is a major risk factor for atherosclerosis (narrowed arteries), retinopathy (eye disease), and diabetic kidney disease in people with diabetes. Long-term studies on large numbers of volunteers have demonstrated that treatment of hypertension is very effective in decreasing the risk of all of these vascular complications of diabetes. While it is hard to make a direct comparison, the magnitude of improvement is at least as great as that achieved by improved blood glucose control. In addition, the effects of treating hypertension appear to be additive to those of improving blood glucose control, and improved blood pressure levels may be easier to achieve.

It has long been believed that even slight elevations of blood pressure may be detrimental in people with

Q   A

diabetes. Evidence suggests that the old criteria for treatment were much too lenient and that more aggressive therapy of hypertension is warranted for many people. Recently, the National Kidney Foundation has recommended a target blood pressure goal for people with diabetes of less than 130/80 mm Hg. Treatment is recommended if either number is consistently elevated.

Most studies suggest that achieving and maintaining blood pressure at the newly recommended level for long periods of time often requires more than one drug. Nevertheless, for most people, aggressive blood pressure lowering appears to offer major benefits for all the vascular complications of diabetes and hypertension.

483.
I had my cholesterol checked at the mall and it was elevated. What are my next steps?

As soon as possible, make an appointment with your doctor. It is important that you tell him the findings. Your doctor will usually do a complete medical assessment, which will include a medical history and a physical examination. There will also be laboratory tests that will give additional information. If it is determined that you indeed do have high cholesterol, your doctor will set up a treatment and management plan for you. After a plan is started, remember to return to your doctor for periodic follow-up visits so he can assess your progress.

There are a number of steps you can take to help improve your cholesterol levels; for example, keeping your blood glucose in the range suggested by your doctor and losing weight if you are overweight. Even a 10% reduction in your weight can result in a significant drop in your cholesterol level. Other ideas for cholesterol management include reducing your intake of dietary fats, especially fats that come from animal sources (saturated fats), reducing high cholesterol foods, limiting processed snack foods, eating more dietary fiber, engaging in regular exercise, and not smoking. However, even after you have made lifestyle changes to reduce your cholesterol level, your doctor may recommend that you take a cholesterol-lowering medicine.

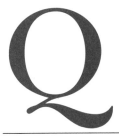 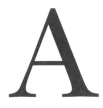

484.
Does being older put me at higher risk for heart disease?

The longer you have had diabetes, the greater your risk for heart disease. Heart disease develops slowly, but people with diabetes are more likely to develop blood vessel disease (also known as atherosclerosis or "hardening of the arteries"). With this condition, blood vessels become narrowed or even blocked by a buildup of plaque—deposits of cholesterol, calcium, cellular waste, and other material—and fat that slows or stops bloodflow. The impeded bloodflow can damage the heart (coronary artery disease), the brain (cerebrovascular disease), or the feet and legs (peripheral vascular disease).

Atherosclerosis is the major cause of death for people with diabetes. The risk of death in diabetic men is two times greater and in diabetic women four times greater than in the nondiabetic population. That's the bad news. The good news is that controlling your blood glucose helps keep you healthy. In addition to diabetes, there are other known risk factors for heart disease: smoking, uncontrolled hypertension, uncontrolled high cholesterol, being overweight, and having a family history of heart disease. While you are not in control of your heredity, you do have a measure of control over the other risk factors listed.

485.
My doctor used the term "lipids profile." What is that?

A lipid is a term for fat circulating in the blood, including particles of cholesterol and triglycerides, which are both produced by the body. They are also found in foods from animal sources—eggs, meat, and milk, for instance. A lipids profile is a measure of these fats. The body uses cholesterol to build cell walls and to make certain vitamins and hormones. Triglycerides are molecules composed of three fatty acids attached to a base of glycerol. Most dietary and body fats exist in the form of triglycerides. As stored fats, triglycerides can be used for future energy use, similar to a car's reserve fuel tank. They are stored chiefly in fat deposits and around organs, where they help to insulate the body from heat loss and pad the organs against injury.

Q A

There are three kinds of blood fats that affect blood vessels: high-density lipoprotein, low-density lipoprotein, and very-low-density lipoprotein. High-density lipoprotein (HDL) carries cholesterol away from the blood vessel walls to the liver. The liver breaks down the cholesterol and sends it out of the body. Low-density lipoprotein (LDL) has a high cholesterol content; it carries cholesterol to parts of the body that need it. However, cholesterol flowing through the bloodstream can stick to blood vessel walls, which can lead to cardiovascular disease. The main function of very-low-density lipoprotein (VLDL) is to carry triglycerides throughout the body, where they are either used for energy or stored as fat. VLDL is then broken down to produce LDL.

It is important to have a lipids profile done annually to make sure that you are maintaining healthy levels of blood fats. Healthy levels are defined as follows:

■ Total cholesterol under 200 mg/dl
■ LDL cholesterol under 100 mg/dl
■ HDL cholesterol over 40 mg/dl for men and over 50 mg/dl for women
■ Triglycerides under 150 mg/dl

The more HDL you have in your blood and the less LDL, the better for your blood vessels.

486.
Will diabetes shorten my life expectancy?

Diabetes that is not well controlled can increase your risk of a shorter life. Complications such as eye disease, kidney disease, nerve damage, and blood vessel disease occur more often in people who have diabetes than in people who do not have diabetes. To reduce your risk of future complications, keep your blood glucose levels as close to normal as possible. Normal levels are the levels of people who do not have diabetes. Major research studies have shown that the closer you can get to normal blood glucose levels, the more likely you are to prevent or delay complications. Persons with diabetes that is under good control are much more likely to enjoy a normal life expectancy. This, too, has been confirmed by large studies.

Q A

487.

I have used insulin for the past 25 years. So far, I have no complications, but I know I don't eat right or exercise enough. I also know it will catch up to me some day. How can I start taking better care of myself when it's so hard to change?

You are absolutely right when you say it's so hard to change. The problem you have is complex, and trying to fix it all at once can be discouraging. The best way to solve such a problem is to break it down into smaller, more manageable parts. Start by looking at your problem as a combination of three issues: poor eating habits, lack of exercise, and negative thinking. Tackling one part at a time can help you to take better care of yourself.

Changing your eating habits can start with examining what you currently eat. For example, if you find you tend to eat foods that are high in saturated fat and cholesterol, which can contribute to insulin resistance and increase the risk of heart disease, you might decide to eat smaller portions of those foods or find lower-fat alternatives for them. If you discover your vegetable intake is very low, you might start by adding a vegetable to your dinner menu every other day, or even every third day. Over time, you can add more vegetable servings more frequently.

If you'd like help or guidance in modifying your diet, consider making an appointment with a registered dietitian who is also a certified diabetes educator.

The second issue is exercise. You probably know a lot about the physical benefits of exercise, but you may not realize that exercising regularly, however moderately, can also give you an emotional boost. People who exercise regularly tend to feel more upbeat. Since you haven't been physically active, start small. Have your doctor assist you in selecting the type and amount of exercise to do at first. With regular exercise, you will be surprised at how quickly you can increase your strength, endurance, and sense of well-being.

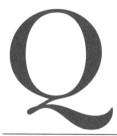 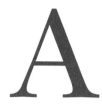

488.
Everything looks slightly cloudy to me. Will I lose my eyesight or go blind as I get older?

People with diabetes are more likely to get an eye disease than people without diabetes. To reduce your risk of eye disease, try to keep your blood glucose levels as close to normal as possible. Uncontrolled diabetes can result in blurred vision, glaucoma, cataracts, or additional eye problems. As with other complications, the keys to prevention are to control your blood glucose level, control high blood pressure, stop smoking, keep your cholesterol at a healthy level, and get yearly eye exams.

The three most common eye diseases in people with diabetes are retinopathy, cataracts, and glaucoma. Of the three, retinopathy is the most common. Retinopathy is damage to the small blood vessels that bring nutrients and oxygen to the retina. The retina is the lining at the back of the eye that senses light. There are two types of retinopathy: nonproliferative and proliferative. In nonproliferative (or background) retinopathy, the small blood vessels in the retina expand and form bulges, which may leak a bit of fluid. This does not usually harm your sight, and often the disease never gets worse. However, background retinopathy can progress to proliferative retinopathy, in which the blood vessels are damaged to the extent that they close off, shutting down circulation to the retina. In response to the retina's need for nutrients and oxygen, many new blood vessels grow, but these new vessels tend to break, releasing blood into the eye, causing dark spots and cloudy vision.

If you are experiencing either of these symptoms, it is very important that you make an appointment with your eye doctor as soon as possible. He will perform an exam and help you treat the damage that may have occurred.

Because of the potential for eye problems associated with diabetes, an annual exam is essential. Proper management of your diabetes will minimize the risk of getting these problems. So remember, to keep your eyes free of disease:

■ Keep your blood glucose levels close to normal. Keeping your blood glucose levels close to normal

Q   A

lowers your risk of getting eye diseases and slows down those that have started.

■ Control high blood pressure. High blood pressure can make eye diseases worse. You may be able to bring blood pressure down by losing weight, eating less salt, and avoiding alcohol. Your doctor can tell you about drugs to lower blood pressure.

■ Quit smoking. Smoking damages your blood vessels.

■ Lower high cholesterol. A high cholesterol level can also damage your other blood vessels.

■ Get yearly eye exams by an eye doctor. Many eye diseases can do damage without any noticeable symptoms. An eye doctor has the tools and tests to find damage early. The earlier damage is found, the greater the chance that treatments can save your sight.

489.
I have been told to check my feet daily, but I have trouble bending over. Why do I need to check my feet, and what am I looking for?

People with diabetes need to take special care of their feet because they are at risk for foot ulcers (approximately 15% develop a foot ulcer) and amputation (about 6 out of every 1,000 people have an amputation). However, nearly three-quarters of all amputations caused by neuropathy and poor circulation could have been prevented with proper foot care.

You need to exam both feet each day. Look all over your feet. If you cannot bend over or see well, have a friend or relative check your feet for you. Or you can use a mirror. During your exam, look for the following:

■ Redness
■ Changes in shape
■ Changes in color
■ Cold spots or hot spots
■ Cuts, cracks, breaks in the skin
■ Ingrown toenails
■ Ulcers
■ Punctures
■ Blisters
■ Calluses
■ Swelling
■ Pain

Q A

- Loss of sensation
- Corns
- Dryness or peeling

Call your doctor if you notice any of these symptoms, no matter how minor. Any injury or opening that does not heal in two days should be reported to your doctor. When you have diabetes, any of these symptoms can get out of control very quickly and cause major problems that are difficult to treat.

490.
I sometimes have trouble walking because I cannot feel the floor. What is happening and what should I do?

Nerve damage can occur in people who have had diabetes for a long time. Although nerve damage can affect many parts of the body, it very commonly affects the feet and legs. Many people with diabetes experience pain in their feet and legs or tingling or numbness. The most common type of peripheral neuropathy damages the nerves of the limbs, especially the feet. Symptoms include the following:

- Numbness or insensitivity to pain or temperature,
- Tingling, burning, or prickling sensations
- Sharp pains or cramp
- Extreme sensitivity to touch (even light touch)
- Loss of balance and coordination

Any of these symptoms can be signs of nerve damage, so let your doctor know so he can start proper treatment. The signs of nerve damage to the feet, legs, or hands tend to worsen at night, but they often get better if you get out of bed and walk around a bit.

With damage to the nerves, a loss of reflexes and muscle weakness may occur. Your foot may become wider and shorter and your gait may change. Foot ulcers may occur due to pressure put on parts of the foot that are not protected. Loss of sensation can cause ulcers to go undetected and become infected. If these infections are not treated in time, the bone may become infected, possibly leading to amputation. However, minor injuries can usually be controlled if detected in time. For these reasons, it is critically important to examine your feet daily and to wear shoes that fit well.

Q A

To prevent or lessen nerve damage, you need to keep blood glucose levels in control, stop smoking, drink less alcohol, keep blood pressure and cholesterol levels under control, and have a yearly check for nerve damage.

491.
I have had symptoms of neuropathy in my feet for eight months or so, but nothing shows up on testing. Why is this? Also, is it inevitable that the affected nerves will die? Or could they recover?

Symptoms of neuropathy may start well before sophisticated nerve conduction testing (which tests whether a nerve can carry a signal) detects any problem. However, there are other tests that may reveal a problem earlier. The American Diabetes Association recommends that people with diabetes have the sensation in their feet checked every year using a simple, painless test in which a doctor touches your feet in a few places with a small, flexible, plastic stick called a monofilament. You simply tell the doctor whether you can feel it.

Another test uses a device that applies a variable amount of pressure to the skin, allowing a doctor to measure how much force is necessary for you to feel the touch. This test can detect neuropathy in the earliest stages, even before the nerve dies.

Research shows that the nerves damaged by diabetes will eventually die. However, identifying the problem early permits sensation to be restored in 80% of people. The first step is to improve your blood glucose control. Then you can ask your doctor to try the drug gabapentin (brand name Neurontin), which is sometimes used to treat pain caused by neuropathy.

If your blood glucose is already under excellent control and drugs don't provide any relief, there is a surgical procedure that may help. The procedure relieves compression on nerves by opening the small tunnels that nerves pass through. Blood flow is restored to the nerves, and that should resolve the pain, tingling, and numbness.

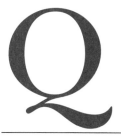 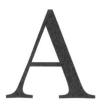

492.
What can I do to prevent damage to my kidneys?

The most important things you can do are to keep your diabetes in good control and keep in contact with your doctor. High blood glucose levels stress your kidneys, which have to work overtime to flush excess blood glucose from your body. If your blood glucose is uncontrolled for a number of years, your kidneys will not be able to continue their work because of the damage done by years of overworking them. So do your best to keep your blood glucose levels normal, eat healthy, and exercise.

There are steps that you can take to prevent or slow down kidney disease:
■ Keep your blood glucose levels as close to normal as possible.
■ Have your doctor check your kidneys periodically by testing your blood urea nitrogen, serum creatinine, creatinine clearance, and albumin excretion rate.
■ Have your eyes checked for eye disease (having one complication increases the chances for others).
■ Keep an eye on your blood pressure.
■ Limit your intake of protein.

493.
How does menopause affect diabetes?

If you finally figured out how to manage your diabetes around the hormonal fluctuations of the menstrual cycle, menopause can really throw your diabetes management plan out of balance.

High levels of progestin can decrease the body's sensitivity to insulin, while high levels of estrogen tend to increase insulin sensitivity. When menopause starts, it proceeds slowly. Ovulation and menstruation become irregular, and blood glucose levels can swing up and down unpredictably. Therefore, you will want to play close attention to the effects this process will have on your blood glucose control.

Estrogen protects against heart disese. When estrogen levels drop off, your total cholesterol level rises and your HDL (good) cholesterol drops, raising the risk of heart disease significantly, particularly in women with diabetes. Other problems associated with menopause include osteoporosis, weight gain, insulin

Q A

resistance, yeast infections, and vaginal dryness. These are problems that you and your doctor should discuss together to tailor your health management to your individual needs over time.

One option some women consider is hormone replacement therapy, which may be beneficial. However, this decision is not one to be made lightly. The decision to use hormone therapy needs to take into account your family history as well as the state of your diabetes management and should be made by both you and your doctor.

494.
Does having diabetes increase my risk of becoming sexually impotent?

Yes, it does. And the prevalence rises with age. About half of all men with diabetes become impotent. When impotence does occur, onset is slow, but the progress is continuous. The most common causes are the nerve damage and blood vessel damage that can occur with diabetes. But there are other causes as well: psychological stress, some medicines, or complications from prostate surgery, for instance.

That's the bad news. The good news is that keeping your blood glucose under control goes a long way toward helping you avoid impotence. If you do experience the beginning symptoms of impotence—a less rigid penis or fewer erections despite having the desire for sexual intercourse—do talk to your doctor about it. Many men are embarrassed to discuss these problems with their doctors—or even with their wives—leading to frustration and no solution. Your doctor can recommend several solutions: a mechanical vacuum device, for instance, or a drug that is injected into the penis before sex. There are also pills that he can prescribe that increase bloodflow to the penis that make it easier to have and maintain an erection.

Although many men prefer to seek treatment alone, most specialists believe that treatment is more likely to be successful if both the man and his partner are involved. The couple is more likely to be satisfied if both partners have a say in deciding on the appropriate treatment.

Q   A

495.
What medical tests should I have to take care of myself? And how often should I get them?

Here are some suggestions for taking charge of your health and health care:

- Blood glucose testing as recommended
- HbA_{1c} test every 3–6 months
- Doctor visits as needed or at least every 3–6 months if your diabetes control is stable
- Physical exam and medical history at every doctor visit
- Microalbumin testing annually
- Electrocardiogram (EKG) yearly
- Yearly eye exam
- Complete foot exam at each visit and a daily self-examination
- Fasting lipids profile yearly
- Urinalysis yearly
- Oral exam yearly

Remember, establishing a good working relationship with your physician is important. Work with your doctor to establish a plan of action to help manage your diabetes and any other health conditions you may have.

496.
I often leave my doctor's office confused and with an unclear memory of what he told me. What can I do about this?

You may want to make a list of questions to take with you and have a pad of paper to write the answers. As soon as possible, talk with the nurse or with the C.D.E. (certified diabetes educator) in the office. Either one of these people will be able to answer your questions or refer you to the person who can. In addition, the pharmacist who fills your prescriptions can also help answer questions, especially those about your prescriptions. Finally, many people find it helpful to have an additional person accompany them to their appointments. Often, an extra pair of ears will make a difference in what you hear and understand.

Q   A

497.
How can I avoid problems with my medications when I seem to take so many different pills?

Make an appointment with your doctor and talk with him about your concerns. Make sure to bring all of the medicines you use, including over-the-counter drugs, diet supplements, herbs, and vitamins—everything. Have him explain what each pill is for and why you need to take it. Tell him about any concerns that you have. Take notes or have a friend or family member come with you so that they also understand about the medicines you take and why you take them. Make sure you always get your prescriptions filled at the same pharmacy. Talking with your pharmacist, who can also describe what each pill is for, can clarify additional questions you may have. He will also be able to let you know of any side effects or possible interactions that can happen between your medicines.

498.
My gums are tender, and they bleed sometimes. Is there any connection between this and my diabetes?

When you have diabetes, you are at risk for gum disease and other oral infections. And people with diabetes can have tooth and gum disease more often if their blood glucose level stays high.

Infections can make your blood glucose levels go up. Furthermore, a high blood glucose level can make your oral infections even worse. You can even lose your teeth. Smoking makes it more likely for you to get a bad case of gum disease, especially if you have diabetes and are older. Red, sore, and bleeding gums are the first sign of gum disease. This can lead to periodontal disease, an infection in the gums and the bone that holds the teeth in place. If the infection gets worse, your gums may pull away from your teeth. You can protect yourself by knowing the signs of gum disease (gingivitis) and other oral infections and contacting your doctor and dentist if they appear, by taking care of your teeth, and by having a dental exam at least every six months. Signs of gum disease include the following:

Q A

- Bad breath
- Swollen or tender gums
- Gums that bleed when you brush or floss
- Red gums
- Gums that pull away from your teeth
- Pus between your teeth and gums when you press on the gums
- Loose teeth
- Teeth that are moving away from each other
- A change in the way your teeth fit together when you bite
- A change in the way your partial dentures fit

There are a number of oral health risks associated with diabetes: gingivitis, periodontal disease, dental cavities, thrush, dry mouth, and loose teeth. You can protect yourself by knowing the signs of gum disease and other oral infections, controlling your blood glucose, not smoking, flossing your teeth daily, brushing your teeth after each meal, keeping your dentures clean, and visiting your dentist regularly.

499.
Does my ethnic background affect my risk of diabetic complications?

If you belong to one of the following ethnic groups, you are at greater risk for diabetic complications and death caused by complications:

- African-American
- Hispanic
- American Indian
- Alaska Native
- Asian and Pacific Islander

Treatment may be different for each ethnic group based on the complication and the usual response to treatment, but the key is to control your blood glucose and to keep it at a level as close to normal as possible. The closer you can get to normal blood glucose levels, the more likely are to prevent or delay complications. Even the very best control may not be able to eliminate all complications, and the risk of complications increases with the length of time you have diabetes. Since genetic background does play a role in diabetes, it would be a good idea to discuss your concerns with your doctor.

Q A

500.
Now that I am older, what do I need to do to take care of my diabetes? Will it make a difference at my age?

Self-care is essential in helping to prevent diabetic complications, and to prevent complications from becoming worse if you already have them. This is important at any age. Self-care means taking charge of your diabetes. You will need to become knowledgeable about your treatment options and the the cost and benefits of these options. You will also need to set personal goals, and evaluate your feelings about your health. You will need to decide what your role is; are you the primary decision-maker, or do you want to share that responsibility with someone else? You can work with your doctor or nurse to help you learn about each of these aspects and learn what you need to know to take the care of your diabetes. These professionals can help you set reasonable goals and learn how to make whatever changes are necessary to optimize your self-care.

501.
I have trouble reading the small print on my drug labels. What can I do about that?

There are several things you can do to get around this problem. A magnifying device can help you read small print. Your pharmacist, doctor, or nurse could read the directions for taking your medicines and write out the information in large letters. Keep this written information with the drug container. Ask questions about anything that you don't understand. You could also have a friend or relative help you in the same manner. Be sure that you double-check the information to make sure that it is correct. You can also ask your pharmacist if large-print prescription labels are available. Again, ask for help if you need it.

Index

target goal, 394
See also High blood pressure
Blood vessel disease, 26, 28
Blurred vision, 14, 21, 28, 52, 69, 79–80, 358
Breath
  bad, 35, 36, 406
  fruity-smelling, 56, 69, 90
Breathing
  deep, 18, 84
  labored, 56
  relaxed, 288
  shortness of breath, 62, 90, 135, 311, 312
  ventilatory threshold, 290, 311
Butter
  alternatives, to, 96–97, 184, 185, 236
  saturated fat in, 235–236

C

Caffeine, 112, 208, 226–227, 371
Calories
  age and, 368
  in alcohol, 213
  burning, 241, 282, 285–286
  from carbohydrates, 155, 156
  daily intake, 103
  from fat, 96, 155, 178, 180
  free foods, 158
  from protein, 155
Candy, 106–107, 370–371
Candy bars, 219–220
Carbohydrate
  absorption, 194–195, 321
  in alcohol, 115
  blood glucose level and, 105, 120, 166, 167, 175, 178, 189, 190
  counting, 120–122, 157, 161, 166, 170–172
  dietary guidelines, 156
  glycemic index of, 175–177
  healthy food choices, 166–167
  during illness, 122–123, 222
  insulin balance, 157, 167, 171–172, 224
  loading, 217
  low-carbohydrate diet, 119–120, 172, 191–192
  servings, 167–169
  in sugar-free foods, 161, 173, 202
  triglyceride levels and, 172
  See also Fiber, dietary; Starches; Sugar
Cataracts, 20, 28, 35, 393, 398
Certified diabetes educator (C.D.E.), 17, 33, 105, 166, 193, 238, 245, 404
Chair exercises, 39, 281, 379
Chest pain, 62, 90, 312
Children
  with diabetes, 164, 344

fat intake, 116
milk consumption, 163
Cholesterol
  defined, 91
  drug treatment for, 61–62, 92
  exercise and, 62, 93, 313
  fiber and, 93, 186, 187
  good and bad types, 91, 312–313
  heart disease and, 26, 27, 60, 92
  insulin resistance and, 60
  lipids profile, 396
  lowering, 61–62, 92–93, 394
  saturated fats and, 94, 178, 179, 180, 181, 236
  target goals, 26, 91, 92, 93
  tests, 26, 38
  trans fats and, 181
  weight loss and, 235
  See also High-density lipoprotein (HDL) cholesterol; Low-density lipoprotein (LDL) cholesterol
Chondroitin, 392
Chromium deficiency, 329
Chromium supplements, 208–209, 293, 342, 343, 366
Circuit training, 41
Clothing
  exercise, 272–273, 377
  insulin injection through, 346–347
Cloudy vision, 21, 29
Commodity Supplemental Food Program (CSFP), 356
Communication
  with coworkers, 15
  about depression, 18, 83
  with doctor, 33, 404, 405
  with family and friends, 14, 16, 83, 122, 365
  for stress management, 18, 81, 82
Complications, diabetes, 392–393
  ethnicity and, 36, 406
  exercise with, 315–322
  preventive measures, 65–66, 406, 407
  See also Foot problems; Gum disease; Heart disease; Kidney disease; Nerve damage; Nerve damage in feet; Vision problems
Confusion, 67, 69, 135, 219, 305, 358
Cooking methods
  low-fat, 17, 95, 97, 115, 118, 185, 236
  low-sodium, 211
Coordination, lack of, 305, 400
Coronary artery disease, 26, 395
Counterregulatory hormones, 308

D

Dairy products, 94, 185
Dawn phenomenon, 308

Deep breathing, 18, 84
Dehydration, 220, 290–291
Denial, 16, 54–55, 83
Dental exams, 36, 66, 77–78
Dental problems. *See* Gum disease; Teeth
Depression, 23, 363
  clinical, 84–85
  talking about, 18, 83
  treatment of, 85
DiaBeta, 300, 325, 349
Diabetes
  changes over time, 54
  defined, 50
  diagnosis of, 53
  living a healthy life with, 53–54
  See also Type 1 diabetes; Type 2 diabetes
Diabetes Control and Complications Trial (DCCT), 21
Diabetes Prevention Program, 163, 362
Diabetic autonomic neuropathy (DAN), 33, 320–321
Diabinese, 300, 349
Diagnosis of diabetes, 53
Diarrhea, 123, 130, 227, 321, 326, 327
Diet
  during illness, 122–123
  low-carbohydrate, high-protein, 119–120, 172, 191–192
  low-fat, 61, 91, 92, 93, 95, 96–97
  protein restriction, 31, 73, 118–119
  See also Meal plan; Nutritional supplements
Dietary Guidelines for Americans, 155
Dietitians
  in health-care team, 25, 87, 152, 362, 404
  meal plan and, 17, 107, 108, 154, 155, 156, 161–162, 166, 172, 192–193, 223
  selecting, 101, 104–105, 166
  weight-loss plan and, 237, 238, 245
Discouragement, 17, 359–360
Distal symmetric polyneuropathy, 31
Dizziness, 62, 67, 69, 291–292
Doctors
  blood glucose records, reviewing, 141
  blood pressure readings by, 70–71
  eye specialist, 88–89
  in health-care team, 25, 87, 152, 362
  as information source, 15, 17
  office visits, 32, 66, 89, 404
  primary-care, 87–88
  specialists, 86–87, 361

during holidays and special occasions, 22, 116–117, 226
individualized, 101–102, 104, 151, 154, 166, 223, 368–369
insulin therapy and, 153, 154–155
mini-vacations from, 82
misconceptions about, 161–162
motivation in following, 17, 160–161
portion size, 58, 153, 184
in restaurants, 117–118
for seniors. *See* Senior meal plan
sodium intake, 110–111, 210–211
for vegetarians, 224–225
See also Beverages; Eating patterns; Snacks; Sweeteners
Meat
cooking methods, 95
lean choices, 95–96, 184
portion size, 184
saturated fat in, 94, 95
Medicaid, 357–358
Medical alert identification, 16
Medical tests
checklist, 404
cholesterol level, 26, 38
dental exams, 36, 66, 77–78
for diabetes, 53, 58
for exercise program, 37–38
eye exams, 20, 21, 29, 34, 80, 88–89, 398, 399
feet check, 19, 29, 65, 401
frequency and types, 32
HbA$_{1c}$ blood test, 27, 75, 89, 127, 141, 175
for kidney disease, 31, 71–72, 402
nerve conduction, 401
Medicare, 357–358
Medications. *See* Drugs; Drugs, diabetes (oral); Insulin therapy; Over-the-counter drugs
Meditation, 75, 242
Meglitinides, 328
Memory, 24, 345, 390
Menopause, 402–403
Menstruation, 58, 402
Metaglip, 349
Metformin, 326, 328, 349, 383
Microalbuminuria, 388
Micronase, 300, 325
Miglitol, 327, 383
Monounsaturated fats, 97, 179–180, 181, 236
Morning blood glucose readings, 220–221, 308, 380, 384–385
Mouth
dry, 14, 36, 56, 77, 90
infections, 35–36, 76–77
numbness, 14, 67, 138, 358
Muscle-building exercises, 278–279, 378
Muscle soreness, morning, 287
Muscle-stretching exercises, 286–289

N

Nail-care practices, 30, 76
Nateglinide, 325, 383–384
Nausea, 14, 51, 56, 62, 123, 130, 135, 222, 227, 326, 358
control of, 339–340
Needles, reuse of, 391
Neotame, 199
Nephropathy. *See* Kidney disease
Nerve damage, 28, 35, 65, 114
alpha-lipoic acid and, 206
autonomic neuropathy, 320–323
exercise and, 275, 280–281, 318–321
gastroparesis, 227–228, 321–322
sexual problems and, 32
urination and, 33
Nerve damage in feet
balance problems, 319
drug treatment for, 75, 401
exercise options, 280–281, 318–320
protection against injury, 275, 318
testing for, 401
warning signs of, 31–32, 74–75, 318
Neuropathy. *See* Nerve damage; Nerve damage in feet
Novolog, 301
NPH insulin, 334
Numbness
in hands and feet, 31, 52, 69, 73, 318, 400
at mouth, 14, 67, 138, 358
Nutritional supplements
alternative therapies, 342–343, 366, 391–392
bodybuilding, 293–294
herbal, 34, 228–229, 330
for osteoarthritis, 391–392
for people with diabetes, 165–166
protein, 196–197
side effects of, 330, 343
See also Vitamin and mineral supplements
Nutrition therapy. *See* Meal plan

O

Omega-3 fatty acids, 179, 182–183
Oral health. *See* Gum disease; Teeth
Over-the-counter drugs
alcohol interaction, 213, 214
for pain, 42, 75
side effects and interactions, 34
Overweight
diabetes risk and, 51, 52
fitness and, 248
health impact of, 79
heart disease risk and, 27
See also Weight loss

P

Pain
chest, 62, 90
during exercise, 39, 41, 42, 258, 275–276, 379
in hands and feet, 30, 31, 41
of heart attack, 62
stomach, 56, 90
Pancreas, in blood glucose regulation, 50–51, 60
Periodontal disease. *See* Gum disease
Peripheral neuropathy. *See* Nerve damage in feet
Peripheral vascular disease, 27, 42, 395
Phenylketonuria, 108, 201
Physical activity. *See* Exercise
Pioglitazone, 327–328, 384
Polyunsaturated fats, 179, 180, 181, 182
Pork insulin, 334
Portion size, 58, 153, 184
Prandin, 325, 349
Precose, 327, 349, 383
Prediabetes, 53, 162–163
Pregnant women
alcohol consumption and, 114, 115, 212
folate supplements for, 204
multivitamins for, 329
PresTabs, 325
Progestin, 402
Protein
blood glucose levels and, 167, 190–191
calories from, 155
with carbohydrate, absorption and, 194–195
high-protein, low-carbohydrate diet, 120, 191–192, 196
kidney disease and, 120, 193–194, 196
low-protein diet, 31, 73, 118–119, 192–193
for resistance (strength) training, 195–196, 294
supplements, 196–197
in urine, 71–72, 193–194, 317, 387–388

R

Registered dietitian (R.D.), 105, 166, 192, 193, 238, 245
Regular insulin, 334
Renal disease. *See* Kidney disease
Repaglinide, 325, 383–384
Resistance (strength) training, 38, 243
circuit training, 41
high blood glucose after, 308–309

Swimming, 280–281, 285, 379
Syringes, reuse of, 347, 391

T

Talk test, 289–290, 381
Teeth
  cavities, 36, 406
  infections, 76
  loose, 35, 36, 406
  preventive measures, 77
Thiazolidinediones, 328
Thirst, excessive, 51, 52, 56, 69
Tingling, in hands and feet, 31, 52, 69, 73, 74–75, 400
Toes
  amputation of, 319–320
  ingrown nails, 29, 30–31, 76
Trans fats, 94, 110, 179, 181–182, 183–184
Transportation services, for seniors, 359
Travel
  exercise during, 298
  insulin therapy during, 388–389
  monitoring supplies/drug storage in, 142–143
Triglycerides, 26, 60, 62, 93, 172, 182, 215, 313, 395
Troglitazone, 328
Type 1 diabetes
  causes of, 51
  illnesses and, 221–222
  insulin regimen for, 350
  ketoacidosis and, 56, 135
Type 2 diabetes
  causes of, 50–51, 59–60, 153, 269
  childhood, 344
  genetic link, 51, 57, 162–163, 267, 362–363
  insulin therapy for, 153, 154, 350
  lifestyle strategies, 58, 152–153, 163, 267, 268, 269, 344
  risk factors for, 51, 52, 53, 57–58, 266–268

U

Ultralente, 334
Urination, frequent, 14, 33, 51, 52, 56, 69, 72, 135, 307
Urine, protein in, 193–194, 317
Urine tests
  for glucose, 134
  for ketones, 57, 134–135, 222, 307, 340, 381
  for protein, 71–72, 387–388

V

Vaginal dryness, 23, 32, 361
Vaginal infections, 23, 361

Vegetables
  choices, 373, 397
  as fiber source, 186, 188, 189
  frozen/canned, 375
  low-fat toppings, 97
  servings, 168
  for weight loss, 237
Vegetarians
  meal plan, 224–225
  multivitamins for, 329
  types of, 225
Ventilatory threshold, 290, 311
Very-low-density lipoprotein (VLDL) cholesterol, 26, 396
Veterans, health-care assistance for, 357
Vision problems
  alcohol use and, 114
  blurred vision, 14, 21, 28, 52, 69, 79–80
  dosage aids and, 19
  drug labels, reading, 407
  exercise and, 21
  checking feet with, 19
  prevention of, 28, 34, 398–399
  risk for, 20, 21, 28
  See also Retinopathy
Vitamin and mineral supplements
  ADA recommendations, 207
  antioxidants, 203, 205–207
  calcium, 204–205, 207, 208
  chromium, 208–209, 293, 342, 343, 366
  folate, 204, 207
  guidelines for using, 229
  magnesium, 293, 366
  megadoses, 203, 205
  negative effects of, 34, 329–330
  nutrient needs of people with diabetes, 202–204, 329
  for seniors, 204–205, 329, 370
VLDL (very-low-density lipoprotein) cholesterol, 26, 396
Vomiting, 51, 56, 90, 123, 222, 227

W

Walking
  brisk, 277
  mall walking, 282–283, 284
  mild to moderate, 312, 314
  as senior activity, 377, 381–382
  shoes for, 273
  starting out, 38, 39, 40, 245
  weight loss and, 243
  with weights, 276
Warning signs, 34–35
  clinical depression, 85
  foot problems, 29–32, 74–75, 318, 399–200
  gum disease, 35–36, 76, 405–406
  heart attack, 62
  heart disease, 312

high blood glucose, 14
ingrown toenail, 30
ketoacidosis, 56, 90
lactic acidosis, 383
life-threatening signs, 90
low blood glucose, 14, 28, 67, 69, 137–138, 219, 301, 305, 358
nerve damage in feet, 31–32, 74–75, 318, 400
overexercising, 258–259
retinopathy, 29, 398
stress, 18
urinary tract infection, 33
Water aerobics, 277–278, 281
Water intake
  benefits of, 111–112
  during exercise, 44–45, 291
  for high glucose levels, 137, 220
  during illness, 222, 339
Water retention, 328
Weakness, 14, 28, 67, 69
Weight gain. *See* Overweight
Weight loss, 51, 93, 225, 345
  blood glucose level and, 233–234, 235, 268
  carbohydrate restriction and, 172
  cholesterol level and, 235
  drugs for, 240
  drug therapy impact of, 345, 347–348, 389–390
  exercise for. *See* Exercise for weight loss
  family support in, 242
  food records in, 242
  gastric reduction surgery for, 240–241
  "grazing" eating pattern and, 237–238
  high blood pressure and, 210, 235
  insulin resistance and, 267
  insulin therapy and, 347
  low-fat cooking methods and, 236
  maintaining, 233, 238–239, 241–242
  meal replacers for, 239
  plateau, 234–235
  rate of, 234
  for seniors, 368, 376, 390
Weight training. *See* Resistance (strength) training
Whole-grain foods, 115, 119, 175, 189
Workplace, rights in, 15

Y

Yoga, 278, 285, 319
Yogurt, 185